Atlas of INFECTIOUS DISEASES

Volume II

SKIN, SOFT TISSUE, BONE, AND JOINT INFECTIONS

Atlas of
INFECTIOUS DISEASES

Volume II

SKIN, SOFT TISSUE, BONE, AND JOINT INFECTIONS

Editor-in-Chief

Gerald L. Mandell, MD

Chief, Division of Infectious Diseases
University of Virginia Health Sciences Center
Charlottesville, Virginia

Editor

Dennis L. Stevens, MD, PhD

Chief, Infectious Diseases Section
Veterans Affairs Medical Center
Boise, Idaho

DEVELOPED BY CURRENT MEDICINE, INC.

PHILADELPHIA

CURRENT MEDICINE
400 MARKET STREET, SUITE 700
PHILADELPHIA, PA 19106

Library of Congress Cataloging-in-Publication Data

Skin, soft tissue, bone, and joint infections/volume editor, Dennis L. Stevens.
      p.   cm.–(Atlas of infectious diseases; v. 2)
  Includes bibliographical references and index.
  ISBN 1-878132-44-X (hardcover)
    1. Musculoskeletal system–Infections–Atlases. 2. Skin–Infections–Atlases.
3. Connective tissues–Infections–Atlases.
I. Stevens, Dennis L. II. Series.
   [DNLM: 1. Skin Diseases, Infectious–atlases. 2.Connective Tissue
Diseases–microbiology–atlases. WR 17 S629 1995]
RC927.S56 1995
616.7–dc20
DNLM/DLC
for Library of Congress   94-33431
                                                 CIP

Development Editor: ....Lee Tevebaugh
Art Director: ....**Paul Fennessy**
Design and Layout: ....**Patrick Whelan and Jerilyn Bockorick**
Illustration Director: ....**Larry Ward**
Illustrators: ....**Liz Carrozza and Weisia Langenfield**
Production: ....**David Myers and Wendy Feinstein**
Typesetting Director: ....**Colleen Ward**

Printed in Hong Kong by Paramount Printing Group Limited.

10 9 8 7 6 5 4 3 2 1

PREFACE

The diagnosis and management of patients with infectious diseases are based in large part on visual clues. Skin and mucous membrane lesions, eye findings, imaging studies, Gram stains, culture plates, insect vectors, preparations of blood, urine, pus, cerebrospinal fluid, and biopsy specimens are studied to establish the proper diagnosis and to choose the most effective therapy. The *Atlas of Infectious Diseases* will be a modern, complete collection of these images. Current Medicine, with its capability of superb color reproduction and its state-of-the-art computer imaging facilities, is the ideal publisher for the atlas. Infectious diseases physicians, scientists, microbiologists, and pathologists frequently teach other health-care professionals, and this comprehensive atlas with available slides is an effective teaching tool.

Dr. Dennis L. Stevens and his team of expert authors have produced a beautifully instructive volume. Depicted are the etiologies and manifestations of infections that involve the skin and underlying soft tissue and bone. The illustrations are remarkable for their breadth and clarity. This atlas will be a heavily used reference for patient care and teaching.

Gerald L. Mandell, MD
Chief, Division of Infectious Diseases
University of Virginia Health Sciences Center
Charlottesville, Virginia

CONTRIBUTORS

Rodolfo M. Abalos, MD

Leonard Wood Memorial Leprosy Research Center
Cebu, Philippines

Jason Calhoun, MD

Chairman
Department of Orthopedic Surgery & Rehabilitation
University of Texas Medical Branch
Galveston, Texas

Roland V. Cellona, MD, DPH

Leonard Wood Memorial Leprosy Research Center
Cebu, Philippines

Michael J. Chiu, MD

Assistant Professor
Department of Internal Medicine
University of Texas Southwestern
Dallas, Texas

Clay J. Cockerell, MD

Associate Professor
Departments of Dermatology and Pathology
University of Texas Southwestern Medical Center
Dallas, Texas

E. Dale Everett, MD

Division Director, Infectious Diseases
University of Missouri Health Science Center
Columbia, Missouri

Tranquilino T. Fajardo, MD, DPH

Leonard Wood Memorial Leprosy Research Center
Cebu, Philippines

Julie S. Francis, MD

Assistant Professor of Pediatrics, Dermatology
Director of Cutaneous Laser Surgery
University of Washington School of Medicine
Seattle, Washington

Robert Gelber, MD

Medical Director, San Francisco Regional Hansen's
  Disease Program
Clinical Professor, University of California-San Francisco
San Francisco, California

Bruce C. Gilliland, MD

Associate Dean for Clinical Affairs
University of Washington School of Medicine
Seattle, Washington

Ellie J.C. Goldstein, MD

Clinical Professor of Medicine, UCLA School of
  Medicine
Director, R.M. Alden Research Lab
Santa Monica, California

Ricardo S. Guinto, MD, MPH

Leonard Wood Memorial Leprosy Research Center
Cebu, Philippines

Jan Hirschmann, MD

Assistant Chief of Medicine, Seattle Veterans Affairs
Professor of Medicine, University of Washington
  School of Medicine
Seattle, Washington

Karen R. Houpt, MD

Assistant Professor
Department of Dermatology
University of Texas Southwestern Medical Center
Dallas, Texas

Elaine C. Jong, MD

Director, Hall Health Primary Care Center
Clinical Professor of Medicine, Department of Medicine
University of Washington School of Medicine
Seattle, Washington

Rajendra Kumar, MD

Professor of Radiology
Director, Musculoskeletal Division
University of Texas Medical Branch
Galveston, Texas

Jon T. Mader, MD

Acting Director, Division of Infectious Diseases
University of Texas Medical Branch
Galveston, Texas

John Neff, MD

Medical Director, Children's Hospital and Medical Center
Associate Dean, Professor of Pediatrics
University of Washington School of Medicine
Seattle, Washington

Justin D. Radolf, MD

Associate Professor
Internal Medicine and Microbiology
University of Texas Southwestern Medical Center
Dallas, Texas

Gregory J. Raugi, MD
Chief of Dermatology
Seattle Veterans Affairs
Seattle, Washington

Daniel J. Sexton, MD
Associate Professor, Division of Infectious Diseases
Assistant Professor, Department of Microbiology
Duke University Medical Center
Durham, North Carolina

David Simmons, PhD
Professor, Department of Surgery
Division of Orthopedics
University of Texas Medical Branch
Galveston, Texas

Dennis L. Stevens, MD, PhD
Chief, Infectious Diseases Section
Veterans Affairs Medical Center
Boise, Idaho

Milan Trpis, PhD
Professor
Department of Molecular Microbiology and Immunology
The Johns Hopkins University School of Hygiene and
  Public Health
Baltimore, Maryland

David H. Walker, MD
Chairman
Department of Pathology
University of Texas Medical Branch
Galveston, Texas

Gerald P. Walsh, PhD
Leonard Wood Memorial Leprosy Research Center
Cebu, Philippines

Mark H. Wener, MD
Associate Professor of Laboratory Medicine and
  Rheumatology
Head of Division of Immunology
University of Washington School of Medicine
Seattle, Washington

Theodore E. Woodward, MD
Professor of Medicine Emeritus, Department of Medicine
University of Maryland School of Medicine and Hospital
Distinguished Physician, Veterans Administration Medical
  Center
Baltimore, Maryland

Herman Zaiman, MD
Editor, A Pictorial Presentation of Parasites
Valley City, North Dakota

CONTENTS

Chapter 15

Joint Infections and Rheumatic Manifestations of Infectious Diseases

Bruce C. Gilliland and Mark H. Wener

Index

CHAPTER 1

Introduction

Dennis L. Stevens

The myriad of microbes that cause infections of skin, soft tissue, and bone is exceeded only by the diverse clinical signs that are manifest in patients. The physician confronted with identifying the cause of infection and prescribing a definitive treatment plan has a formidable task. Understanding the anatomical relationships within the soft tissues and bone will help the clinician develop a differential diagnosis and to understand the pathogenic mechanisms that are so characteristic of many infectious agents. Disruption of the stratum corneum by burns, bites, abrasion, or foreign bodies, including needles, allows penetration of bacteria to the deeper structures. Similarly, the sweat gland and hair follicle can serve as portals of entry for either normal flora (staphylococci) or extrinsic bacteria (pseudomonads, as in hot tub folliculitis). Intracellular infection of the squamous epithelium with vesicle formation may arise from cutaneous inoculation with viruses (herpes simplex 1), from the dermal capillary plexus with viruses associated with viremia (varicella), or from cutaneous nerve roots (herpes zoster). *Streptococcus pyogenes* may infect the epidermis alone but may also be translocated laterally to deeper structures via lymphatics, resulting in the rapid superficial spread of erysipelas. Engorgement or obstruction of lymphatics causes flaccid edema of the epidermis, another characteristic of erysipelas.

The rich plexus of capillaries beneath the dermal papillae provides nutrition to the stratum germinativum, and physiologic responses of this plexus provide important clinical signs and symptoms. For example, infective vasculitis of the plexus may result in Osler's nodes, Janeway lesions, petechiae, and palpable purpura, which are important clues to the existence of endocarditis. Hematogenous seeding of this plexus can result in cutaneous clues to disseminated fungal infection as well as gonococcal, salmonella, pseudomonas (ie, ecthyma gangrenosum), meningococcal, and staphylococcal infection. This plexus also may provide access for bacteria to the circulation, thereby facilitating local spread or bacteremia. Postcapillary venules of this plexus are the major site of polymorphonuclear leukocyte sequestration, diapedesis, and chemotaxis to the site of cutaneous infection. In normal hosts, all the cardinal manifestations of inflammation— rubor, dolor, calor, tumor, and functio laesa—are usually present. In compromised patients these manifestations may be attenuated or absent. Bacterial cell wall components, bacterial toxins, or excessive cytokine production may cause dysregulation of these physiologic mechanisms, resulting in leukostasis and subsequent venous occlusion causing marked pitting edema. Edema associated with the appearance of purple bullae and ecchymosis suggests loss of vascular integrity and requires exploration of the deeper structures for evidence of necrotizing fasciitis or myonecrosis. Infection of the joints and bones may occur as a consequence of transient, discontinuous, or continuous bacteremia, from direct inoculation as a result of trauma, or from iatrogenic causes such as joint injection.

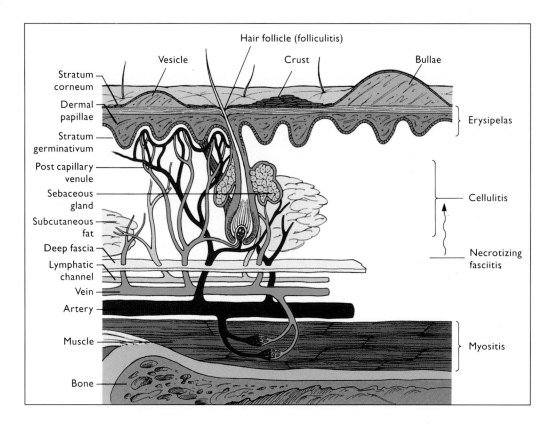

FIGURE 1-1 The structural components of the skin and soft tissue are illustrated on the *left* of the figure. Superficial infections are depicted on the *top* of the figure, and infections of the deeper structures of the soft tissue are located on the *right edge* of the figure. The rich capillary network beneath the dermal papillae plays a key role in localizing infection and in the development of the acute inflammatory reaction. (*Illustration by* Michael Wyett.)

INFECTIONS ASSOCIATED WITH VESICLES

Infections associated with vesicles

Variola (smallpox)
Varicella (chickenpox)
Herpes zoster (shingles)
Herpes simplex types 1 and 2
Coxsackie A-16
    (hand, foot, and mouth disease)
Orf

FIGURE 1-2 Infectious diseases associated with vesicle formation are caused by viral proliferation within the epidermis (*see* Chapter 7). Variola has not been seen in humans since 1977. Vesicles of varicella have a "dewdrop on a rose petal" appearance and occur in crops randomly about the trunk, extremities, and face over the course of 3–4 days. Herpes zoster occurs in a single dermatome and is preceded by pain several days before the appearance of vesicles. Vesicles due to herpes simplex virus are found on or around the lips (herpes simplex 1) or genitals (herpes simplex 2) but may appear on the head and neck in young wrestlers (herpes gladiatorum) or on the digits (herpetic whitlow) in health-care workers. Coxsackie virus A-16 characteristically causes vesicles on the hands, feet, and mouth in children. Orf occurs primarily in veterinarians and goat and sheep ranchers (*see* Chapter 5).

INFECTIONS ASSOCIATED WITH BULLAE

Infections associated with bullae

Staphylococcal scalded skin syndrome
Necrotizing fasciitis
Gas gangrene
Halophilic vibrio infection

FIGURE 1-3 Staphylococcal scalded skin syndrome (SSSS) occurs predominantly in neonates and is caused by a toxin from phage group II *Staphylococcus aureus*. SSSS must be distinguished from toxic epidermal necrolysis, which occurs primarily in adults, is drug-induced, and has a higher mortality (*see* Chapter 2). Punch biopsy with frozen section is useful because the cleavage plane in SSSS is the stratum corneum (*see* Fig. 1-1), whereas in toxic epidermal necrolysis, it is the stratum germinativum. Necrotizing fasciitis and gas gangrene also induce bullae formation early in their course (*see* Chapters 3, 5, and 13).

INFECTIONS ASSOCIATED WITH CRUSTED LESIONS

Infections associated with crusted lesions

Impetigo
Superficial dermatophyte infection
Systemic dimorphic fungal infection
Cutaneous leishmaniasis
Cutaneous tuberculosis
Nocardiosis

FIGURE 1-4 Impetigo contagiosa may be caused by *Streptococcus pyogenes* (*see* Chapter 3) or *Staphylococcus aureus* (*see* Chapter 2). It is important to recognize impetigo because of its relationship to poststreptococcal glomerulonephritis. Superficial dermatophyte infections (ringworm) and primary dimorphic fungal infections, such as *Blastomyces* and *Sporothrix schenckii*, usually appear as crusted skin lesions with raised borders (*see* Chapters 5 and 6). Patients with disseminated *Coccidioides immitis* infection may also present with crusted skin lesions, and biopsy and culture should be performed on such lesions in patients from a cocci-endemic area.

FOLLICULITIS

Etiologies of folliculitis

Staphylococcus aureus
Pseudomonas aeruginosa
  (hot tub folliculitis)
Schistosoma (swimmer's itch)
Acne vulgaris

FIGURE 1-5 The most common cause of localized folliculitis is *Staphylococcus aureus* (*see* Chapter 2). Sebaceous cysts may resemble staphylococcal abscess or become secondarily infected. Hidradenitis suppurativa can also mimic infected hair follicles, particularly in the axillae. Diffuse folliculitis occurs in two distinct settings. The first, "hot tub folliculitis," is caused by *Pseudomonas aeruginosa* in waters that are insufficiently chlorinated and maintained at temperatures between 37° and 40° C. The second type of diffuse folliculitis, swimmer's itch, occurs when a skin surface is exposed to water infested with freshwater avian schistosomes (*see* Chapters 5 and 10). Free-swimming cercariae readily penetrate human hair follicles or pores but quickly die. These dead cercariae elicit a brisk allergic reaction, causing intense itching and erythema.

ULCERS WITH OR WITHOUT ESCHARS

Ulcers with or without eschars

Anthrax
Cutaneous diphtheria
Ulceroglandular tularemia
Bubonic plague
Mycobacterial infections
Syphilis
Chancroid
Miscellaneous

FIGURE 1-6 Cutaneous anthrax progresses to an enlarging ulcer with a black eschar. Patients with cutaneous diphtheria may present with chronic nonhealing ulcers with an overlying dirty-gray membrane, and lesions may mimic psoriasis, eczema, or impetigo. Ulceroglandular tularemia may have associated ulcerated skin lesions but usually also have associated painful regional adenopathy. Classically, *Mycobacterium ulcerans* causes chronic skin ulcers on the extremities of individuals living in the tropics, and *M. leprae* may be associated with cutaneous ulcerations in patients with lepromatous leprosy associated with the Lucio phenomenon or during reversal reactions (*see* Chapter 11). *M. tuberculosis* may also cause ulcerations, papules, or erythematous macular lesions of the skin in normal and immunocompromised patients. Decubitus lesions and diabetic ulcers are invariable due to tissue hypoxia secondary to vascular insufficiency caused by pressure or intrinsic microcirculatory disease, respectively. Each may become secondarily infected with skin and gastrointestinal flora, including anaerobes. Ulcerative lesions on the anterior shins may be due to pyoderma gangrenosum, which must be distinguished from an infectious etiology based upon histologic evaluation of biopsy sites. Ulcerations on the genitals should arouse suspicion regarding syphilis or chancroid (*see* Chapter 12).

ERYSIPELAS

Erysipelas is caused exclusively by *Streptococcus pyogenes* and is characterized by an abrupt onset of fiery, red swelling of the face or extremities. Distinctive features are its well-defined margins, particularly along the nasolabial fold, its rapid progression, and intense pain. Flaccid bullae may develop during the second to third day of illness, but extension to deeper soft tissues is uncommon (*see* Chapter 2).

CELLULITIS

Cellulitis of the skin is an acute inflammatory condition characterized by localized pain, erythema, swelling, and heat. Infection may be caused by group A, B, C, or G streptococci (*see* Chapter 3) or *Staphylococcus aureus* (*see* Chapter 2). *Streptococcus agalactiae* infection is rare in adults except those with diabetes mellitus or peripheral vascular disease. Periorbital cellulitis caused by *Haemophilus influenzae* occurs in children in association with sinusitis, otitis media, or epiglottitis.

Exogenous bacteria may be introduced into the skin by various means as follows: *Pasteurella multocida* from cat bites; *Streptococcus intermedius* from dog bites (*see* Chapter 4); *Aeromonas hydrophila*, cuts in freshwater; *Pseudomonas aeruginosa*, sweaty tennis shoe syndrome; *Erysipelothrix rhusiopathiae*, fish monger's cellulitis; *Mycobacterium marinum*, fish tank exposure; and gram-negative rod cellulitis, compromised hosts (*see* Chapters 4, 5, 11, and 13 for additional information not associated with an obvious portal of entry).

Bacterial diagnosis is difficult in acute cellulitis, and several studies have demonstrated that needle aspiration or even punch biopsy yields positive cultures in only 20% of cases. The low number of bacteria suggests that toxins or host response to infection may be largely responsible for the signs and symptoms of cellulitis.

NECROTIZING FASCIITIS

Causes of necrotizing fasciitis

Streptococcus pyogenes
Mixed aerobic/anaerobic infection

FIGURE 1-7 Necrotizing fasciitis was formerly called streptococcal gangrene, but it may be associated not only with group A streptococci but also with mixed aerobic-anaerobic bacteria or as part of gas gangrene caused by *Clostridium perfringens* (*see* Chapters 2 and 14). Early diagnosis may be difficult, because pain or unexplained fever may be the only presenting symptom and sign. Next, swelling followed by brawny edema and tenderness develop. With progression, dark red induration of the epidermis appears along with bullae filled with blue or purple fluid. Later, skin becomes friable and takes on a bluish, maroon, or black color. By this stage, extensive thrombosis of blood vessels supplying the dermal papilla has already occurred. Infection extends down to the level of the deep fascia, which when infected has a brownish-gray appearance. Rapid spreading of infection occurs along fascial planes, through venous channels and lymphatics. Patients in the later stages are toxic and frequently manifest shock and multiorgan failure.

MYOSITIS

Myositis

Pyomyositis
Streptococcal necrotizing myositis
Gas gangrene
Nonclostridial (crepitant) myositis
Synergistic nonclostridial anaerobic
Myonecrosis

FIGURE 1-8 Muscle involvement can occur in relation to virus infection—influenza, dengue, or Coxsackie virus B (pleurodynia)—or parasitic invasion—*Trichinella spiralis* (trichinosis), *Taenia solium* (cysticercosis), and *Toxoplasma gondii* (toxoplasmosis). Although myalgia can occur in most of these infections, severe muscle pain is the hallmark of pleurodynia, trichinosis, and bacterial infection. Acute rhabdomyolysis predictably occurs with clostridial and streptococcal myositis but may also be associated with influenza, echovirus, coxsackievirus, Epstein-Barr virus, and *Legionella* infection. Pyomyositis is usually due to *Staphylococcus aureus*, is common in tropical areas and rare in temperate climates, and commonly has no known portal of entry. Infection remains localized, and unless strains produce toxic shock syndrome toxin 1 or certain enterotoxins, shock does not occur. In contrast, *Streptococcus pyogenes* may induce a primary myositis referred to as streptococcal necrotizing myositis, which is associated with severe systemic toxicity. Such infections have been described recently as part of the streptococcal toxic shock syndrome. Gas gangrene usually occurs following severe penetrating injuries that result in interruption of blood supply and introduction of soil into wounds. Such cases of traumatic gangrene are usually caused by *Clostridium perfringens*, *C. septicum*, or *C. histolyticum*. Recently, spontaneous nontraumatic gangrene caused by *C. septicum* has also been recognized among patients with neutropenia, gastrointestinal malignancy, diverticulosis, or recent radiation therapy to the abdomen. Synergistic nonclostridial anaerobic myonecrosis, also known as necrotizing cutaneous myositis and synergistic necrotizing cellulitis, is a variant of necrotizing fasciitis caused by mixed aerobic and anaerobic bacteria with the exclusion of clostridial organisms (*see* Chapter 14).

SELECTED BIBLIOGRAPHY

Hook EW, *et al.*: Microbiologic evaluation of cutaneous cellulitis in adults. *Arch Intern Med* 1986, 146:295.

Simmons RL, Ahrenholz DH: Infections of the skin and soft tissue. *In* Howard RJ, Simmons RL (eds.): *Surgical Infectious Diseases*, 2nd ed. Norwalk, CT: Appleton & Lange; 1988:377–441.

Stevens DL: Invasive group A streptococcus infections. *Clin Infect Dis* 1992, 14:2.

Stevens DL, *et al.*: Spontaneous, nontraumatic gangrene due to *Clostridium septicum*. *Rev Infect Dis* 1990, 12:286.

CHAPTER 2

Staphylococcal Soft Tissue Infections

Jan Hirschmann

IMPETIGO

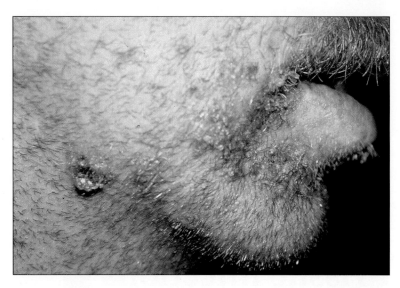

FIGURE 2-1 Impetigo. Thick, adherent, golden ("honey-colored") crusts surmounting an erythematous base are present around the mouth and on the jaw. These findings are characteristic of non-bullous impetigo, which typically occurs on the face or extremities. More common in children than adults, impetigo often follows minor trauma, such as abrasions and insect bites, and is more prevalent in tropical climates, crowded living conditions, and circumstances of poor hygiene. Cultures of impetigo most frequently yield *Staphylococcus aureus* alone, less commonly a mixture of *S. aureus* and *Streptococcus pyogenes* (group A streptococci), and, least often, streptococci alone. Treatment is topical mupirocin or an oral antistaphylococcal antibiotic.

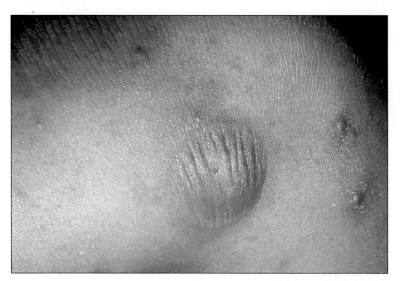

FIGURE 2-2 Bullous impetigo. On the knee, a large flaccid bulla on an erythematous base is surrounded by numerous small pustules. Bullous impetigo occurs with infections caused by some strains of *S. aureus*, usually group II phage type 71, that produce a toxin causing cleavage in the epidermis just below the stratum corneum. Treatment is with an oral antistaphylococcal antibiotic.

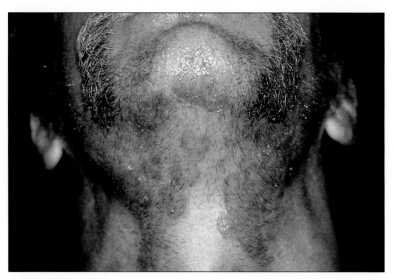

FIGURE 2-3 Bullous impetigo. Numerous erythematous erosions with well-delineated borders appear on the face, chin, and neck. Because the epidermal cleavage is so superficial in bullous impetigo, the vesicles, bullae, and pustules produced are fragile and easily rupture to form erosions, with the exudate often drying into a thin brown crust that resembles lacquer. The lesions commonly spread and coalesce to create large rounded areas of involvement. Frequently, as in this patient, no intact blisters or pustules are present.

ECTHYMA

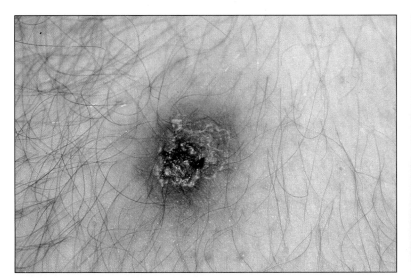

FIGURE 2-4 Ecthyma. Erythematous ulcerations with adherent crusts, most commonly on the lower extremities, characterize ecthyma. It begins as vesicles or bullae, which rupture to form scabs. Unlike impetigo, the infection penetrates to the dermis to produce ulcerations below the crust and heals with scarring. As in nonbullous impetigo, ecthyma often follows skin trauma in patients with poor hygiene, and the cause may be *Staphylococcus aureus*, *Streptococcus pyogenes*, or both. Treatment is topical mupirocin or an oral antistaphylococcal antibiotic.

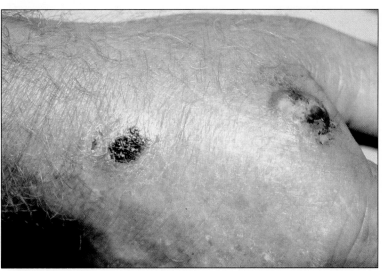

FIGURE 2-5 Ecthyma. An erythematous lesion on the proximal hand has an overlying adherent crust, which, if removed, would reveal an ulceration. Distal to it is an earlier stage of ecthyma, demonstrating an erythematous, pustular lesion.

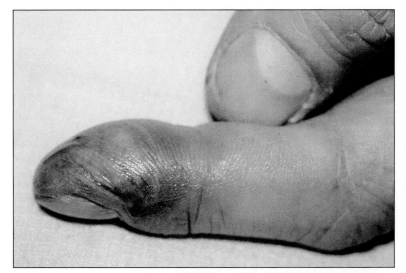

FIGURE 2-6 Blistering distal dactylitis. A large tender blister is present on the finger pad of the left forefinger. Most cases of blistering distal dactylitis have occurred in children, and *Streptococcus pyogenes* has been the usual isolate, but *Staphylococcus aureus* can produce the same disorder. Cases due to streptococci respond to oral penicillin, whereas those caused by staphylococci require an oral antistaphylococcal antibiotic. Incision and drainage may be helpful for large, tender, or purulent bullae.

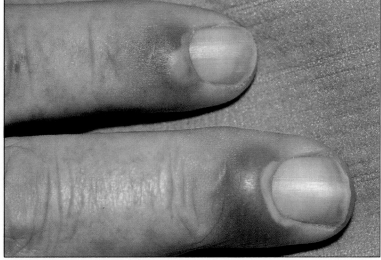

FIGURE 2-7 Paronychia. Erythema, swelling, and accumulated pus are present proximal to the nail plates on these fingers. *S. aureus* is the isolate in about 60% of finger paronychia. Predisposing factors include trauma, finger sucking, and protracted or repeated exposure to water. Streptococci and mouth anaerobes are frequent isolates in those not due to *S. aureus*. Gentle separation of the cuticle from the underlying nail plate with a scalpel blade provides drainage of the pus. Topical or systemic antimicrobials are rarely necessary.

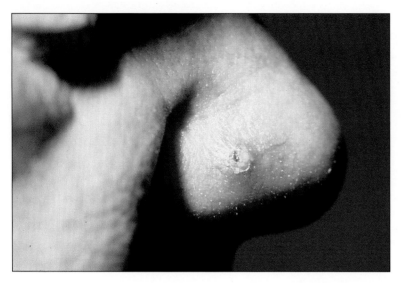

FIGURE 2-8 Pustule. A small pustule is present on the nose. A culture revealed a pure growth of *S. aureus*. Often such pustules originate in hair follicles (folliculitis), and numerous lesions may occur. Folliculitis, however, may develop from infections with other organisms, such as *Pityrosporum orbiculare*, or from noninfectious causes such as chemicals, physical trauma, and over-hydration of the skin. Incision and drainage suffice when only a few lesions are present, but with numerous pustules, an oral antistaphylococcal antibiotic may be necessary, if *S. aureus* is the cause.

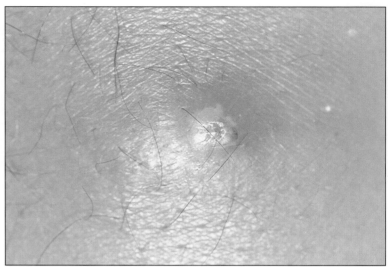

FIGURE 2-9 Furuncle. A furuncle (boil) is a deeper infection of the hair follicle than folliculitis and consists of an inflammatory nodule with a pustular center through which a hair emerges. By contrast, a carbuncle (*see* Fig. 2-10) involves several adjacent hair follicles, creating an inflammatory mass with pus discharging from several follicular orifices. Furuncles commonly occur on the face, neck, upper extremities, and buttocks. Treatment is incision and drainage, with oral antistaphylococcal antibiotics reserved for those with numerous lesions, substantial surrounding cellulitis, or fever. Some patients develop recurrent episodes of furunculosis. Occasionally, a white cell disorder such as Job's syndrome may be responsible, but most victims are otherwise healthy and have colonization of the anterior nares with *S. aureus*, as does about 30% of the general population. Why some nasal carriers develop skin infections and others do not is unknown, but trauma to the skin is often an important factor.

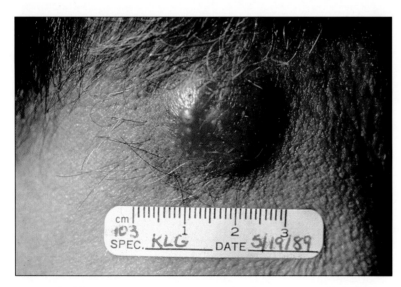

FIGURE 2-10 Carbuncle. A large violaceous nodule has formed on the back of the neck with a pustule near its left border. A carbuncle is a staphylococcal infection involving several adjacent hair follicles. It typically occurs on the posterior neck, especially in diabetics, and begins as a nodule that enlarges to form an inflammatory mass with pus discharging from several follicular openings. Other common sites are the shoulders, hips, and thighs. Treatment consists of incision and drainage. Systemic antibiotics are unnecessary unless substantial surrounding cellulitis or fever is present.

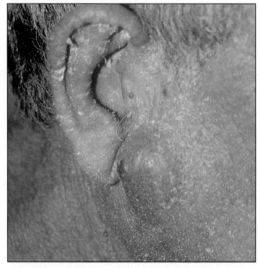

FIGURE 2-11 Cutaneous abscess. An erythematous mass with a pustular head is present on the mandibular area anterior to the ear. *S. aureus*, usually in pure growth, causes about 25% of all cutaneous abscesses and is especially common in those involving the axillae, breasts of puerperal women, and hands. Abscesses in other locations usually yield mixed cultures—without *S. aureus*—containing the aerobic and anaerobic organisms that constitute that area's normal regional flora. Treatment is incision and drainage. Systemic antibiotics are unnecessary unless substantial surrounding cellulitis or fever is present.

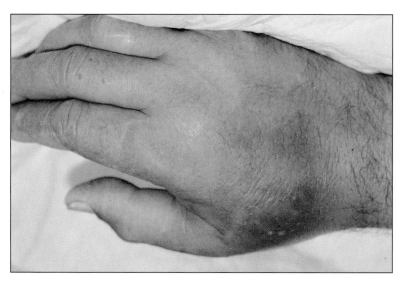

FIGURE 2-12 Subcutaneous abscess. A large area of erythema involves the dorsum of the hand, which is diffusely swollen, and several pustules are present just distal to the thumb. Such abscesses are usually secondary to trauma, as in this case, which followed penetrating injury in an industrial accident. Thorough incision and drainage are required, and an antistaphylococcal antibiotic is usually given orally or parenterally, depending on the severity of the infection.

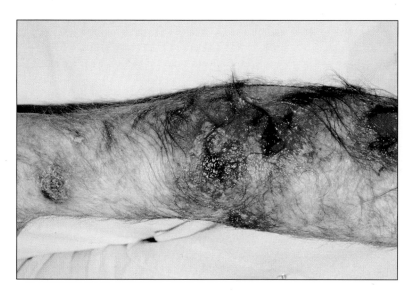

FIGURE 2-13 Infected superficial trauma. Abrasions to the forearm incurred in a fall preceded this infection, which consists of areas of erythema, crusting, ulcerations, and pustules. *S. aureus* is a common cause of infection in diffusely damaged skin, as well as in small areas of trauma. Treatment is an antistaphylococcal antibiotic given orally or parenterally, depending on the severity of infection.

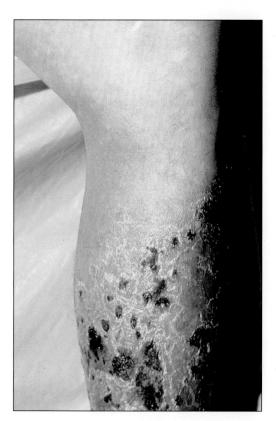

FIGURE 2-14 Infected eczema. Erythema, crusts, and proximal lymphangitis developed in this patient with preceding eczema caused by venous disease of his right lower extremity. *S. aureus* is very commonly present on the skin of patients with eczema. Distinguishing between nonpathogenic colonization and superinfection can be difficult, because erythema, exudation, and crusting are frequent in uninfected eczema. The presence of cellulitis (a substantial area of adjacent erythema and warmth), lymphangitis, lymphadenitis, fever, or pustules clearly indicates superinfection that warrants therapy with an oral antistaphylococcal antibiotic.

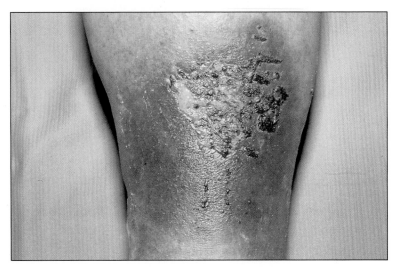

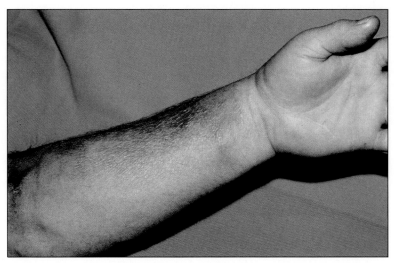

FIGURE 2-15 Staphylococcal cellulitis. A dusky, edematous erythema extends from purulent erosions on the shin of this patient. Most cases of substantial cellulitis are due to *Streptococcus pyogenes* or other streptococci, which produce enzymes that allow infection to spread widely along tissue planes. *S. aureus*, on the other hand, tends to produce localized pus and abscesses with a small amount of circumferential cellulitis, rather than diffuse soft tissue inflammation. Staphylococcal cellulitis, therefore, is most commonly associated with cutaneous abscesses, open wounds, or damaged skin, where it appears as a relatively small area of erythema and edema surrounding the suppurative focus.

FIGURE 2-16 Suppurative thrombophlebitis. A band of erythema extends from the wrist to the antecubital area. Surgical exploration revealed suppurative thrombophlebitis. This infection, most commonly due to *S. aureus*, may occur from intravascular injection of an illicit drug, as in this patient, or as a complication of intravenous catheters. Often, a scab is present at the entry site of the infection, and, if the scab is removed, pressure on the vein proximal to it may cause pus to appear. Most of these infections resolve with parenteral antistaphylococcal antibiotic therapy, but incision and drainage or excision of the infected vein may be necessary when substantial purulence is present.

STAPHYLOCOCCAL PYOMYOSITIS

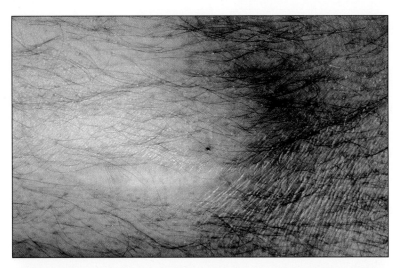

FIGURE 2-17 Staphylococcal pyomyositis. A fluctuant bulge without overlying erythema or pustules is present on the right thigh. Most commonly seen in children in tropical countries, where *S. aureus* causes over 90% of the cases, pyomyositis is an uncommon disease in temperate climates, where *S. aureus* is responsible for about 70% of reported cases. In nontropical areas, trauma, diabetes mellitus, connective tissue disorders, and immunodeficiency may be predisposing factors. Large muscle groups, especially of the lower extremity, are most commonly affected. Pain and swelling of the area, often with tenderness, are the usual findings. The overlying skin often feels indurated but is typically normal in temperature and color. Needle aspiration of the area will usually yield pus. Treatment is incision and drainage of the pus plus a parenteral antistaphylococcal antibiotic. Early in the course of the infection, before pus has formed, antibiotic therapy alone may suffice.

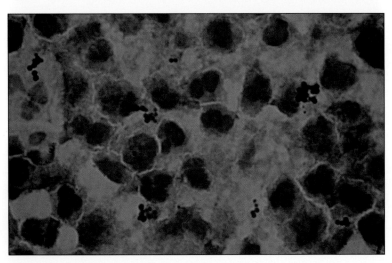

FIGURE 2-18 Staphylococcal pyomyositis. A Gram stain of pus obtained by needle aspiration of the thigh lesion of the patient in Fig. 2-17 demonstrates numerous neutrophils and large gram-positive cocci in pairs, chains, and clusters. This appearance is typical of *S. aureus*, which grew in pure culture.

STAPHYLOCOCCAL PAROTITIS

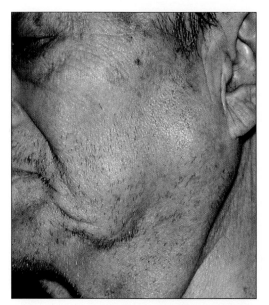

FIGURE 2-19 Staphylococcal parotitis. A fluctuant mass with slight overlying erythema is present in the parotid area of an elderly patient who recently underwent abdominal surgery. Suppurative parotitis most commonly occurs in patients with diminished salivary flow because of volume depletion, atropine-like medications, decreased oral intake, recent surgery, or underlying parotid disease, such as Sjögren's syndrome. Organisms probably ascend from the oral cavity through Stensen's duct to reach the gland. Usually, the infection is unilateral and begins abruptly with swelling, pain, and induration in the parotid area. Overlying cutaneous erythema is common. *S. aureus* is the most frequent single pathogen, but isolation of anaerobes alone or mixed with aerobic bacteria is common. Similar infections can occur in the submandibular salivary glands. Treatment consists of systemic and oral hydration plus a parenteral antistaphylococcal antibiotic. Massage of the gland may promote drainage of pus through Stensen's duct, but surgery is rarely necessary.

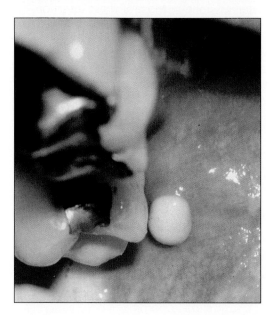

FIGURE 2-20 Staphylococcal parotitis. Examination of the oral cavity following massage of the parotid gland of the patient shown in Fig. 2-19 demonstrates pus exuding from the orifice of Stensen's duct. A Gram stain of this material revealed numerous neutrophils and gram-positive cocci in clusters; the culture yielded a pure growth of *S. aureus*.

STAPHYLOCOCCAL SCALDED SKIN SYNDROME

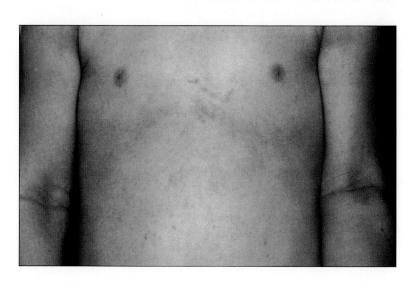

FIGURE 2-21 Staphylococcal scalded skin syndrome. A faint macular erythema is present on the trunk and arms of a febrile 4-year-old girl. The redness is accentuated in the skinfolds of the upper arms and the antecubital area. This disease occurs from the effects of epidermolytic toxins produced by some strains of *S. aureus*, most commonly group II phage types. The patients are usually children less than 5 years of age, in whom the staphylococci commonly colonize the mucous membranes of the nasopharynx, vagina, or conjunctivae, from which the toxin is readily absorbed. This disorder is rare in adults, apparently because they can inactivate or eliminate the toxins by immunologic mechanisms or urinary excretion. Affected adults usually have had suppurative infections, rather than just mucosal colonization, and severely compromised renal or immune function.

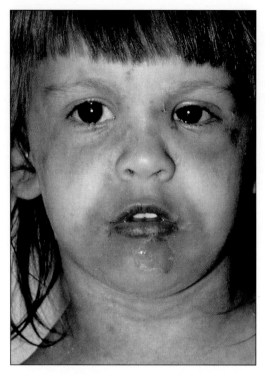

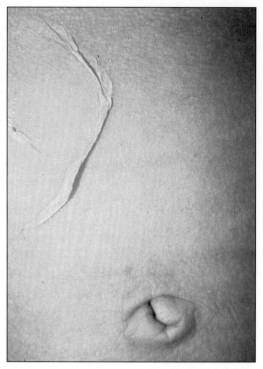

Figure 2-22 Staphylococcal scalded skin syndrome. Erythema is prominent on the neck and around the eyes and mouth. Crusting is also apparent in the periorificial areas. Over the chin, a bulla has ruptured, leaving a moist erosion. The usual sequence of this disease is cutaneous erythema, the development of superficial vesicles and bullae, and, finally, skin separation in sheets and ribbons, leaving a moist red base that dries quickly. The toxins responsible for this disease cause intraepidermal cleavage, typically at the granular layer. Toxic epidermal necrolysis, a rare complication of therapy with certain medications, also causes diffuse blistering and skin separation, but the split occurs lower, at the dermal–epidermal junction. Furthermore, target lesions and mucous membrane involvement are characteristic of toxic epidermal necrolysis but are absent in the staphylococcal scalded skin syndrome.

Figure 2-23 Nikolsky's sign in staphylococcal scalded skin syndrome. Nikolsky's sign—shearing of the skin with firm rubbing—is demonstrated on the trunk of this patient. Because the skin separation is superficial, fluid loss is usually minor, and most affected children are not very ill. A parenteral antistaphylococcal antibiotic is the appropriate therapy, combined with intravenous fluids for those with volume depletion. Patients (primarily adults) with suppurative infections rather than just mucosal colonization may require drainage of purulent collections.

STAPHYLOCOCCAL TOXIC SHOCK SYNDROME

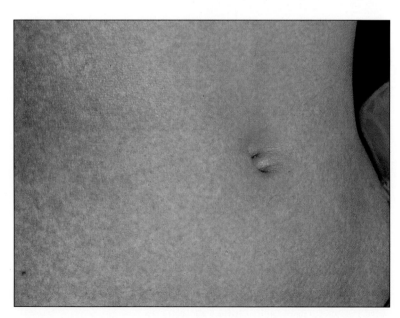

Figure 2-24 Staphylococcal toxic shock syndrome. A diffuse morbilliform erythema that blanches on pressure is present on the trunk of a young woman who developed a high fever, vomiting, myalgias, watery diarrhea, and hypotension during menstruation. This disorder is caused by strains of *S. aureus* that produce certain toxins, including toxic shock syndrome toxin 1 and enterotoxins B or C. The responsible organisms may be present in the vagina, especially during menstruation when highly absorbent tampons are used. In nonmenstrual cases, the source of the staphylococci has included cutaneous and surgical wound infections, soft tissue suppuration, pneumonia, empyema, sinusitis, osteomyelitis, and postpartum genital tract infections. The eruption that occurs with this disease is an erythema that may be macular, resembling measles, or confluent, simulating a sunburn, and often contains tiny papules that give the skin a "sand-paper" texture. It is frequently more intense around the site of the staphylococcal infection, is accentuated in flexural areas, and is absent in locations of pressure such as under a waistband. It usually fades within 3 days. Petechiae may occur within the rash, and nonpitting edema is sometimes present, especially in periorbital and periarticular areas. Treatment includes intravenous volume repletion, vasoactive agents for those with hypotension unresponsive to fluid replacement, and an intravenous antistaphylococcal antibiotic. Those with a suppurative focus of infection may require drainage of pus.

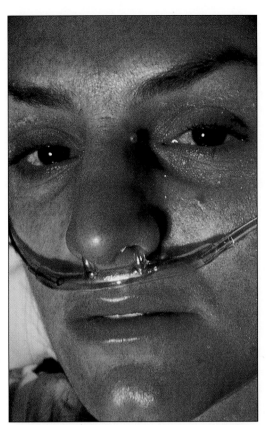

FIGURE 2-25
Staphylococcal toxic shock syndrome. The bulbar conjunctivae are reddened in this young woman with menstrual-related toxic shock syndrome. Hyperemia of the mucous membranes, including the vagina, pharynx, and conjunctivae is common in this disorder. Sometimes, subconjunctival hemorrhages occur, and erosions can develop in the oral cavity and vagina.

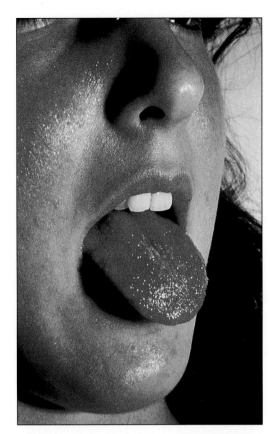

FIGURE 2-26
"Strawberry tongue" in staphylococcal toxic shock syndrome. Hyperplastic, erythematous lingual papillae produce a markedly red tongue (strawberry tongue), a common finding in this disease.

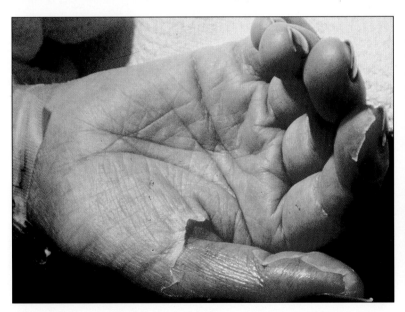

FIGURE 2-27 Staphylococcal toxic shock syndrome. Desquamation of the skin, especially on the palms and soles, occurs 10 to 21 days after the onset of the disease. Another late finding is a pruritic, generalized maculopapular eruption developing on days 9 to 13. Patients can lose their nails and hair after 4 to 16 weeks, with resolution of these abnormalities by 5 to 6 months.

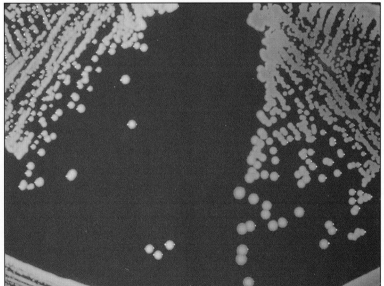

FIGURE 2-28 Staphylococcus on blood agar culture plate. Colonies of *S. aureus* have several characteristic morphologic features on blood agar plates. Like colonies of most gram-positive bacteria, those of staphylococci are smaller and less moist than those of gram-negative organisms. The distinction between staphylococci and streptococci is that the former are translucent and the latter opaque. β-Hemolysis does not discriminate between them because this phenomenon occurs frequently with *S. aureus* as well as streptococci. Compared with coagulase-negative staphylococci, colonies of *S. aureus* are creamier in color and stick more tenaciously to a metal loop when lifted from the agar surface.

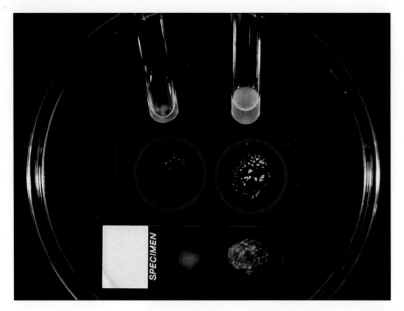

FIGURE 2-29 Coagulase test. *S. aureus* has two coagulant factors—coagulases—that cause plasma to clot. One is a diffusible substance produced by the organism; the other is a fixed material present on the cell membrane that converts fibrinogen to fibrin and causes the cell membrane to become sticky. Detection of these coagulases distinguishes *S. aureus* from other staphylococci. This slide shows three methods of demonstrating these coagulases, with negative tests on the *left* and positive ones on the *right*. At the *top* is the tube coagulase method, which requires up to 4 hours of incubating the organisms in plasma before the test can be declared negative. This method has been replaced in most laboratories by a slide test. At the *bottom* of the picture is one method that involves adding plasma to a suspension of organisms. In the *center* is a commercial latex agglutination preparation that detects both coagulase and protein A, also present on the cell membrane of *S. aureus*.

SELECTED BIBLIOGRAPHY

Barton LL, Friedman AD: Impetigo: A reassessment of etiology and therapy. *Pediatr Dermatol* 1987, 4:185–188.

Wortman PD: Bacterial infections of the skin. *Curr Prob Dermatol* 1993, 6:197–208.

Meislin HW, Lerner SA, Graves MH, *et al*.: Cutaneous abscesses: Anaerobic and aerobic bacteriology and outpatient management. *Ann Intern Med* 1977, 87:145–149.

Christin L, Sarosi GA: Pyomyositis in North American: Case reports and review. *Clin Infect Dis* 1992, 15:668–667.

Brook I, Frazier EH, Thompson DH: Aerobic and anaerobic microbiology of acute suppurative parotitis. *Laryngoscope* 1991, 101:170–172.

Resnick SD: Staphylococcal toxin-mediated syndromes in childhood. *Semin Dermatol* 1992, 11:11–18.

CHAPTER 3

Streptococcal Infections of Skin and Soft Tissues

Dennis L. Stevens

MICROBIOLOGY

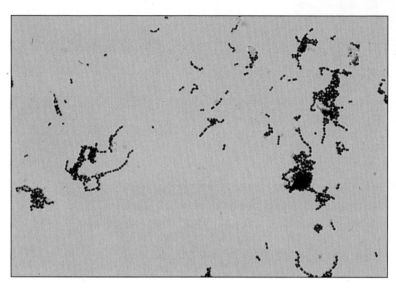

FIGURE 3-1 Gram stain of *Streptococcus pyogenes* grown in Todd-Hewitt broth, showing characteristic chains of Gram and cocci.

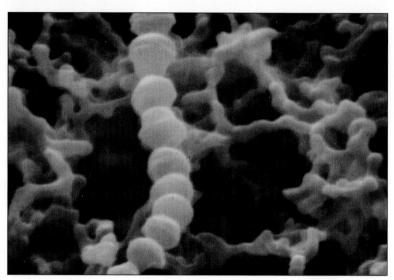

FIGURE 3-2 Scanning electron micrograph of *S. pyogenes*, clearly showing the elongated chain of cocci.

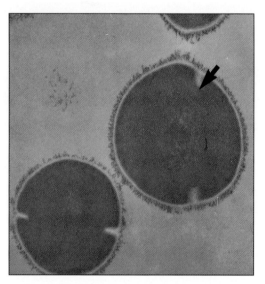

FIGURE 3-3 Transmission electron micrograph of an ultrathin section of *S. pyogenes* demonstrates M-protein (fuzzy material projecting through the outer cell wall, *arrow*). M-protein, a cell surface component, plays a key role in the pathogenesis of group A streptococci by inhibiting phagocytosis. Following infection with a particular M-protein, individuals develop type-specific immunity. Over 70 antigenically distinct varieties of M-protein are known to occur in strains of *S. pyogenes*. (*Courtesy of* E. Beachey, MD, and J. Dale, MD.)

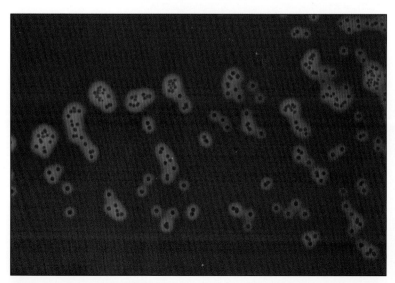

FIGURE 3-4 β-Hemolysis is apparent on a sheep-blood agar plate after overnight incubation. Hemolysis is due to the extracellular toxins streptolysins O and S.

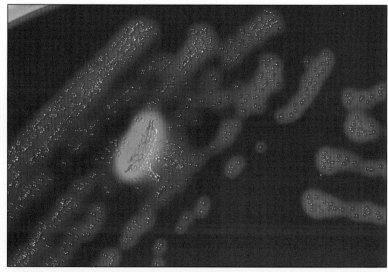

FIGURE 3-5 β-Hemolysis can be accentuated by "stab" inoculation. This enhancement is due to increased production or stability of the oxygen-labile streptolysin O.

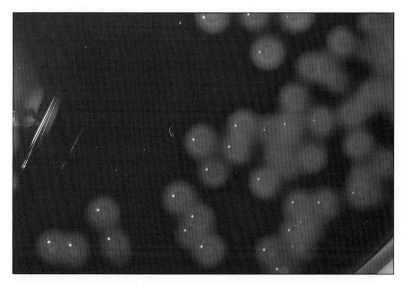

FIGURE 3-6 Mucoid colony of *S. pyogenes*. The larger size of the colony is related to increased hyaluronic acid production and may occur with many M-types, although recently mucoidity has been associated with M-type 18. Mucoid colony type may be associated with rheumatic fever.

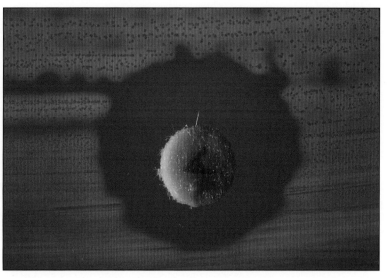

FIGURE 3-7 Inhibition of growth of β-hemolytic colonies by bacitracin is a presumptive test for identification of an organism as group A streptococcus, as only about 5% of nongroup A hemolytic streptococci are susceptible to bacitracin.

CLINICAL CONDITIONS

Major streptococcal infections of skin, soft tissues, and mucous membranes

Scarlet fever
Pharyngitis
Impetigo (pyoderma)
Erysipelas
Cellulitis
Lymphangitis
Myositis
Bacteremia
Toxic shock syndrome

FIGURE 3-8 Major streptococcal infections of skin and soft tissues. Different strains of *S. pyogenes* can affect any or all of these sites, although M-types 1–40 are associated with pharyngitis and scarlet fever and M-types 49–61 are associated with impetigo.

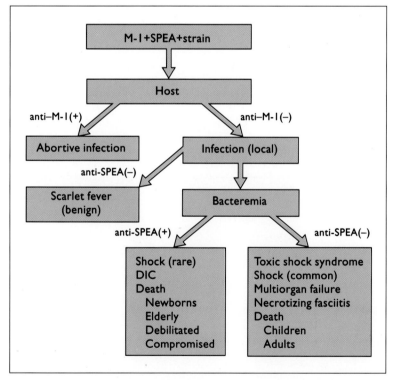

FIGURE 3-9 Pathogenesis of scarlet fever, bacteremia, and toxic shock syndrome. Various features of the group A streptococci, including M-1 type protein, streptococcal pyogenic exotoxin A (SPEA), and strain, combine with host, susceptibility factors to enable the development of local streptococcal infection, which then progresses to more severe forms. Bacteremia may progress along two courses, depending on the individual's antibody status to SPEA. Bacteremia may develop in patients lacking anti–M-protein antibody. Streptococcal toxic shock syndrome may develop in those patients lacking antibody to SPEA. (DIC—disseminated intravascular coagulation.)

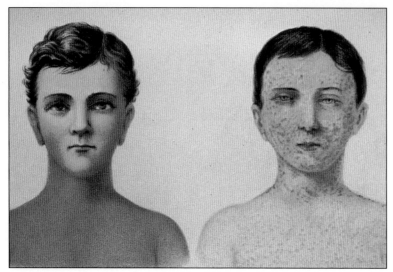

FIGURE 3-10 Historically, scarlet fever was a common epidemic ailment of childhood, although it is now uncommon in the United States. The primary site of infection is usually the pharynx, with the distinctive rash resulting from an erythrogenic toxin produced by the streptococcus. The rash appears soon (within 2 days) after the onset of the sore throat and disappears in 6–10 days. This illustration is of a boy with scarlet fever (*left panel*) compared with measles (*right panel*), showing diffuse erythema and circumoral pallor characteristic of scarlet fever. (*From* Rotch TM: *Pediatrics*. Philadelphia: J.B. Lippincott; 1896; with permission.)

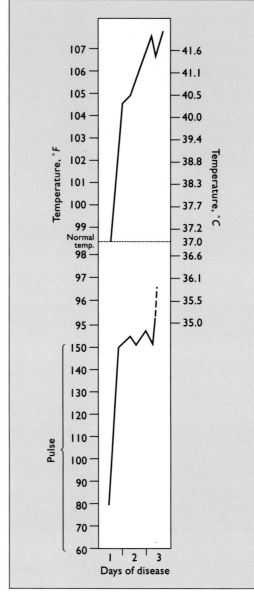

FIGURE 3-11 Typical fever curve of an 11-year-old girl with scarlet fever. Untreated, scarlet fever may lead to serious complications of acute rheumatic fever, rheumatic heart disease, and acute glomerulonephritis. (*From* Rotch TM: *Pediatrics*. Philadelphia: J.B. Lippincott; 1896; with permission.)

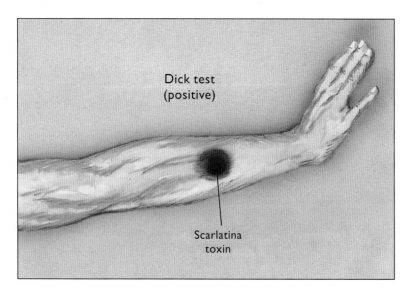

FIGURE 3-12 Dick test. Culture supernatant from a strain of group A streptococcus isolated from the throat of a child with acute scarlet fever was injected into the arm of a subject who never had scarlet fever. The erythema surrounding the injection site was considered a positive Dick test. (*Illustration by* Michael Wyett.)

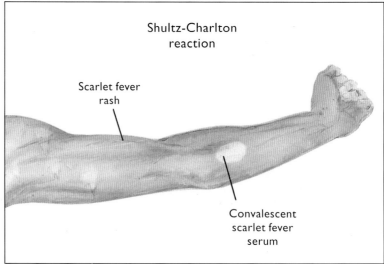

FIGURE 3-13 Schultz-Charlton reaction. Convalescent serum from a scarlet fever patient blanches the rash of a patient with scarlet fever. (*Illustration by* Michael Wyett.)

Three types of scarlet fever

Type	Clinical findings	Outcome
Benign	Red rash Pharyngitis	

Septic	Red rash
	Pharyngitis
	Local invasion
	  of vital structures of
	  the neck
		Slow, lingering death
		due to bleeding,
		suffocation

Toxic	Red rash Pharyngitis Profound fever (> 108 ° F) Dehydration Convulsions	High mortality rate; rapid death due to status epilepticus, dehydration, etc.

FIGURE 3-14 Three types of scarlet fever, categorized by severity.

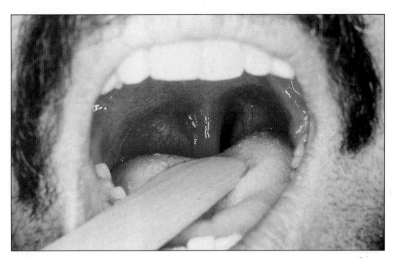

FIGURE 3-15 Pharyngitis. The most common of the group A streptococcal infections, streptococcal pharyngitis typically affects school-aged children, although adults are still highly susceptible. Transmission is through close personal contact, via saliva droplets produced during sneezing or coughing, with infection rates peaking in the winter months. This slide demonstrates the cardinal manifestations of erythema, pharyngeal exudate, and lymphoid enlargement. This patient also has peritonsillar abscess, an infrequent complication of streptococcal pharyngitis. Note the unilateral displacement of the tonsil to the midline.

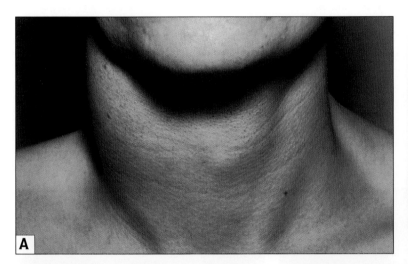

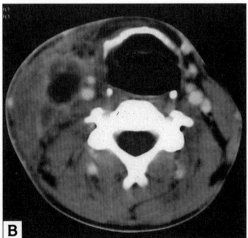

FIGURE 3-16 A patient's neck clearly shows peritonsillar abscess with extension to deep tissues of the neck. **A**, Swelling of the neck with loss of definition of the sternocleidomastoid muscle is shown. **B**, A computed tomography scan of the neck shows a deep collection of inflammatory material.

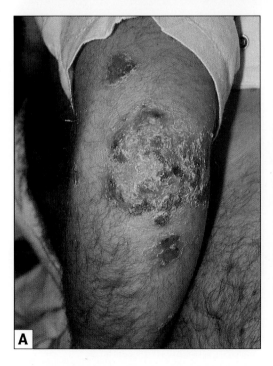

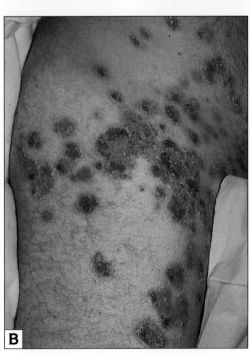

FIGURE 3-17 Impetigo (pyoderma). Group A β-hemolytic streptococci have been the most frequent cause of impetigo, although *Staphylococcus aureus* is now more common and must be distinguished from the streptococcal form. The disease is endemic in the warmer southern states and most tropical areas. It primarily affects younger and preschool-aged children, in summer months, usually appearing on faces, hands, legs, and other exposed areas. **A**, The dry, crusty lesions of impetigo sometimes have a straw-colored appearance like dried serum. **B**, Impetigo can occur as a single lesion or be widespread, as seen in this homeless, malnourished man. Acute glomerulonephritis had been a serious complication of streptococcal impetigo, but its occurrence has declined because of accessibility to antibiotics and a decreasing prevalence of nephrotoxic strains of streptococci.

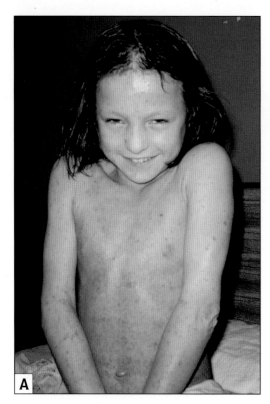
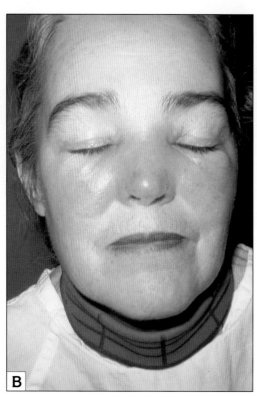

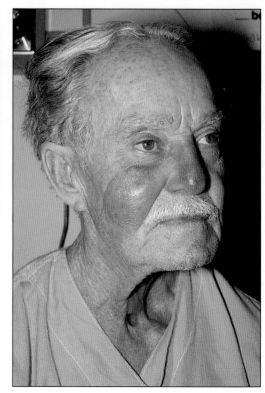

FIGURE 3-18 Streptococcal infection is transmitted by close personal contact, and a single strain may have different manifestations in different people. **A,** As this case illustrates, a young girl developed scarlet fever. **B,** A few days later, her mother developed erysipelas. The same strain of group A streptococcus caused both types of infection. (*Courtesy of* P. Quie, MD.)

FIGURE 3-19 Erysipelas. In the characteristic appearance of erysipelas, a brilliant red or salmon red, painful confluent erythema in a "butterfly" distribution involves the nasal eminence, cheeks, and nose with abrupt borders along the nasolabial fold. The erythema increases over a course of 3–6 days and usually resolves in 7–10 days. Erysipelas has been associated with high fevers, bacteremia, and possible death, even in modern times. The fluctuation in severity may reflect cyclical changes in the virulence of group A-β hemolytic streptococci.

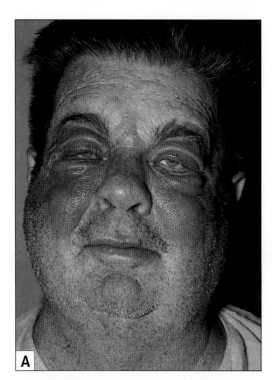
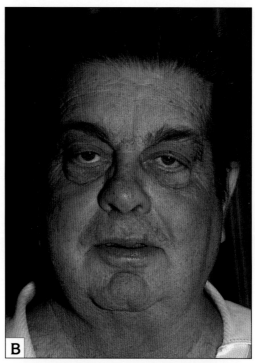

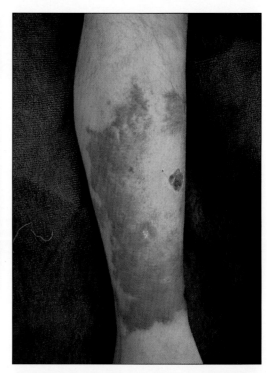

FIGURE 3-20 Erysipelas responds quickly to penicillin. **A** and **B,** Photographs were taken 5 days apart and demonstrate that scarring or loss of tissue is rare because infection occurs above the stratum germinativum. The patient was not "toxic."

FIGURE 3-21 Erysipelas usually occur on the face, although any skin surface, such as the leg, can be affected. Note the sharp line of demarkation and bright red color, features that distinguish it from cellulitis.

Streptococcus strains causing soft tissue infection associated with unique clinical settings	
Surgical incision	Group A
Childbirth (puerperal sepsis)	Groups A, B
Peripheral vascular disease	Group B
Diabetes	Group B
Saphenous vein donor site	Groups C, G
Venous insufficiency	Groups A, C, G
Chronic lymphedema	Groups A, C, G

FIGURE 3-22 Streptococcus strains causing soft tissue infection associated with unique clinical settings.

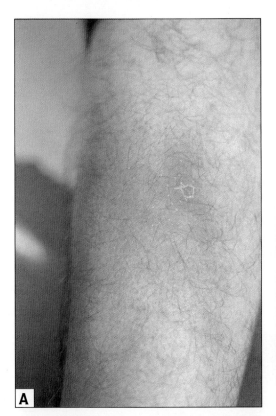 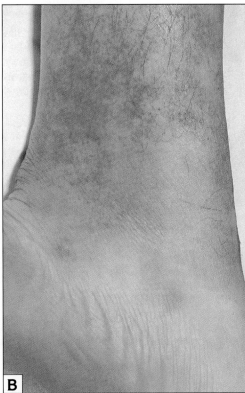 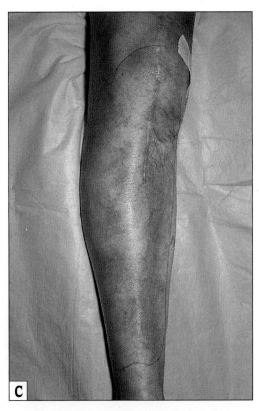

FIGURE 3-23 A, B, and **C,** Cellulitis of the skin. Erythema, swelling, heat, and pain are cardinal features of cellulitis. The erythema may be pink or red but lacks the intense, fiery-red or salmon-colored appearance of erysipelas. Small breaks in the skin are associated with streptococcal infection, whereas staphylococcal cellulitis is often associated with larger wounds, ulcers, or abscesses. Fever is suggestive of streptococcal infection.

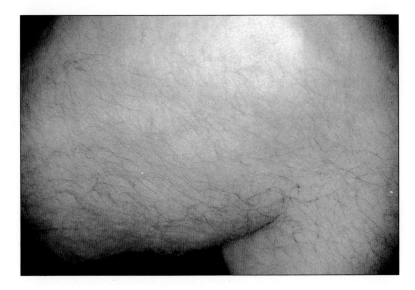

FIGURE 3-24 Lymphangitis. Reddened streaks extending proximally from an infected wound or cellulitis are invariably caused by group A streptococcus. Prompt antibiotic treatment is mandatory because bacteremia and systemic toxicity develop rapidly.

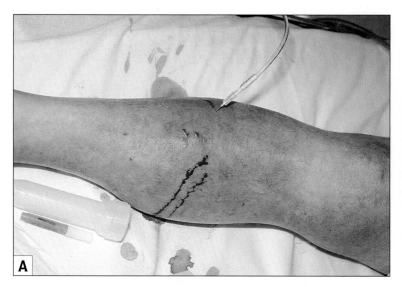

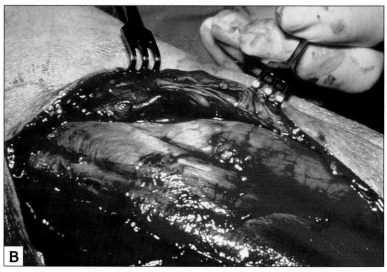

FIGURE 3-25 Necrotizing fasciitis and myositis. The patient had sudden onset of excruciating pain and signs of systemic toxicity. **A,** Note the swelling of the leg and two small purple or violaceous bullae on the anterior shin, whereas the adjacent skin appears healthy. The pressures in the anterior and lateral compartments were measured by placing a needle in the deep tissue (hence the blood at the sampling site). Pressures were elevated and surgical exploration was performed. **B,** The fascia overlying the deep musculature was friable and brownish to dishwater-gray in appearance, establishing a diagnosis of necrotizing fasciitis. Deeper exploration of muscle compartments is warranted in such cases.

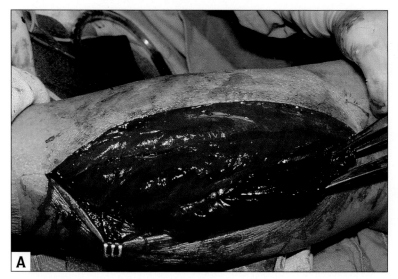

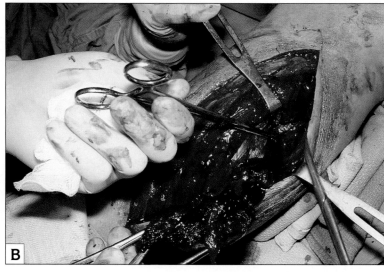

FIGURE 3-26 **A,** Musculature in streptococcal myositis is deep red, reddish-blue, or black. **B,** Necrotic muscle must be aggressively debrided.

FIGURE 3-27 Histopathologic examination of myonecrotic tissue demonstrates an absence of acute inflammatory cells in the areas of degenerative muscle bundles. When present, infiltrating granulocytes can be seen at the interface between normal and necrotic tissue and are often massed within small postcapillary venules.

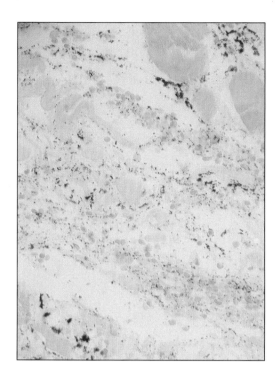

FIGURE 3-28 Tissue Gram stain of an area of myonecrosis shows absence of inflammatory cells and the presence of gram-positive cocci.

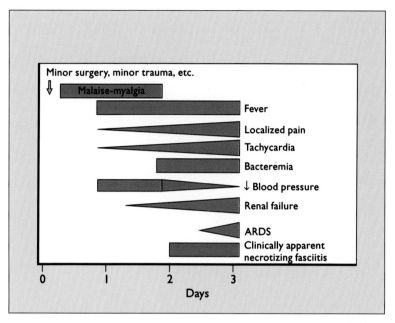

FIGURE 3-29 Clinical signs and symptoms of streptococcal toxic shock syndrome. (ARDS—adult respiratory distress syndrome.)

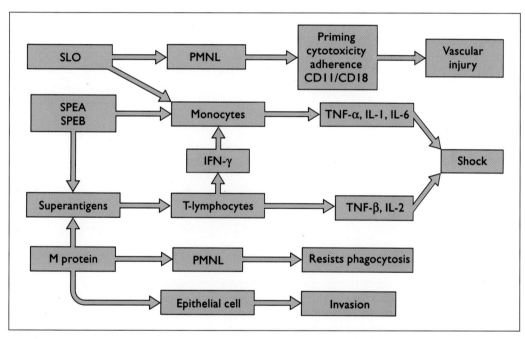

FIGURE 3-30 Pathogenesis of streptococcal toxic shock syndrome. Vascular injury, capillary leak, acute respiratory distress syndrome, and multiorgan failure are common features. Although direct effects of the streptolysin O toxin (SLO) on eukaryotic cells cause some of the pathology, it is the intimate interaction of cells of the host immune system with specific streptococcal toxins and cell wall components that causes activation and release of cytokines in sufficient concentration to have detrimental effects on host organ function. (SPEA—streptococcal pyogenic exotoxin A; SPEB—streptococcal pyogenic exotoxin B; PMNL—polymorphonuclear leukocyte; TNF—tumor necrosis factor; IL—interleukin; IFN-γ—interferon-γ.)

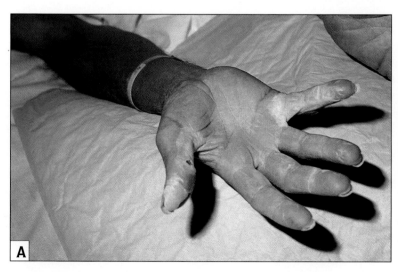

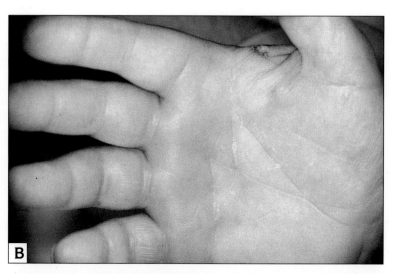

FIGURE 3-31 **A**, Desquamation of skin in streptococcal toxic shock syndrome occurs 10–14 days after infection at sites that were erythematous during the initial phase. **B**, Swelling of the hand is acutely due to diffuse capillary leak, which may be induced directly by bacterial toxins or by endogenous cytokines produced in response to infection.

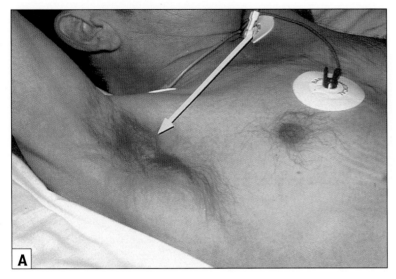

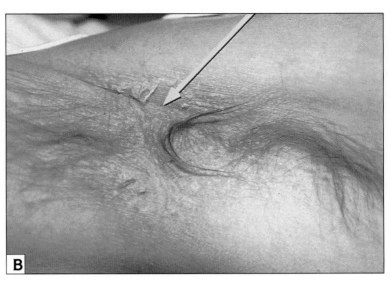

FIGURE 3-32 Erythematous rash in streptococcal toxic shock syndrome may occur anywhere and is transient. **A** and **B**, *Panel 32A* illustrates erythema of the axillae in such a patient, followed by *panel 32B* by desquamation of the erythematous skin 10–14 days after the rash appeared.

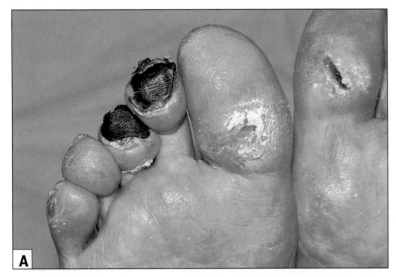

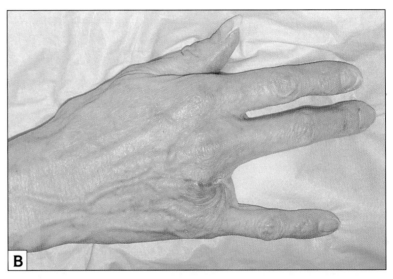

FIGURE 3-33 Vascular compromise in patients with streptococcal toxic shock syndrome. **A**, Blackened toes are apparent in a patient who survived streptococcal toxic shock syndrome. **B**, Concomitant therapy with potent vasoconstrictors, such as epinephrine, phenylephrine (Neo-Synephrine), or metaraminol bitartrate (Aramine), can greatly exacerbate this condition, leading to symetrical necro-sis of hands and feet. Mechanisms contributing to vascular compromise in this infection are poorly understood but may involve bacterial toxin-induced leukostasis within small venules, leading to regional tissue ischemia. Cytokines produced by the host may also contribute to this condition.

FIGURE 3-34 Localized cutaneous gangrene in a patient with group A streptococcal bacteremia. The well-circumscribed necrotic areas are likely due to vascular occlusion and tissue infarction.

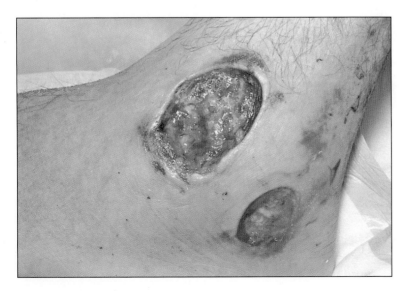

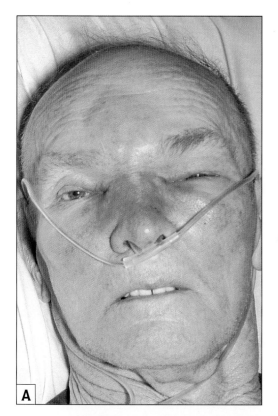

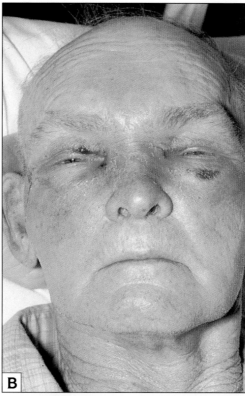

FIGURE 3-35 Cellulitis due to mixed *Staphylococcus aureus* and group A streptococcus infection in a patient with diabetes mellitus. Diabetes also predisposes to cellulitis due to *Streptococcus agalactiae*. **A**, The patient is shown at 4–5 hours after onset of intense pain, erythema, and swelling. Antibiotics were begun just prior to this picture. **B**, The symmetric distribution had characteristics of erysipelas without the intense red color. **C**, Progression of lesions continues with evidence of tissue necrosis 72 hours after onset. **D**, The patient following plastic surgical repair.

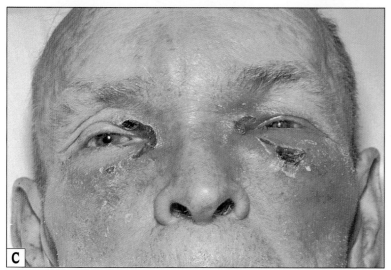

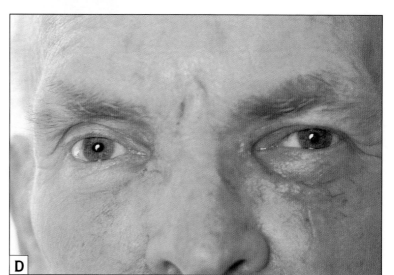

ACKNOWLEDGMENTS

All photographs, unless otherwise noted, were taken by the author and John Mangan. Illustrations were prepared by Kelly Thompson, Amy Bryant, and Michael Wyett.

SELECTED BIBLIOGRAPHY

Bisno AL: Group A streptococcal infections and acute rheumatic fever. *N Engl J Med* 1991, 325:783–793.

Fischetti VA: Streptococcal M protein. *Sci Am* 1991, 264(6):58–65.

Stevens DL, Tanner MH, Winship J, *et al.*: Reappearance of scarlet fever toxin A among streptococci in the Rocky Mountain West: Association with severe streptococcal soft tissue infection, sepsis and the toxic shock-like syndrome. *N Engl J Med* 1989, 321:1–7.

CHAPTER 4

Animal Bite Infections

Ellie J.C. Goldstein

	Pets	Bites/yr
Household pets and yearly incidence of bite wounds in the United States		
Dogs	52 million (38% of households)	1–2 million
Cats	56 million (31% of households)	400,000
Small mammals	125 million	Unknown
Snakes	Unknown	45,000

FIGURE 4-1 Incidence of animal bite wounds. Animal bites injuries are frequent worldwide. One out of every two Americans will be bitten by an animal, usually a dog, in their lifetime. Most patients (approximately 80%) suffer only minor injuries and do not seek, nor do they require, medical care. However, for the other 20%, complications are frequent, and residual disability may be lifelong. Patients who seek care < 8 hours after injury are usually concerned about wound care or the need for rabies or tetanus prophylaxis. Patients who seek care > 8 hours after injury usually do so because of established infection.

Infections associated with human and animal bites

Abscess	Cellulitis
Tenosynovitis	Periostitis
Necrotizing fasciitis	Septic arthritis
Osteomyelitis	Collar-button abscess
Sepsis	Compartment syndrome
Hepatitis A, B	Syphilis
HIV	Tuberculosis
Mycobacterium marinum	*Mycobacterium fortyitum*
Herpes simplex 1 or 2	Simian herpes B
Cat scratch disease	Actinomycosis
Brucellosis	Tularemia
Histoplasmosis	Leptospirosis
Rat bite fever	Rabies

FIGURE 4-2 Infections associated with human and animal bites.

DOG BITES

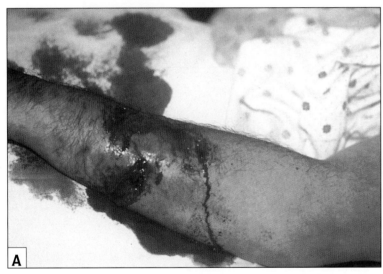

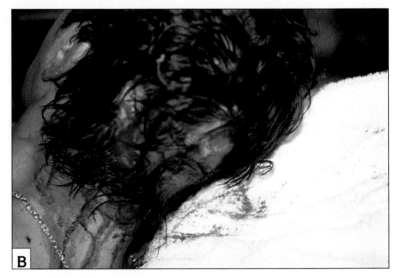

FIGURE 4-3 Dog bite victim. **A**, Arm of a dog bite victim 2 hours after injury. There are several types of bite wound injuries: tears, evulsions, punctures, and scratches. In addition, crush injury and resultant swelling may be prominent and predispose to the subsequent development of infection. Approximately 80% of these early-presenting wounds harbor potential bacterial pathogens. **B**, Head wound in the same patient. Bite wounds may be to any part of the body and involve nerves and blood vessels. (*From* Goldstein EJ: Infection secondary to cat and dog bites. *Infect Med* 1991, 8(Aug):30; with permission.) *(continued)*

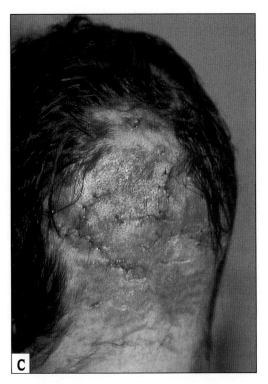

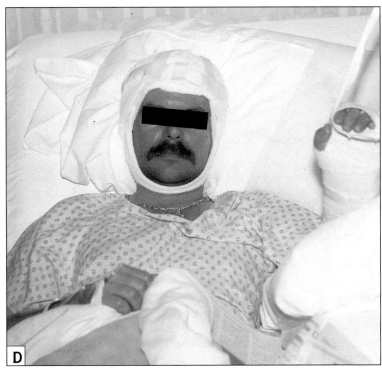

FIGURE 4-3 *(continued)* **C,** Head wound in the same patient after cleansing and suturing. The extent of wounds needs to be delineated accurately. The role of primary closure of early-presenting wounds has not been adequately studied to date. In most cases, bite wounds to the face and head may be closed after copious irrigation, if "prophylactic" antibiotics are also used. Wounds to the face and head may be exceptions among bite wounds in allowing early closure; unlike other sites, they have a superior blood supply and dependent edema rarely develops from the injury. (*From* Goldstein EJC, Richwald GA: Human and animal bite wounds. *Am Fam Physician* 1987, 36(Jul):101–109; with permission.) **D,** The same patient during recovery. The patient's left hand was also injured. The tendon was severed during the attack and required exploration and splinting. Joint range of motion as well as tendon nerve function must be evaluated in all hand injuries.

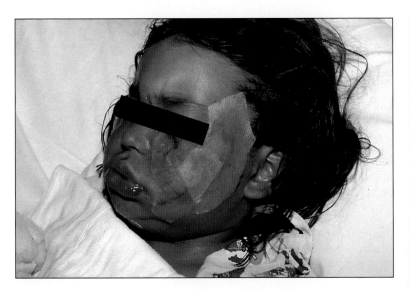

FIGURE 4-4 Facial wounds in a child. Approximately five children die from dog bite wounds each year in the United States, usually due to exsanguination when a major blood vessel is injured. Note the extensive edema and careful plastic surgical reconstruction.

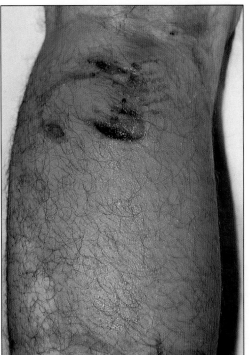

FIGURE 4-5 Infected dog bite wound to the leg. The patient's extensive cellulitis arises from the area of the eschar, under which several drops of pus act as an abscess. This abscess grew *Pasteurella multocida* and three anaerobic bacteria (*Peptostreptococcus, Prevotella* sp., and *Fusobacterium* sp.). Anaerobes are present in approximately 33% of dog bite wounds. When anaerobes are present, the infections tend to be more serious and have a propensity for abscess formation. (*From* Goldstein EJC: Infectious complications and therapy of bite wounds. *J Am Podiatr Med Assoc* 1989, 79:486–491; with permission.)

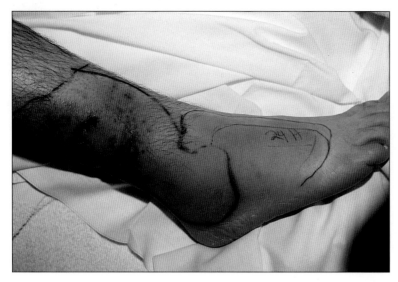

FIGURE 4-6 Leg wound infection, which developed during ampicillin therapy. Despite ampicillin therapy, the cellulitis extended (note marks on leg). *Staphylococcus aureus* was grown from this wound and is present in approximately 25% of dog bite wounds. *Staphylococcus intermedius* is an animal-infecting species, which can be coagulase-positive and mistaken for *S. aureus*, though it is often penicillin-susceptible.

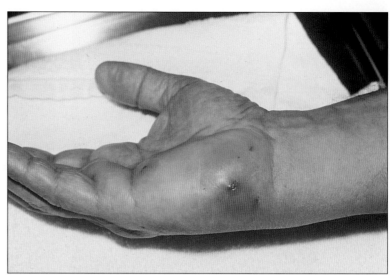

FIGURE 4-7 Dog bite wound to the hand. Two days after injury, the hand shows swelling of the hypothenar eminence with surrounding cellulitis and underlying abscess formation. This patient's wound grew seven isolates: α-streptococci, EF-4, *Pasteurella multocida*, *Moraxella* sp., *Fusobacterium nucleatum*, *Prevotella oralis*, and *Peptostreptococcus* sp.

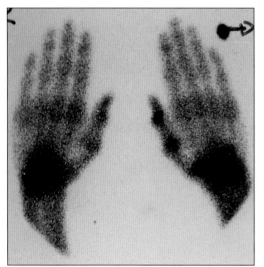

FIGURE 4-8 Bone scan showing septic arthritis. Because many bite wounds are to the hands, there is ample potential for joint penetration and inoculation of bacteria into the bone. Septic arthritis and osteomyelitis are two of the more frequent complications of bite wounds and can result in permanently stiff joints.

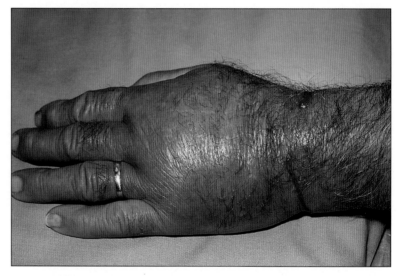

FIGURE 4-9 Dog bite to the hand. Swelling spreads proximally and not distally. Rings may need to be removed to maintain circulation.

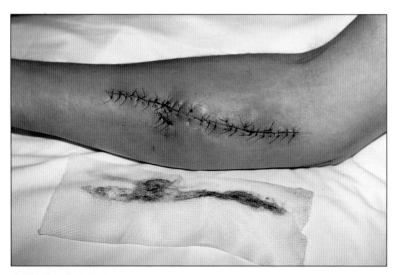

FIGURE 4-10 Infection in a sutured wound of the forearm. No controlled, prospectively studied data exist as to the advisability of suturing early-presenting animal bite wounds. In this anecdotal case, a *Bacteroides fragilis* infection developed in such a sutured wound. My recommendation is to approximate wound edges and close them by either delayed primary or secondary intent (except for facial wounds).

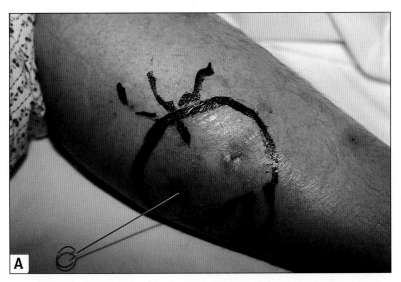

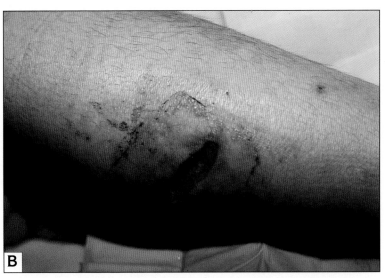

FIGURE 4-11 Chronically draining dog bite wound after 4 months of therapy. **A**, This patient received antibiotics for 4 months for a presumed persistently infected dog bite wound. Note insertion of a minitipped swab into the wound and demonstration of a fistulous tract. The patient was a kennel owner who was bitten by one of her own dogs. More than 80% of bite victims are bitten by their own pet or an animal known to them. **B**, The patient was cured by unroofing the wound and allowing it to granulate from the bottom out. (*From* Goldstein EJ: Infection secondary to cat and dog bites. *Infect Med* 1991, 8:30; with permission.)

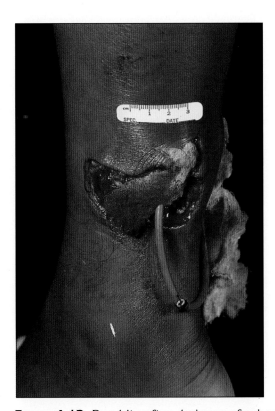

FIGURE 4-12 Dog bite after drainage of subcutaneous abscesses. Subcutaneous abscess is a relatively frequent complication of dog bites. Removal of debris and excision of necrotic tissue are sometimes required. (*From* Goldstein EJ: Infection secondary to cat and dog bites. *Infect Med* 1991, 8:30; with permission.)

Bacteriology of dog bite wounds

Aerobes	Anaerobes
α-Streptococci	*Actinomyces* sp.
β-Streptococci, group A and others	*Bacteroides* sp.
γ-Streptococci, including enterococci	*Bacteroides fragilis*
	Clostridium perfringens
Actinobacillus actinomycetemcomitans	*Eubacterium lentum*
Capnocytophaga canimorsus (DF-2)	*Eubacterium moniliforme*
	Fusobacterium nucleatum
Capnocytophaga cynodegmi	*Fusobacterium russii*
Eikenella corrodens	*Leptotrichia buccalis*
Haemophilus aphrophilus	*Porphyromonas asaccharolytica*
Micrococcus sp.	*Prevotella bivia*
Neisseria canis	*Prevotella intermedia*
Neisseria weaveri (M-5)	*Prevotella melaninogenica*
Pasteurella multocida	*Prevotella oris*
Pseudomonas aeruginosa	*Prevotella oris-buccae*
Staphylococcus aureus	*Peptostreptococcus* sp.
Staphylococcus epidermidis	*Peptostreptococcus anaerobius*
Staphylococcus intermedius	*Peptococcus magnus*
	Veillonella parvula

FIGURE 4-13 Bacteriology of dog bite wounds.

CAT BITES

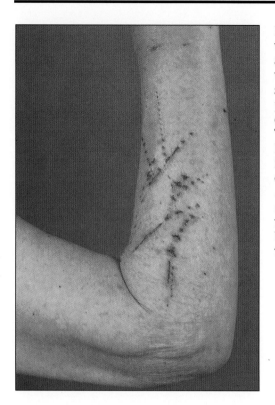

FIGURE 4-14 Arm with cat scratches and infection at the wrist. Although dog scratches are not prone to infection, cat scratches are. This is because cats lick themselves and inoculate oral flora onto their claws. *Pasteurella multocida* can be isolated from > 50% of cat bite wound infections.

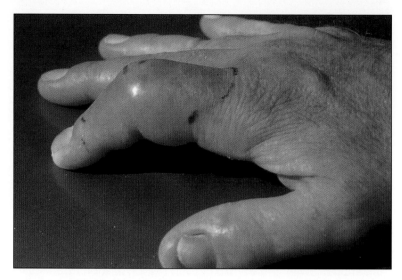

FIGURE 4-15 Septic arthritis due to cat bite. Cat teeth may seem small but can easily penetrate into a joint and cause septic arthritis. This patient received cephalexin as early empiric therapy but had a therapeutic failure and developed permanent diminished range of motion. Although the *Pasteurella multocida* isolated from the wound was reported as susceptible to cephalosporins, susceptibility breakpoints are determined by the relationship to levels achieved with maximal parenteral dosage of an antibiotic; such high levels are often not achieved by use of oral agents. The same has been true of erythromycin, which also has been associated with therapeutic failure in bite wounds. (Goldstein EJC, Citron DM, Richwald GA: Lack of *in vitro* efficacy of oral forms of certain cephalosporins, erythromycin, and oxacillin against *Pasteurella multocida. Antimicrob Agents Chemother* 1988, 32:213–215.)

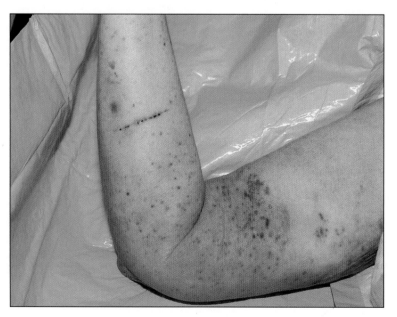

FIGURE 4-16 Cat scratch leading to *Staphylococcus aureus/Pasteurella multocida* sepsis in a patient with chronic upper extremity edema resulting from modified radical mastectomy. Patients with edema of an extremity, due to any reason, may have more severe infections and a greater risk of bacteremia associated with bite wounds and scratches. This is particularly true of women who have undergone radical and modified-radical mastectomy. Not only is there edema, but radiation decreases vascularity and node dissection alters local host defenses. These patients should be treated more aggressively with antibiotics when they are bitten on an affected extremity.

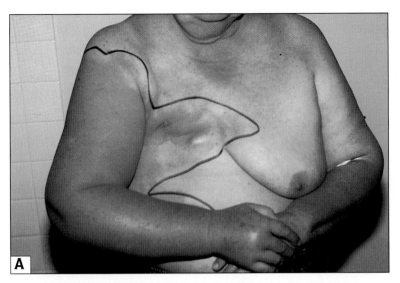

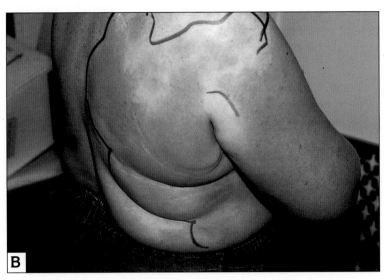

FIGURE 4-17 A and **B**, A woman with a cat bite and cephalexin failure. This patient had a previous mastectomy with resultant chronic edema of the arm. After being bitten by her cat, she developed a fever and cellulitis and was treated with oral cephalexin. After 72 hours of therapy, the infection spread all over her torso, and she became septic due to *Pasteurella multocida*.

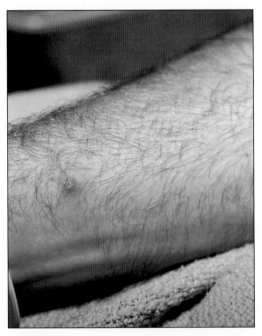

FIGURE 4-18 Primary inoculation papule of cat scratch disease. The primary inoculation papule (3–5 mm) may develop 3–10 days after injury and is often unnoticed by the patient. The papule disappears by the time the patient presents with typical symptoms of cat scratch disease.

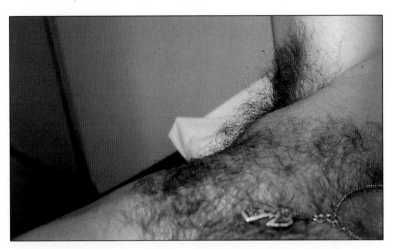

FIGURE 4-19 Adenopathy due to cat scratch disease. Cat scratch disease is thought to be due to a gram-negative rod, *Bartonella* (*Rochalimaea*) *henselae* and *B.* (*Rochalimaea*) *quintana*. Some cases may be associated with *Afipia felis*. The disease is predominant in the cool weather months and often presents with unilateral or more generalized adenopathy.

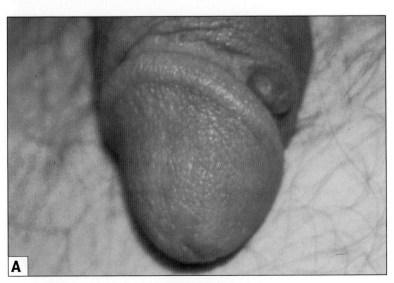

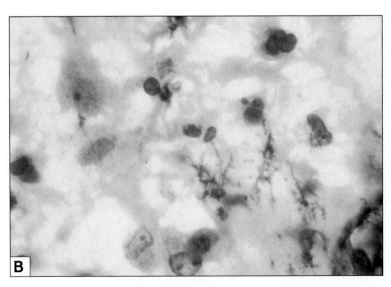

FIGURE 4-20 A, Bacillary angiomatosis lesion of the penis due to *Bartonella* (*Rochalimaea*) *henselae* is shown in an AIDS patient.

B, Warthin-Starry stain of biopsy specimen of lesion shows *B. henselae*. (*Courtesy of* W.A. Schwartzman, MD.)

RABIES

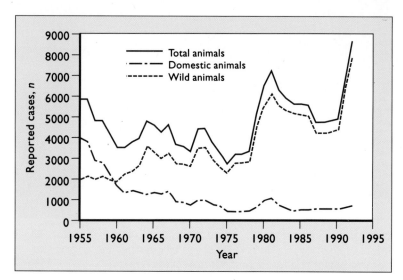

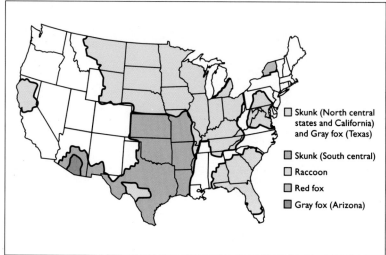

FIGURE 4-21 Incidence of rabies from wild and domestic animals, 1955–1992. Since the 1950s, there has been a decline of dog and cat rabies and an increase in wild animal rabies in the United States and Puerto Rico. Currently, there is a dramatic rise in epizootic raccoon rabies in the Middle Atlantic and Northeastern states. Raccoon rabies is now enzootic from Florida to Maine. Despite the increase in animal rabies, only 18 human cases have been reported from 1980 through 1993, mostly associated with bat rabies strains but not bat exposure. The last three human cases were from California, Texas, and Arkansas. (Centers for Disease Control and Prevention: Summary of notifiable diseases, United States—1992. *MMWR* 1993, 41(55):47.)

FIGURE 4-22 Distribution of rabies virus strains, United States, 1988. Five antigenically distinct rabies virus strains, specific to different animal species, have been isolated in the contiguous United States. Since 1980, seven of nine human cases of rabies acquired in the United States have been associated with bat rabies strains. Dog-associated rabies strains were the cause of all eight imported cases. No cow-to-human rabies transmission has been reported since before 1946. Dog rabies is a significant problem in Mexico and parts of the United States (Texas)–Mexican border. Human-to-human transmission has occurred only in corneal transplant-associated cases. (*Courtesy of* the Centers for Disease Control and Prevention.)

FIGURE 4-23 Therapy after rabies exposure.

Therapy after rabies exposure
Wash wound with soap and water immediately
Vaccine administration
Two types available in the United States
Human diploid cell vaccine
Rabies vaccine adsorbed
Give 1-mL dose, intramuscularly (deltoid)
Administer on days 0, 3, 7, 14, 28
Rabies immune globulin (RIG)
Inject 20 IU/kg intramuscularly
Half of dose is infiltrated around wounds, if possible
Half of dose is given intramuscularly at a different site from the vaccine
Failure to give RIG has been associated with vaccine failure
If the patient was previously vaccinated against rabies, give 1 mL vaccine intramuscularly at days 0 and 3 and no RIG

UNUSUAL ANIMAL BITES

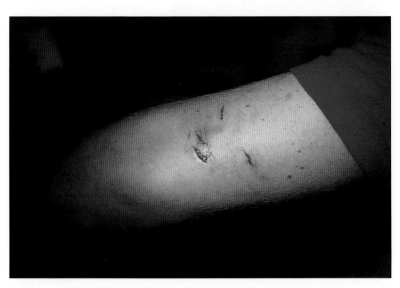

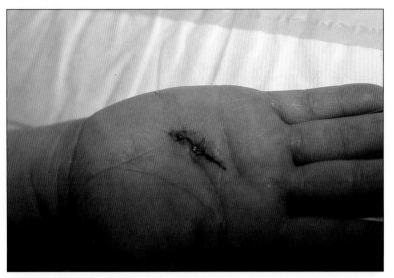

FIGURE 4-24 Young boy with seal bites to the elbow. Wild animals should not be approached, as they will defend themselves.

FIGURE 4-25 Pig bite to the hand. This woman was bitten by a pig at a petting zoo. Despite treatment with cephalexin, she developed a stricture and continued infection due to a previously undescribed *Flavobacterium* IIb–like organism and micrococcus. More than 55 million pigs are kept in the United States. They are aggressive animals and can gore and bite people. Among bacteria isolated from pig bite wounds are *Pasteurella multocida*, *Staphylococcus* spp., and *Bacteroides fragilis*. (Goldstein EJC, Citron DM, Merkin TE, Pickett JJ: Recovery of an unusual *Flavobacterium* IIb–like isolate from a hand infection following pig bite. *J Clin Microbiol* 1990, 28:1709–1711.)

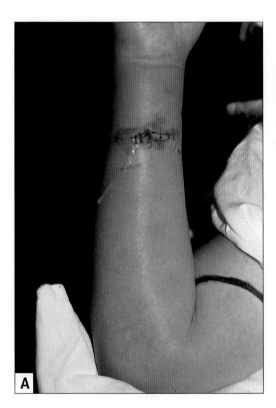

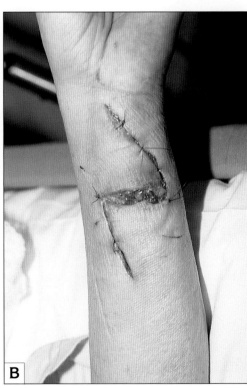

FIGURE 4-26 Monkey bite to the arm. This patient was visiting Bali when she was bitten by a local monkey. She was treated with ampicillin, and the wound was sutured. Within 48 hours, she became febrile, developed a spreading cellulitis, and flew back to the United States for further care. She had a "compartment syndrome" and required surgery. The wound grew *Streptococcus sanguis II*, *Streptococcus intermedius*, *Enterococcus durans*, and *Klebsiella pneumoniae*. **A**, Preoperative view. **B**, Postoperative view.

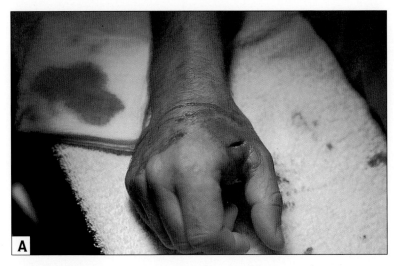 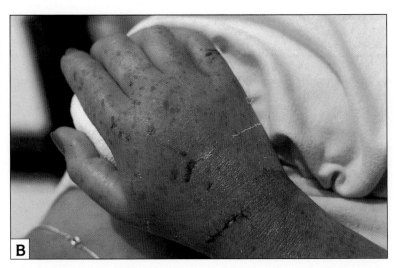

FIGURE 4-27 Monkey bite to the hand. **A,** This patient came to the emergency department and stated he had been bitten by a dog. The characteristics of the wound suggested this was not true. The patient had sustained a monkey bite from his own pet, which had not gone through quarantine on importation. Old world monkeys can harbor a herpes B virus that is fatal to humans. Some suggest treating these bites with acyclovir in addition to antibiotics. The bacteriology of monkey bites has not been defined and often these seem innocuous; however, clinically, these bites result in severe infections. **B,** The wound was sutured, and cultures grew *Streptococcus agalactiae, Streptococcus mitis, Streptococcus sanguis, Staphylococcus epidermidis,* and *Neisseria sicca/subflava* group. Marked swelling, obscuring the knuckles, developed despite persistent elevation and amoxicillin–clavulanate therapy.

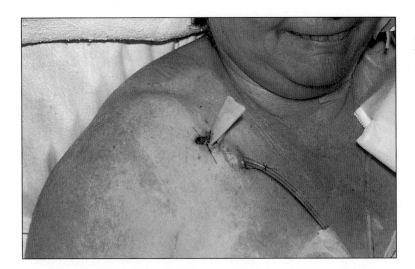

FIGURE 4-28 Septic arthritis after rabbit exposure. This patient, on steroids for systemic lupus erythematosus, bought a pet rabbit for her daughter. She denied any contact with the animal but developed septic arthritis in both shoulders and hips due to *Pasteurella multocida.* This was initially mistaken for "hand-shoulder" syndrome.

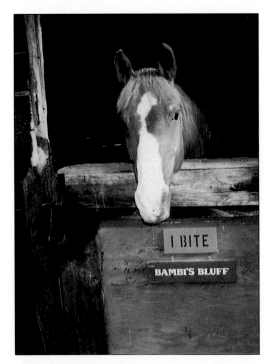

FIGURE 4-29 Horse bites. More than 6.6 million horses are kept as pets in the United States, and 2.5 million are kept as farm animals. Most horse bites are crush injuries and do not break the skin. Infections have been reported due to *Actinobacillus lignieresii* (often mistakenly identified as *Pasteurella multocida*), *A. equii,* and *A. equii*–like organisms. Anaerobes, including *Bacteroides ureolyticus, Prevotella melaninogenica,* and *Bacteroides fragilis* have also been isolated from horse bite wound infections.

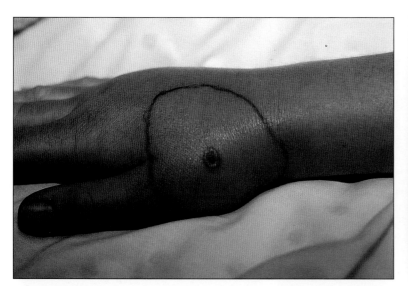

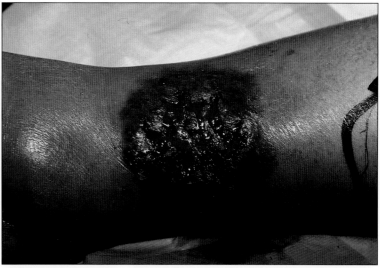

FIGURE 4-30 Brown recluse spider bite. This minor bite shows the typical necrotic center, surrounding ridge, and large amount of edema due to allergic reaction. Often, the necrotic area must be debrided. Dapsone has been recommended as therapy.

FIGURE 4-31 Pyoderma gangrenosa. Patients often report any unusual skin lesion as a "spider bite." The diagnosis of spider bite should only be made when the patient brings in the dead spider or one of its compatriots. This patient claimed to have a spider bite but actually has pyoderma gangrenosa, which is associated with diabetes and ulcerative colitis. Note the purple color and the sharp margins with central breakdown. Secondary infection is present.

HUMAN BITES

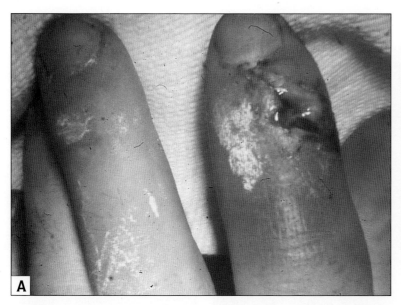

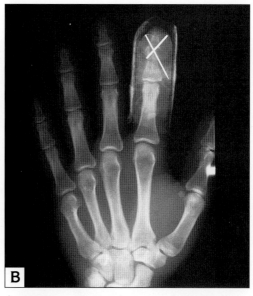

FIGURE 4-32 Occlusional human bite to the finger. **A,** This patient was bitten a week previously around the proximal interphalangeal (PIP) joint. Self-therapy was attempted with ampicillin. **B,** There was an underlying osteomyelitis with tuft destruction and pinning was attempted. Cultures grew both aerobic and anaerobic bacteria characteristic of the normal human oral flora. (*From* Goldstein EJC, Miller TA: Bites. *In* Spitell J (ed.): *Clinical Medicine.* Philadelphia: Harper & Row; 1987:1–12; with permission.)

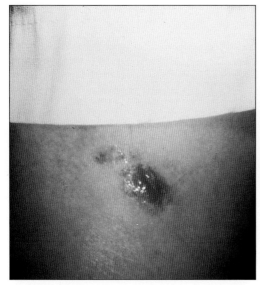

FIGURE 4-33 Occlusional human bite to the arm. This hospital orderly was bitten while trying to restrain an elderly patient. Patients' biting of hospital personnel, including physicians, has become an increasingly common event. HIV has been transmitted by human bites in several instances. This orderly refused "prophylactic" antimicrobial therapy, and despite being seen within 2 hours of injury and a thorough irrigation and cleansing of the wound, severe bacterial infection developed within 24 hours. (*From* Goldstein EJC: Infections following human bite. *Infect Surg* 1985, 4:849–852; with permission.)

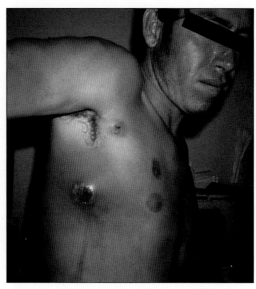

FIGURE 4-34 Multiple occlusional human bites to the torso. This patient stated he was walking on the street, minding his own business, when someone came up to him and bit him in multiple locations. Obviously, the stories given by patients are not always true. Approximately, 60 mL of pus was drained from the axillary wound and yielded a pure growth of *Streptococcus pyogenes* (group A). (*From* Goldstein EJC: Infections following human bite. *Infect Surg* 1985, 4:849–852; with permission.)

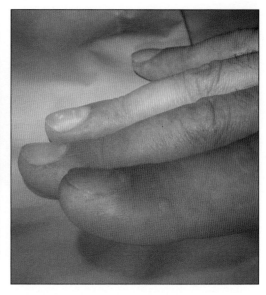

FIGURE 4-35 Herpetic whitlow. This orthodontist did not like to wear gloves when examining patients' mouths. Infection comes from cutaneous inoculation, often through inapparent (microscopic) breaks in the skin, by orally carried virus. These wounds should not be punctured, as infection may spread. In addition, there were several recurrences of the infection. (*From* Goldstein EJC: Infections following human bite. *Infect Surg* 1985, 4:849–852; with permission.)

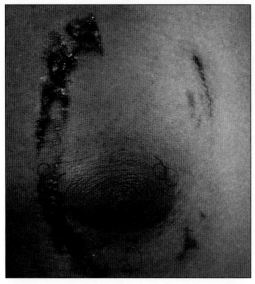

FIGURE 4-36 Love nip to the breast. This patient was seen 9 hours after his lover bit him in the breast area. One study of forensic bites in Los Angeles County noted that men are most often bitten on the extremities, but women are often bitten on the breasts. In children, human bites may be signs of sexual abuse or harbingers of general abuse. (Vale G, Noguchi I: *J Forensic Sci* 1983, 28:61–69.)

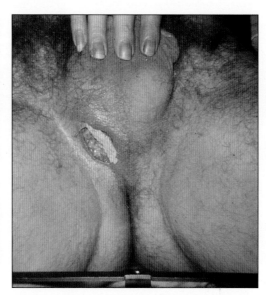

FIGURE 4-37 Love nip to the groin. This patient developed a groin abscess due to a human bite, which occurred during sexual intimacy. Both oral flora and fecal flora isolates were recovered from the abscess. Appropriate antimicrobials plus surgical drainage were required for cure. (*From* Goldstein EJC: Infections following human bite. *Infect Surg* 1985, 4:849–852; with permission.)

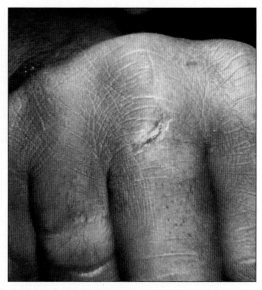

FIGURE 4-38 Clenched fist injury. The most serious of all bite wounds is the clenched fist injury, which occurs when the clenched fist of one person strikes the teeth of another during a fight. The wound may only be a few millimeters in length, but the tooth edge may break the skin, penetrate into the tendon space, joint capsule, and even the bone, and inoculate oral bacteria into the areas. When the hand is relaxed, the tendon potentially can carry bacteria into deeper spaces and compartments of the hand. (*From* Goldstein EJC, Richwald GA: Human and animal bite wounds. *Am Fam Physician* 1987, 36(Jul):101–109; with permission.)

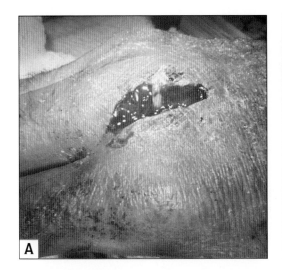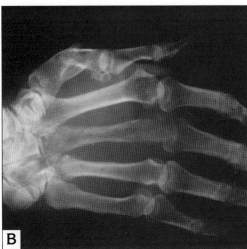

FIGURE 4-39 Clenched fist injury with osteomyelitis. **A**, The patient had undergone several operations and had been on 6 weeks of intravenous antibiotic therapy when this photograph was taken. **B**, A radiograph showed osteomyelitis. Routine aerobic culture had yielded only a coagulase-negative staphylococcus. Anaerobic culture yielded *Eikenella corrodens*, which when treated appropriately led to healing. (*From* Goldstein EJC: Clenched-fist injury infections. *Infect Surg* 1986; 5(Jul):384–390; with permission.)

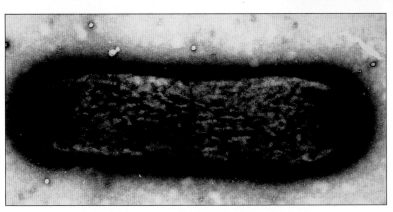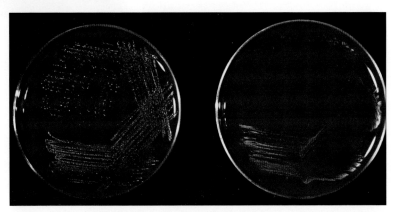

FIGURE 4-40 Electron micrograph of *Eikenella corrodens*. This capnophilic gram-negative rod is present in 30% of dental plaque samples (Goldstein EJC, Tarenzi LA, Agyare EO, Berger JR: Prevalence of *Eikenella corrodens* in dental plaque. *J Clin Microbiol* 1983, 17:636–639) and in 20% of clenched-fist injury infections (Goldsetin EJC, Barones MF, Miller TA: *Eikenella corrodens* in hand infections. *J Hand Surg* 1983, 8:563–567.) It can be missed easily on routine (aerobic) culture and, in conjunction with α-streptococci (*Streptococcus viridans*), causes insidious infection and leads to amputation. It is susceptible to penicillin G, cefoxitin, sulfamethoxazole-trimethoprim, tetracycline, and fluoroquinolones but resistant to oxacillin, cefazolin, clindamycin, and erythromycin. (Goldsetin EJC, Gombert ME, Agyare EO: Susceptibility of *Eikenella corrodens* to newer beta-lactam antibiotics. *Antimicrob Agents Chemother* 1980, 18:832–833. Goldstein EJC, Citron DM: Comparative susceptibilities of 173 aerobic and anaerobic bite wound isolates to sparfloxacin, temafloxacin, clarithromycin, and older agents. *Antimicrob Agents Chemother* 1993, 37:1150–1153.) (*From* Goldstein EJC, Gombert ME: *Eikenella corrodens*: A new perspective. *In* Bottone EJ (ed.): *Unusual Microorganisms: Fastidious Gram-Negative Species.* New York: Marcel Dekker Inc; 1983:1–43; with permission.)

FIGURE 4-41 Comparative growth of *E. corrodens* after 48 hours of CO_2 and anaerobic incubation. *E. corrodens* requires blood supplementation to grow in an aerobic environment. It grows best in a CO_2 environment with blood supplementation, and the colonies "pit" or "corrode" the agar (*left plate*). Colonies also grow, though less well, under anaerobic conditions (*right plate*). Small colonies (0.5 mm) may take 5–7 days to grow and can be missed if plates are not held longer than the third day. (*From* Goldstein EJC, Gombert ME: *Eikenella corrodens*: A new perspective. *In* Bottone EJ (ed.): *Unusual Microorganisms: Fastidious Gram-Negative Species.* New York: Marcel Dekker Inc; 1983:1–43; with permission.)

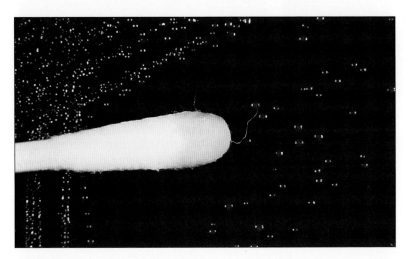

FIGURE 4-42 Yellow pigment of *E. corrodens*. *E. corrodens* is a nonmotile, nonsaccharolytic, oxidase-positive, catalase-negative, gram-negative rod. A yellow pigment is produced, as seen on the swab, and an odor similar to that of hypochlorite bleach is produced. (*From* Goldstein EJC, Gombert ME: *Eikenella corrodens*: A new perspective. *In* Bottone EJ (ed.): *Unusual Microorganisms: Fastidious Gram-Negative Species.* New York: Marcel Dekker Inc; 1983:1–43; with permission.)

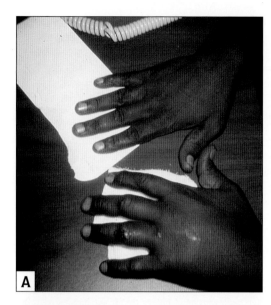

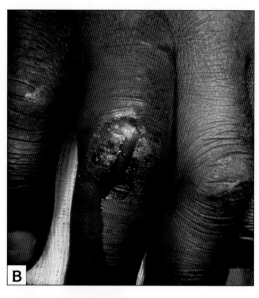

FIGURE 4-43 Presentation of clenched fist injury. **A**, Patients often awaken 6–10 hours after the injury with throbbing pain and edema of the affected extremity. The metacarpophalangeal third joint (metacarpal phalangeal joint, knuckle) of the dominant hand is the usual location. **B**, This slide shows injury to the fourth proximal interphalangeal joint, with purulent drainage due to aerobic and anaerobic bacteria with a septic arthritis. Note that swelling occurs proximally but not distally. There is diminished range of motion. Fever, adenopathy, and lymphangitis are uncommon. (*From* Goldstein EJC: Clenched-fist injury infections. *Infect Surg* 1986, 5(Jul):384–390; with permission.)

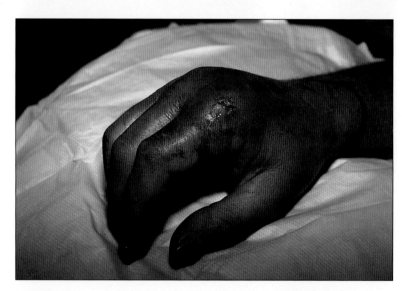

FIGURE 4-44 Clenched fist injury. This patient was seen 24 hours after injury with established infection due to *Streptococcus viridans*, *Eikenella corrodens*, *Moraxella* sp., *Neisseria* sp., *Prevotella* (*Bacteroides*) *melaninogenica*, *Fusobacterium nucleatum*, and *Peptostreptococcus* sp. Fifty-five percent of clenched fist injury infections involve anaerobes. Therapy includes evaluation by an experienced hand surgeon, determination if the joint capsule has been violated, elevation, and intravenous antibiotics. (*From* Goldstein EJC, Richwald GA: Human and animal bite wounds. *Am Fam Physician* 1987, 36(Jul):101–109; with permission.)

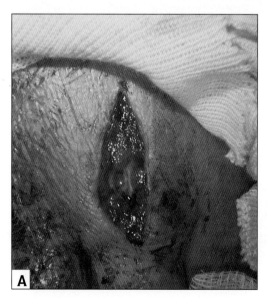

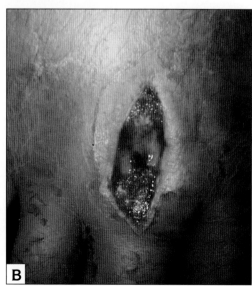

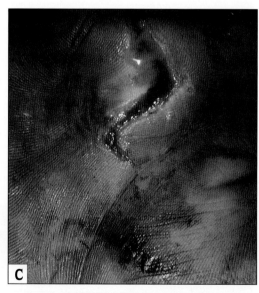

FIGURE 4-45 Complication of clenched fist injury. **A**, Despite appropriate antibiotics active against aerobes and anaerobes, joint exploration and elevation, this patient's infection continued. **B**, It led to destruction of the tendon (*dark area*) and its subsequent rupture. **C**, A second operation was required using a palmar approach to drain a collar button abscess. The wound then healed, but the patient required tendon transfer and reconstruction. (*From* Goldstein EJC: Clenched-fist injury infections. *Infect Surg* 1986, 5(Jul):384–390; with permission.)

A. Bacteriology of human bite wounds and clenched fist injuries: Aerobes

Streptococcus sp., α, β, and γ	*Moraxella* sp.
Staphylococcus aureus	*Moraxella catarrhalis*
Staphylococcus epidermidis	*Neisseria* sp.
Corynebacterium sp.	*Nocardia* sp.
Acinetobacter sp.	*Haemophilus influenzae*
Eikenella corrodens	*Haemophilus parainfluenzae*
Enterobacter cloacae	*Haemophilus aphrophilus*
Klebsiella pneumoniae	

B. Bacteriology of human bite wounds and clenched fist injuries: Anaerobes

Acidaminococcus sp.	*Bifidobacterium* sp.
Actinomyces sp.	*Clostridium* sp.
Bacteroides sp.	*Eubacterium* sp.
Bacteroides brevis	*Fusobacterium* sp.
Bacteroides ureolyticus	*Fusobacterium nucleatum*
Prevotella buccae	*Peptostreptococcus magnus*
Prevotella disiens	*Peptostreptococcus micros*
Prevotella intermedia	*Peptostreptococcus prevotii*
Prevotella loeschii	*Peptostreptococcus anaerobius*
Prevotella melaninogenica	*Veillonella parvula*
Prevotella oralis	*Spirochetes*
Prevotella ruminocola	

FIGURE 4-46 Bacteriology of human bite wounds and clenched fist injuries. **A**, Aerobes. **B**, Anaerobes.

MANAGEMENT OF BITE WOUNDS

Indications for hospitalization with bite wound infection

Fever/sepsis
Spread of cellulitis
Compromised host (asplenia, liver disease, mastectomy, lupus, steroids)
Patient noncompliance
Bone/joint involvement

FIGURE 4-47 Indications for hospitalization of patients with bite wound infections.

Outline of therapy for human bite wounds

Evaluation of function (nerve, tendon), blood supply (pulses)
Diagram wound (especially joint proximity)
Irrigation
Cautious debridement
Antibiotics
  3–5 days for prophylaxis
  Longer for established infection
Elevation of injured limb/area
Immobilization/exercise program
Culture (if infected, aerobic and anaerobic)
Baseline radiograph
Tetanus toxoid
Suture (?)
Rabies therapy (as needed)
Health department report (if required)

FIGURE 4-48 Outline of therapy for human bite wounds.

FIGURE 4-49 Causes of clinical failure in therapy for bite wound infections.

Causes of clinical failure

Failure to elevate
Failure to recognize joint penetration
Selection of incorrect antibiotic

Antibiotic activity: Animal bites

	P. multocida	*S. aureus*	*S. intermedius*	*Capnocytophaga*	Anaerobes
Penicillin	+	–	V	++	V
Dicloxacillin	–	+	+	–	–
Amoxicillin/clavulanate, Ampicillin/sulbactam	+	+	+		+
First-generation cephalosporins	–	+	+	V	–
Cefuroxime	+	+	+	+	–
Cefoxitin	+	+	+	+	+
Quinolones	+	V	+	+	–
Erythromycin	–	V	+	+	–
Azithromycin	RP	RP	RP	RP	RP
Clarithromycin	RP	RP	RP	RP	RP
Tetracycline	+	V	U	V	V

FIGURE 4-50 Susceptibilities of animal bite wound pathogens to antimicrobial agents. (+ —active; – —not active; RP—results pending; U—unknown; V—variable activity.)

Antibiotic activity: Human bites

	S. aureus	*Eikenella*	*Haemophilus*	Anaerobes
Penicillin	–	+	–	–
Dicloxacillin	+	–	–	–
Amoxicillin/clavulanate Ampicillin/sulbactam	+	+	+	+
First-generation cephalosporins	+	–	–	–
Cefuroxime	+	+	+	–
Cefoxitin	+	+	V	+
Quinolones	V	+	+	–
Erythromycin	V	–	+	–
Azithromycin	NT	NT	NT	NT
Clarithromycin	NT	NT	NT	NT

FIGURE 4-51 Susceptibilities of human bite wound pathogens to antimicrobial agents. (+ —active; – —not active; NT—not tested; V—variable activity.)

SELECTED BIBLIOGRAPHY

Goldstein EJC: Bite wounds and infection. *Clin Infect Dis* 1992, 14:633–640.

Brook I: Microbiology of human and animal bite wounds in children. *Pediatr Infect Dis J* 1987, 6:29–32.

Goldstein EJC: Bite wound infections. *In* Mandell GL, Bennett JE, Dolin R (eds.): *Principles and Practice of Infectious Diseases*, 4th ed. New York: Churchill Livingstone; 1994.

Weber DJ, Hansen AR: Infections resulting from animal bites. *Infect Dis Clin North Am* 1991, 5:662–680.

Chuinard RG, D'Ambrosia RD: Human bite infections of the hand. *J Bone Joint Surg* 1977, 59A:416–418.

CHAPTER 5

Infections Associated With Animal Contact

E. Dale Everett

BACTERIAL INFECTIONS

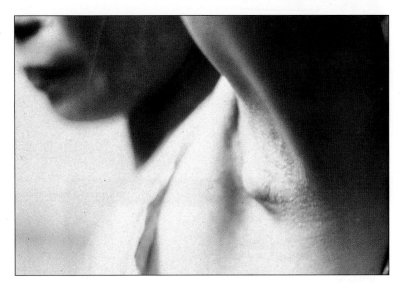

FIGURE 5-1 Plague. An axillary bubo of bubonic plague is shown in a patient. Usually plague is a febrile illness with regional lymphadenopathy. Its incubation period is 1–6 days. Patients may become septicemic and develop pneumonic plague, during which time they may transmit the illness to others by cough-generated aerosols. Diagnosis may be confirmed by culture, fluorescent antibody stain of pus from a bubo, or serologic testing. Streptomycin, tetracyclines, or chloramphenicol is considered appropriate therapy.

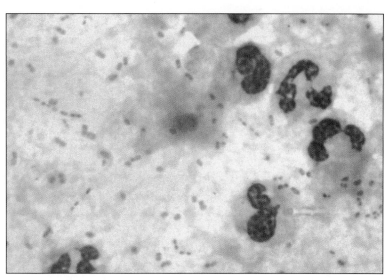

FIGURE 5-2 Plague. Gram stain shows small gram-negative rods of *Yersinia pestis*, the etiologic agent of plague. The bacillus is transmitted primarily by the bite of infected fleas (*Xenopsylla cheopis*) but, on rare occasions, has been transmitted to humans by bites, scratches, or other means from domestic animals. (Human plague—United States, 1993–1994. *MMWR* 1994, 43:242–246.)

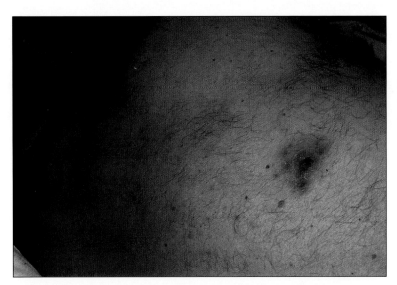

FIGURE 5-3 Tularemia. An eschar with several small satellite lesions appears at the site of a tick bite. The most common syndrome caused by *Francisella tularensis* is a febrile illness with regional lymphadenopathy, which occurs following a tick bite or handling of infected rodents or lagomorphs. Other than ulceroglandular disease, tularemia also may occur as pneumonic, oculoglandular, typhoidal, or oropharyngeal disease.

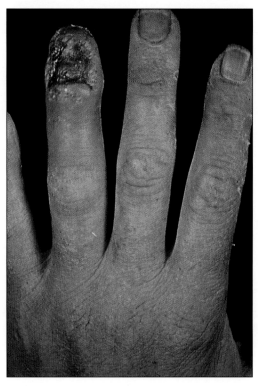

FIGURE 5-4 Tularemia. A finger ulcer in a patient who skinned a wild rabbit. The patient also had epitrochlear and axillary lymphadenopathy. The incubation period for tularemia is usually 2–10 days. Streptomycin, other aminoglycosides, tetracyclines, chloramphenicol, and probably fluroquinolones are considered effective therapy.

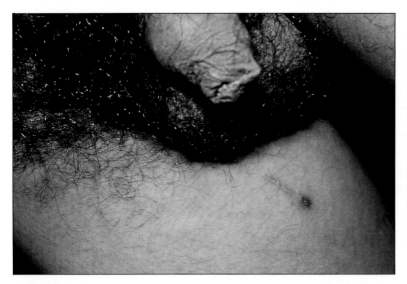

FIGURE 5-5 Cat scratch disease. A primary papule of cat scratch disease is associated with skin erythema overlying enlarged inguinal lymph nodes. The syndrome usually consists of regional lymphadenopathy and minimal to no systemic symptoms, following a history of cat exposure. Most cases are thought be caused by a bacterial agent, *Rochalimaea henselae*, or a closely related organism. Most patients resolve their illness over a few weeks to a few months. A clear response to antimicrobial agents remains to be demonstrated.

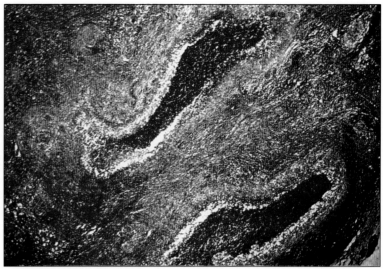

FIGURE 5-6 Cat scratch disease. Histologic section of a lymph node, stained with hematoxylin-eosin, shows necrotic, pus-filled areas and a granulomatous reaction. Visualization of organisms with Warthin-Starry silver stain is sometimes possible, and organisms have been isolated from biopsy materials. The most useful test at present for confirming the diagnosis appears to be a serologic test using an indirected fluorescent-antibody method to *R. henselae* antigen. (Zangwill KM, *et al.*: Cat scratch disease in Connecticut. *N Engl J Med* 1993, 329:8–12.)

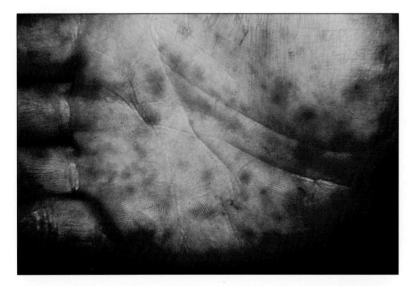

FIGURE 5-7 Rat bite fever. Hemorrhagic palmar rash associated with rat bite fever. The illness is transmitted by rat bites (occasionally by carnivores) and caused by two different organisms, *Streptobacillus moniliformis* or *Spirillum minus*. The clinical syndromes differ depending on the species of infecting organism. *S. moniliformis* is the most common cause in the United States and results in a characteristic flulike illness, arthritis, exanthem, and, occasionally, endocarditis 3–10 days after the bite. Diagnosis is by culture or seroagglutination tests. Penicillin or tetracyclines are considered effective therapy.

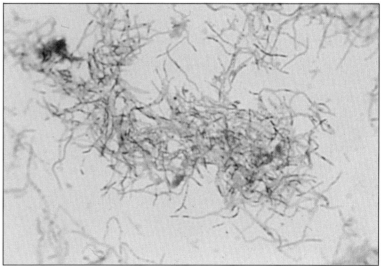

FIGURE 5-8 Rat bite fever. Gram stain discloses filamentous gram-negative rods, *S. moniliformis*, isolated from the blood of a patient.

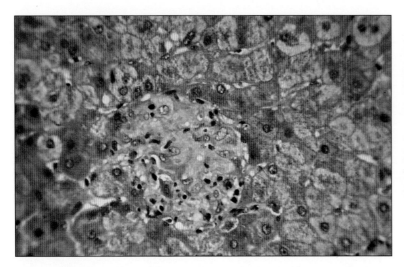

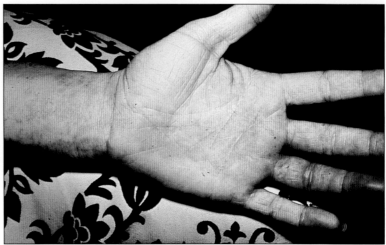

FIGURE 5-9 Brucellosis. A liver biopsy specimen from a patient with brucellosis shows a noncaseating granuloma. Brucellosis, or undulant fever, is caused by several species, including *Brucella abortus*, *B. melitensis*, *B. suis*, and *B. canis*. It is a nonspecific febrile illness, which may affect virtually any organ system, especially the reticuloendothelial system. Most cases in the United States are seen in animal handlers and abattoir workers. It can also be acquired from unpasteurized milk. Diagnosis can be made from blood or bone marrow cultures or from bone or serologic testing. The organism is one of the many causes of granulomatous hepatitis. (*Courtesy of* T.E. Woodward, MD.)

FIGURE 5-10 Erysipeloid. A violaceous finger lesion with proximal spread of an erythematous rash. Erysipeloid is caused by a gram-positive pleomorphic rod, *Erysipelothrix rhusiopathiae*, and usually occurs in animal and fish handlers. It may occasionally cause systemic disease such as endocarditis. Diagnosis is by culture of aspirated or biopsy specimens. Penicillin, cephalosporins, erythromycin, or clindamycin is considered appropriate therapy. (Reboli AC, Farrar WE: *Erysipelothrix rhusiopathiae*: An occupational pathogen. *Clin Microbiol Rev* 1989, 2:354–359.)

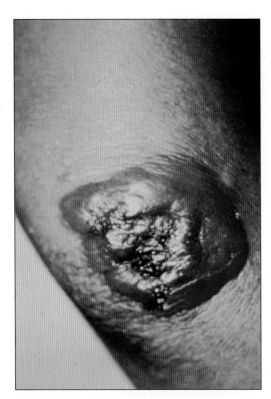

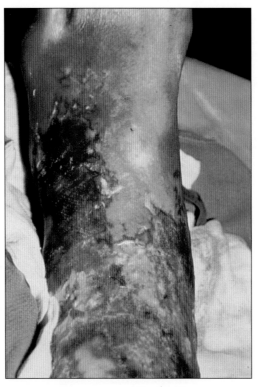

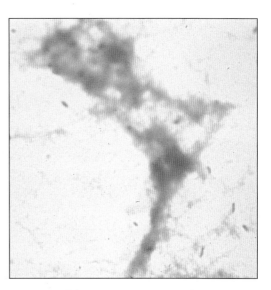

FIGURE 5-11 Cutaneous anthrax. An ulcerated lesion with heaped-up edematous margins due to a gram-positive rod, *Bacillus anthracis*. The disease is seen most commonly in animal handlers, especially sheep and goat handlers, or hide processors. Evolution of the lesion is usually from a papule, to a bulla, followed by ulceration. Septicemia may result. Diagnosis is confirmed by culture. Penicillin is considered appropriate therapy.

FIGURE 5-12 *Vibrio vulnificus*. An erythematous lesion with hemorrhagic bulla developed in an immunocompromised patient who injured his leg while swimming in the Chesapeake Bay. *V. vulnificus* is a halophilic vibrio, which is associated with cellulitis. It may be acquired by direct contact with contaminated water or sea creatures or by ingestion of improperly cooked seafood. The ingestion syndrome may produce septicemia with secondary skin lesion and tends to occur in patients with chronic liver disease or immunocompromise. Diagnosis is usually by culture.

FIGURE 5-13 *Vibrio vulnificus*. Gram stain (× 1000) of material from a bullous lesion shows proteinaceous material and gram-negative rods. The organism is susceptible *in vitro* to several antimicrobial agents. Tetracyclines are often considered the "drug of choice," but substantial data for optimum antimicrobial therapy are lacking. Surgical debridement of cutaneous lesions is frequently needed. (*Courtesy of* T. Flynn, MD.) (Case Records of the Massachusetts General Hospital: Case 41-1989. A 65-year-old man with fever, bullae, erythema, and edema of the leg after wading in brackish water. *N Engl J Med* 1989, 321:1029–1038.)

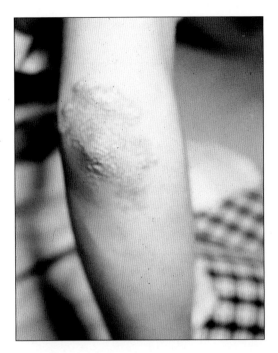

FIGURE 5-14 Swimming pool granuloma. Nodular, slightly erythematous cutaneous lesions appearing over the elbow due to *Mycobacterium marinum*. *M. marinum* is an atypical mycobacterium, and disease is usually seen in swimmers, fish handlers, and aquarium keepers. Nodules may be ulcerated. Diagnosis is accomplished by culture of abscess and/or biopsy material. Fluoroquinolones, doxycycline, amikacin, rifampin, ethambutol, and clarithromycin, often in some combination, have been reported as effective therapy.

FUNGAL INFECTIONS

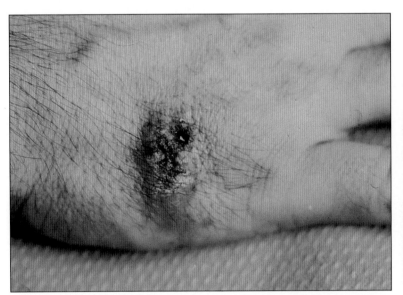

FIGURE 5-15 Sporotrichosis. A solitary sporothrix cutaneous chancre. The disease is caused by a dimorphous fungus, *Sporothrix schenckii*, which is acquired most commonly from the soil, but occasionally from animals, especially cats. (Reed KD, *et al.*: Zoonotic transmission of sporotrichosis: Case report and review. *Clin Infect Dis* 1993, 16:384–387.)

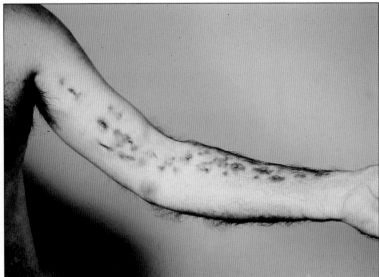

FIGURE 5-16 Sporotrichosis. Lymphocutaneous sporotrichosis, the most common clinical syndrome caused by *S. schenckii*, usually begins with a solitary lesion followed by red nodules ascending along superficial lymphatics. It has no systemic symptoms. Diagnosis is by culture; the organism is rarely seen in biopsy material. Saturated solution of potassium iodide administered orally or itraconazole is considered effective therapy.

VIRAL INFECTIONS

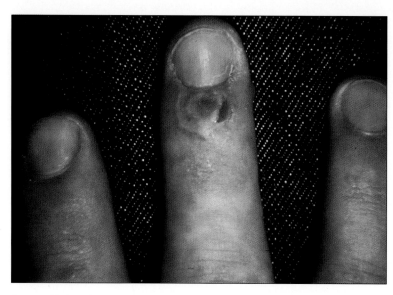

FIGURE 5-17 Orf (contagious ecthyma). A papulopustular lesion on the finger of a goat rancher. Seen primarily in sheep and goat handlers, orf is caused by Parapoxvirus (a DNA virus), which causes scabby mouth disease in sheep and goats. In humans, lesions usually occur on the hands and there are no systemic symptoms. It may occasionally be accompanied by lymphangitis, a diffuse pruritic vesiculopapular eruption, or erythema multiforme. Lesions heal in 2–4 weeks.

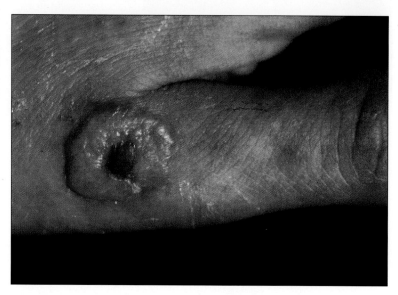

FIGURE 5-18 Milker's nodule. An umbilicated cutaneous lesion occurring on a finger. Lesions are caused by a DNA virus, Parapoxvirus, and usually are acquired by those handling the udders and teats of cows. Lesions heal spontaneously in 7–10 days without scarring or systemic symptoms. (*Courtesy of* E.L. Overholt, MD.)

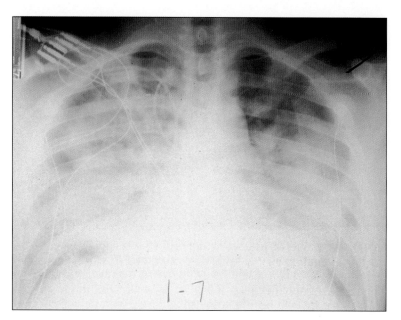

FIGURE 5-19 Korean hemorrhagic fever. A chest radiograph shows pulmonary hemorrhage and/or edema occasionally associated with Korean hemorrhagic fever. The disease is caused by Hantaan virus and clinically manifested by hemorrhagic tendencies and renal failure. It is thought to be acquired from aerosols of rodent urine, feces, or saliva. Diagnosis may be confirmed by serologic testing.

PARASITIC DISEASES

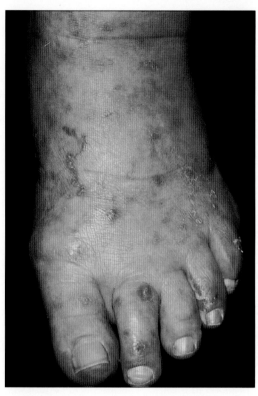

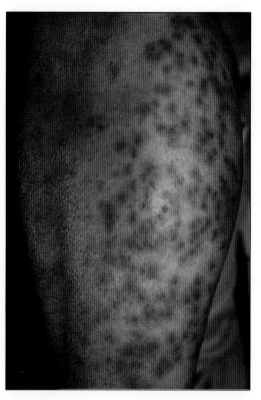

FIGURE 5-20 Creeping eruption (cutaneous larva migrans). Papular and linear erythematous lesions associated with cutaneous larva migrans. Creeping eruption is caused by larvae of cat or dog hookworms, *Ancylostoma braziliense* and *A. caninum*. It usually is seen in workers or children having contact with soil contaminated by dog and cat feces. Effective therapy has been accomplished with freezing of lesions with topical ethylene chloride or liquid nitrogen, topical thiabendazole, oral albendazole, and oral ivermectin. (Davies HD, Sakuls P, Keystone JS: Creeping eruption. *Arch Dermatol* 1993, 129:588–591.)

FIGURE 5-21 Swimmer's itch. A pruritic, erythematous, papular rash is acquired by exposure to water contaminated by avian schistosomal species. It usually occurs in swimmers or fishermen. A rash occurs 5–14 days after water exposure and is caused by an allergic response to disintegration of cercariae in the skin. The rash is self-limited.

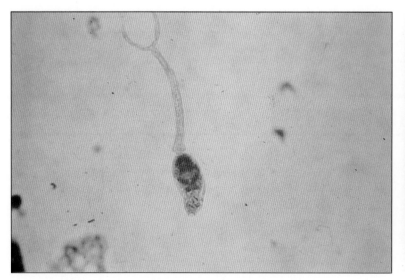

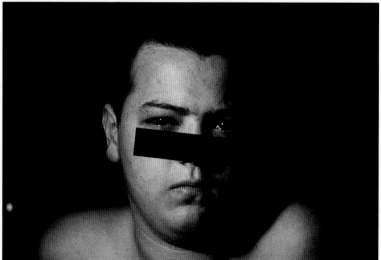

FIGURE 5-22 Swimmer's itch. Cercariae of a *Schistosoma sp*. This is the stage of schistosoma that penetrates the skin.

FIGURE 5-23 Trichinosis. Periorbital and eyelid edema associated with acute trichinosis. Humans acquire the disease by ingestion of raw or insufficiently cooked meat (pork, bear, and walrus are the most common) that contains encysted larvae of *Trichinella spiralis*. Heavy infestation may result in an illness with fever, myalgias, eyelid edema, splinter hemorrhages, and eosinophilia. Diagnosis is by serologic studies or muscle biopsy. (*Courtesy of* T.E. Woodward, MD.)

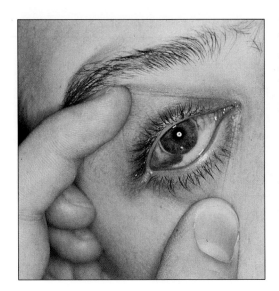

FIGURE 5-24
Trichinosis. Subconjunctival hemorrhages in a patient with trichinosis. This patient acquired trichinosis from eating "hamburger," but investigation revealed that some pork had been added to the ground beef. (*Courtesy of* T.E. Woodward, MD.)

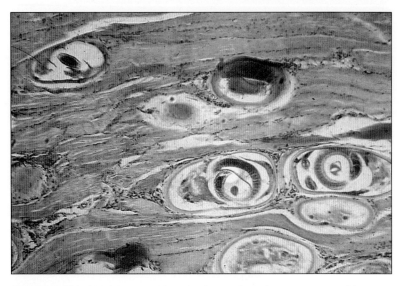

FIGURE 5-25 Trichinosis. Histologic section shows encysted larvae of *T. spiralis* in skeletal muscle.

CHLAMYDIAL INFECTION

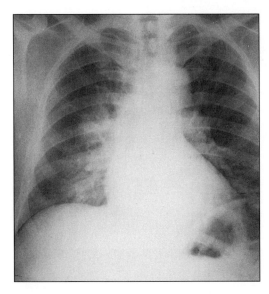

FIGURE 5-26 Ornithosis (psittacosis). A chest radiograph shows a right lower lobe infiltrate in a patient with ornithosis. Although frequently associated with exotic (psittacine) birds, actually many bird species may harbor the agent. This patient acquired his illness infection while trapping pigeons in a barn. The infectious agent is *Chlamydia psittaci* and is acquired by inhalation. Symptoms usually include fever, chills, myalgias, and upper or lower respiratory complaints. Although the organism can be grown in egg or tissue cultures, diagnosis is usually confirmed serologically. (*Courtesy of* T.E. Woodward, MD.)

SELECTED BIBLIOGRAPHY

Beneson AS (ed.): *Control of Communicable Diseases in Man,* 15th ed. Washington, DC: American Public Health Association; 1990.

Achar PN, Szyfres B: *Zoonoses and Communicable Diseases Common to Man and Animals,* 2nd ed. Washington, DC: Pan American Health Organization; 1987.

CHAPTER 6

Fungal and Yeast Infections of the Skin, Appendages, and Subcutaneous Tissues

Gregory J. Raugi

TINEA VERSICOLOR AND VARIANTS

Characteristics of tinea versicolor	
Etiology	*Pityrosporon orbiculare*
Onset	Adolescence (usually)
Appearance	Individual small, circular pink, light brown, or hypopigmented macules with distinctive fine branny or furfuraceous scale
Site	Neck, upper back, shoulders, upper chest

FIGURE 6-1 Characteristics of tinea versicolor. Tinea versicolor (Latin *versicolor*, of many colors) is a common superficial lipophilic yeast infection of the skin caused by *Pityrosporon orbiculare*. Colonization of the skin with this organism occurs shortly after birth, yet clinical disease is uncommon until adolescence, probably because of greater sebaceous gland activity. Individual lesions are characteristic and begin as small circular pink, light brown, or hypopigmented macules with distinctive fine branny or furfuraceous (Latin *furfur*, bran or scurf) scale. The lesions may progress over a period of weeks to months to become patchy or confluent. The lesions begin around the neck, upper back, shoulders, and upper chest and may extend distally to the antecubital fossa and caudally to the abdomen or lumbar area. Occasionally, lesions occur in the groin. Pruritus is uncommon. Considerable variation in color is observed from patient to patient, yet individuals express only one color variant.

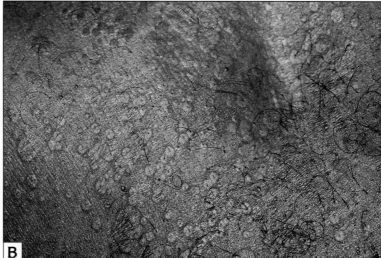

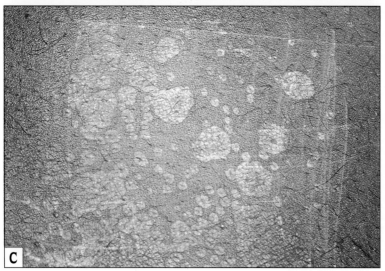

FIGURE 6-2 Hyperpigmented tinea versicolor. **A**, Round, hyperpigmented, barely palpable plaques and some perifollicular patches are evident on the upper abdomen. **B**, Perifollicular round patches of hyperpigmented lesions are tightly grouped on the upper back. **C**, The fine, branny scaling is not readily evident until lesions are gently scraped with the end of a glass microscope slide.

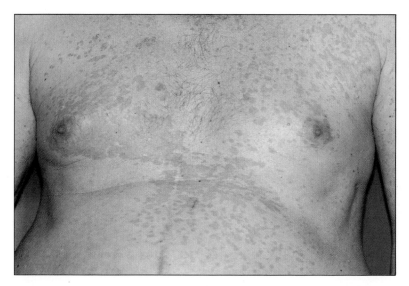

FIGURE 6-3 Inflammatory tinea versicolor. The reddish, fine scaly patches of this variant are associated with pruritus, whereas symptoms are rarely mentioned by patients with the hyper- and hypopigmented variants. The clinical diagnosis may be confused with nummular eczema, pityriasis rosea, or drug eruption.

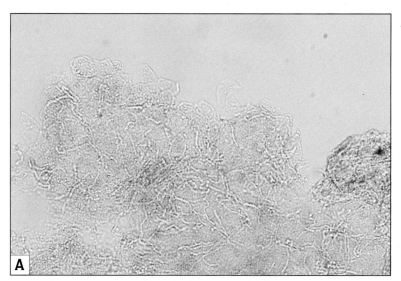

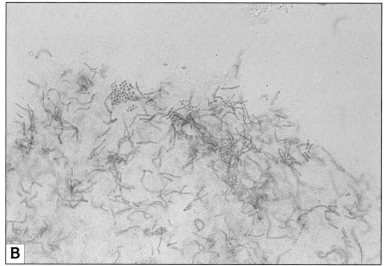

FIGURE 6-4 KOH wet mount of tinea versicolor. **A,** Abundant short hyphae and round spores, so-called spaghetti and meatballs are apparent. **B,** Adding a small amount of Parker's blue-black ink to the KOH stains *Pityrosporon* organisms blue and facilitates their identification from skin scrapings.

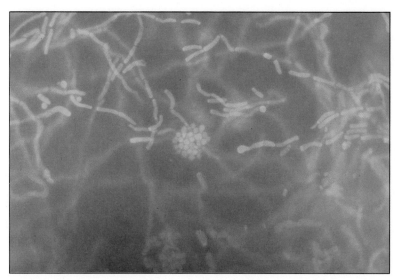

FIGURE 6-5 Calcifluor of *Pityrosporon*. Very small numbers of organisms are identifiable with calcifluor, a very sensitive and specific reagent. The extraordinary sensitivity of the reagent, taken with the fact that *Pityrosporon* is part of the normal skin flora, makes clinicopathologic correlation essential in interpreting preparations with only a few organisms.

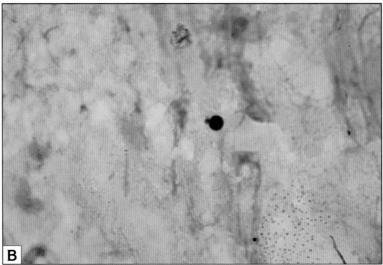

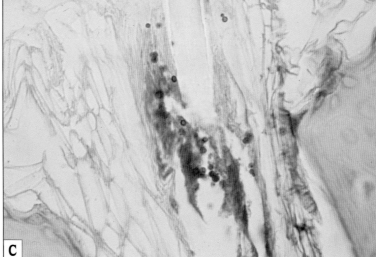

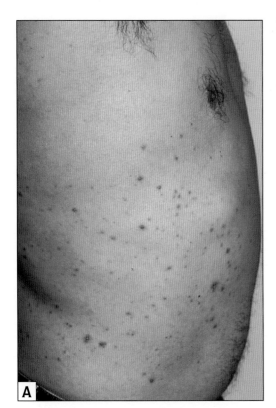

FIGURE 6-6 *Pityrosporon* folliculitis. This variant often occurs in young or middle-aged patients. **A,** Sometimes, tinea versicolor or seborrheic dermatitis coexists, but usually this fine follicular, pustular eruption occurs on the upper back and chest in isolation. Differential diagnosis includes miliaria pustulosa, bacterial folliculitis, mild acne vulgaris, or pustular drug eruption. **B,** Diagnosis is easily made by Gram stain of pus. Because *Pityrosporon* is a normal inhabitant of the hair follicle, clinicopathologic correlation is required to make the diagnosis from a skin biopsy. **C,** Periodic acid–Schiff stain of the skin biopsy specimen shows organisms in the follicle.

CANDIDA INFECTIONS

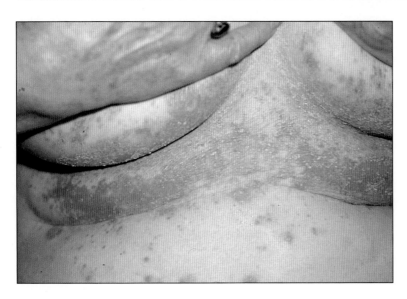

FIGURE 6-7 Intertriginous candidiasis. The typical appearance of candidiasis is with bright red erythema and satellite papules and pustules, occurring in the axillae, groin, or other skin folds, as beneath pendulous breasts in this woman. The vigorous neutrophilic response is thought to be due to release of complement-derived chemotactic factors by fungal polysaccharides.

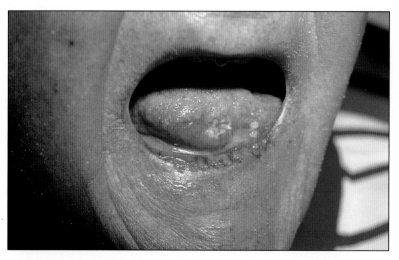

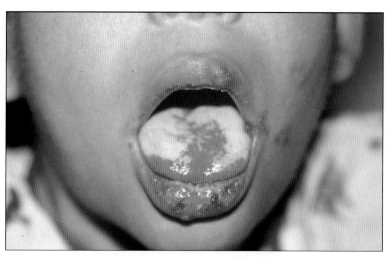

FIGURE 6-8 Oral candidiasis (thrush or acute pseudomembranous candidiasis). The cheesy or curdlike adherent white patches on the mucous membranes are composed of desquamated epithelial cells, necrotic keratinocytes, food, leukocytes, and bacteria and are held in place by hyphae of *Candida* organisms. When the pseudomembrane is removed, the exposed surface is tender and friable. This edentulous patient also has mild angular cheilitis (perlèche). Candida may be present in the cutaneous lesion, but noninfective factors play a more important role in the pathogenesis of angular cheilitis. (*Courtesy of* K. Abson, MD.)

FIGURE 6-9 Oral candidiasis in HIV infection. This child with HIV-1 infection has extensive involvement of the lingual mucosa. (*Courtesy of* J. Hirschmann, MD.)

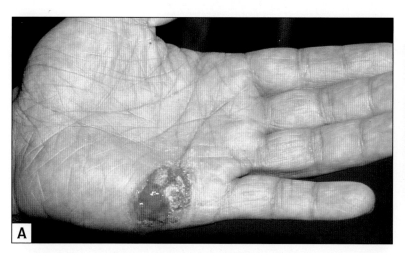

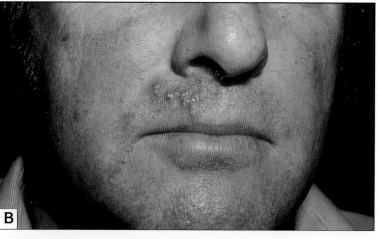

FIGURE 6-10 Candida granuloma. The solitary indolent lesion of candida granuloma typically contains organisms only in the cornified cell layer of the epidermis, but the reactive inflammatory infiltrate may extend into the subcutaneous fat. **A** and **B**, Two examples, on the hand (*panel 10A*) and the upper lip (*panel 10B*), demonstrate part of the clinical spectrum of this condition. (*Courtesy of* K. Abson, MD.)

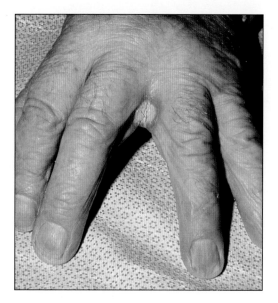

FIGURE 6-11 Erosio blastomycetica interdigitale. Interdigital candidiasis usually occurs between the middle and ring fingers. Moisture trapped under a ring macerates the epidermis and predisposes to infection. (*Courtesy of* J. Hirschmann, MD.)

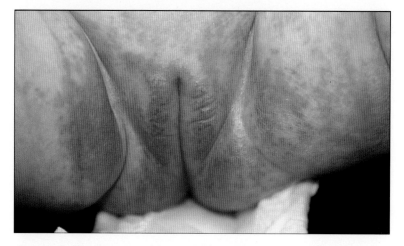

FIGURE 6-12 Diaper candidiasis. This child had an irritant diaper dermatitis (note the characteristic sparing of the depths of the creases) with secondary colonization and infection with candida. (*Courtesy of* J. Francis, MD.)

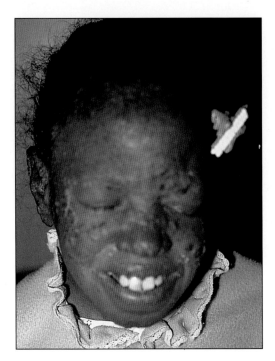

FIGURE 6-13
Chronic mucocutaneous candidiasis. This distinctive clinical syndrome occurs in patients with defective cellular immunity. Multiple acral and periorificial sites are involved with nonhealing, verrucous, hyperkeratotic plaques. Biopsy shows invasion of organisms into the dermis and subcutaneous fat, in contrast to the superficial invasion in other cutaneous forms of candidiasis. (*Courtesy of* J. Francis, MD.)

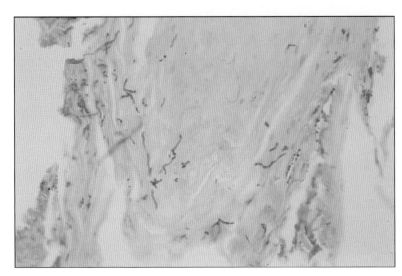

FIGURE 6-14 Histopathologic stain in candidiasis. Periodic acid–Schiff–stained sections of tongue epithelium show short pseudohyphae in the cornified cell layer. Unless the host is immunocompromised, *Candida* does not invade to deeper levels. (*Courtesy of* K. Abson, MD.)

SUPERFICIAL DERMATOPHYTE INFECTIONS OF THE SKIN

Inflammatory Dermatophyte Infections

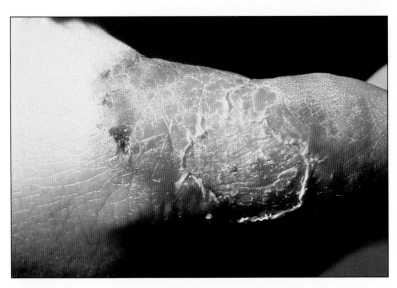

FIGURE 6-15 Vesicular inflammatory tinea manuum. The host response to the first infection by dermatophytes is often very inflammatory and is easily mistaken for eczema or allergic contact dermatitis. Inadvertent treatment with topical corticosteroids results in a prompt but transient decrease in inflammation, followed in a week or two by rapid spread of disease.

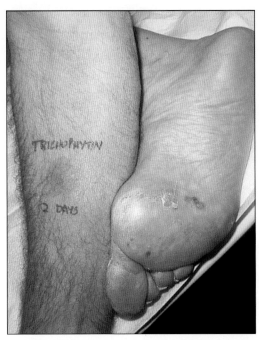

FIGURE 6-16
Vesicular inflammatory tinea pedis. The multiloculated vesicles typical of inflammatory tinea pedis contain abundant fungal elements in the blister roof, but not in the blister fluid. A trichophytin intradermal skin test placed on the forearm is strongly positive after 2 days.

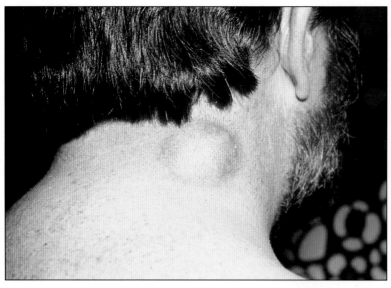

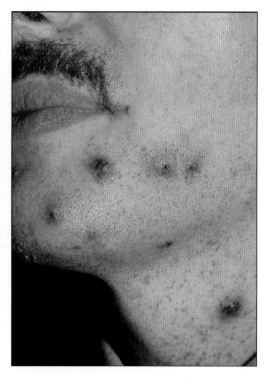

FIGURE 6-18
Inflammatory tinea barbae. The exudative crusted lesions in the beard area of this man were initially misdiagnosed as impetigo or folliculitis.

FIGURE 6-17 Inflammatory tinea corporis. The edematous indurated border, accompanied by minimal scaling and central clearing, is typical of early infection with dermatophytes. *Trichophyton verrucosum*, an etiologic agent for cattle "ringworm," was recovered from the lesion on this veterinarian.

Chronic Stable Dermatophyte Infections

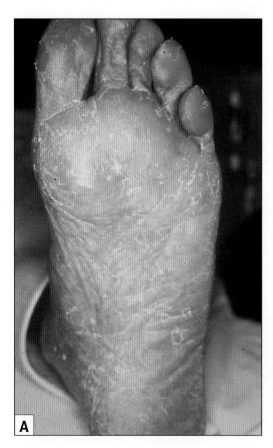

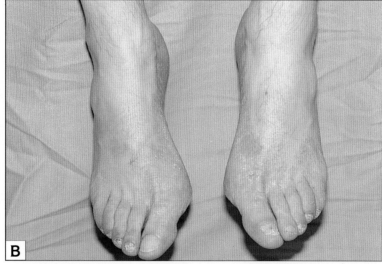

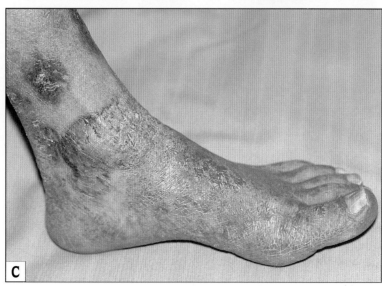

FIGURE 6-19 Chronic tinea pedis. The typical, mildly erythematous, scaly dermatosis is limited to the "moccasin" distribution of the foot. **A**, Abundant loose scaling is evident in this example. A KOH wet mount of scrapings of this scale will have many visible long branching hyphae (*see* Fig. 6-31). **B**, Note the extension of the affected area onto the medial aspects of the feet, but with relative sparing of the hair-follicle–bearing skin. **C**, Infection progressed beyond the sole to the hair-bearing skin of the lower extremity in this corticosteroid-dependent man. The slate-gray areas of pigmentation surrounding the residual scars from pyoderma gangrenosum are due to minocycline therapy. Note the concomitant nail infection.

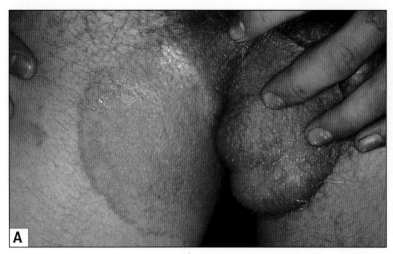

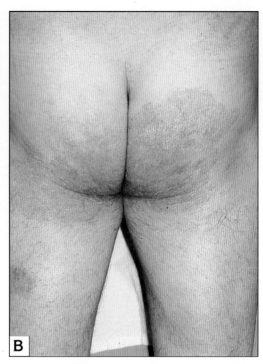

FIGURE 6-20 Chronic tinea cruris. **A**, Asymmetrical distribution on the medial thighs, lack of scrotal skin involvement, and the papular erythematous border are characteristic of chronic tinea cruris. The best area to sample for a wet mount is the scaling just central to the papular erythematous border. **B**, Extension of tinea cruris to the buttock area occurred in this patient. Note that little inflammation accompanies this chronic stable infection.

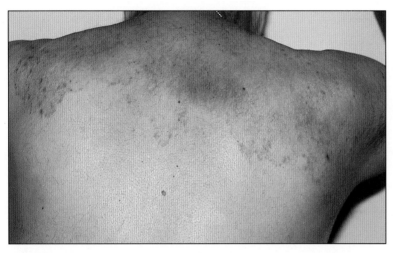

FIGURE 6-21 Tinea corporis. Extensive infection in the mantle area of the trunk is evident in this patient. Note the serpiginous, mildly inflammatory, papular border and the hyperpigmentation in the relatively clearer central areas. Fungi are most easily recovered from scales taken from the leading border of the clinical lesion.

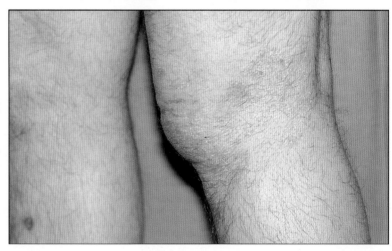

FIGURE 6-22 Tinea corporis. Scarcely any inflammation is present in this subtle, irregularly shaped, scaly patch with the serpiginous border.

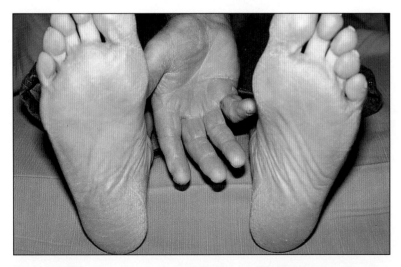

FIGURE 6-23 Two-foot, one-hand disease. Stable tinea pedis may be accompanied by unilateral infection of the hand. Nail infection may be present in all three sites. Note the subtle desquamating scale and prominent, yellowish, diffuse hyperkeratosis on the feet.

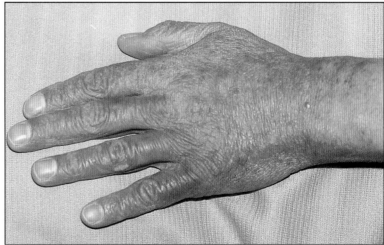

FIGURE 6-24 Tinea manuum. The dusky erythema and scaling on the dorsal aspect of the hand are accompanied by hyperkeratosis and mild erythema on the palm, yet the nails are unaffected.

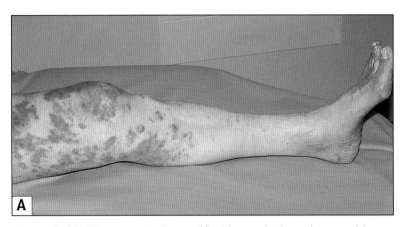

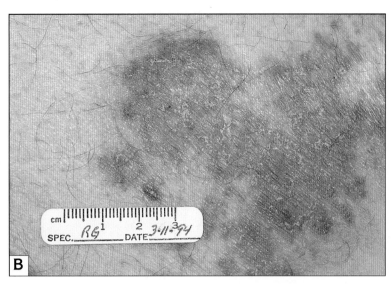

FIGURE 6-25 Tinea corporis modified by topical corticosteroid treatment. **A**, Note the typical indolent infection of the foot and the patchy, erythematous, minimally scaling dermatitis on the leg and thigh. Wet mounts from the dermatitic areas showed abun-

dant fungal elements. **B**, A close-up view of a patch on the thigh shows papular eruption, no tendency to central clearing, and indistinct borders characteristic of "tinea incognito."

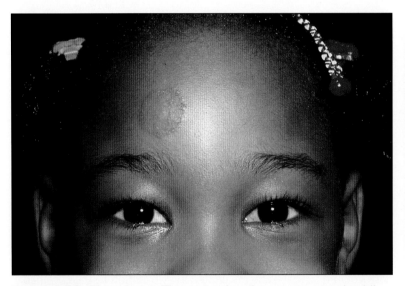

FIGURE 6-26 Tinea faciei. These annular plaques are seen in children when transmission from an infected pet occurs. (*Courtesy of E. Rasmussen, MD.*)

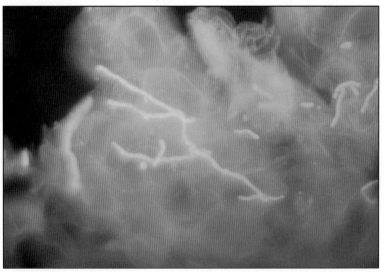

FIGURE 6-27 Calcifluor stain. Skin scrapings show brightly staining branching hyphae.

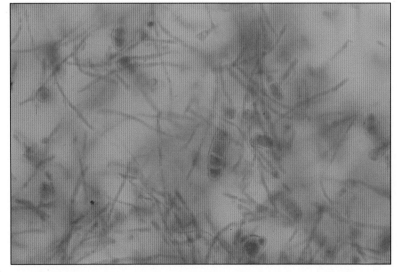

FIGURE 6-28 *Epidermophyton floccosum.* Abundant smooth-walled, club-shaped macroconidia arise from hyphae. Microconidia are not present.

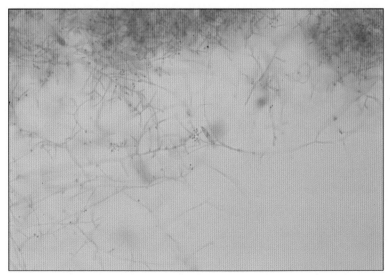

FIGURE 6-29 *Trichophyton mentagrophytes.* Clusters of teardrop-shaped microconidia arising from hyphae are accompanied by smooth-walled elongated macroconidia.

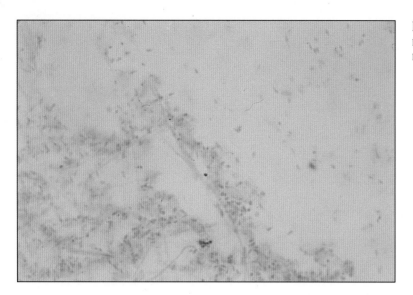

FIGURE 6-30 *Trichophyton rubrum.* Most isolates produce few microconidia. Some isolates, such as this one, produce abundant microconidia clustered on the hyphae.

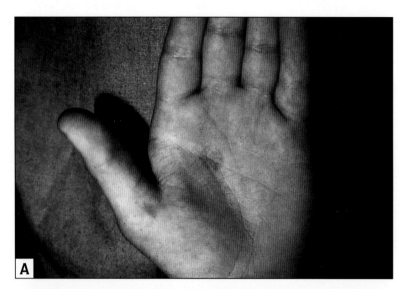

A

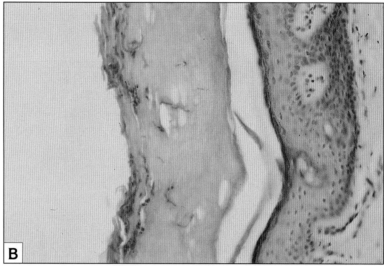

B

FIGURE 6-31 Tinea nigra. This superficial dermatophyte infection is caused by the parasitic mold *Exophiala werneckii.* Most patients acquire this infection in tropical or subtropical regions. The often-cited differential diagnosis of lentigo, junctional nevus, or acral melanoma is easily dismissed by finding fungal elements in a wet mount of skin scrapings. **A,** The characteristic lesion color is a property of the dark-colored fungus. (*Courtesy of* F. Abson, MD.) **B,** Hematoxylin-eosin–stained sections of palmar skin show abundant dark-colored fungal elements limited in distribution to the cornified cell layer. (*Courtesy of* P. Goodkin, MD.)

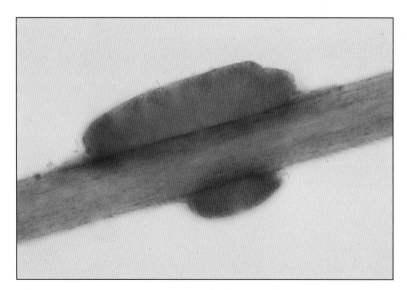

FIGURE 6-32 Black piedra. This superficial mold infection of the hair is characterized by dark-colored, hard (Spanish *piedra,* stone) irregular nodules on the hair shaft. The causative organism, *Piedraia hortae,* is found in humid, wet, tropical areas and infects animals and humans. (*Courtesy of* K. Abson, MD.)

DERMATOPHYTE INFECTIONS OF THE HAIR AND FOLLICLES

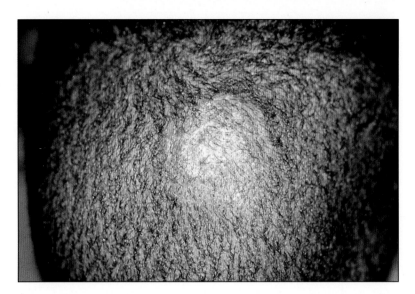

FIGURE 6-33 Tinea capitis. An area of scaling and broken-off hair on the scalp of a child is characteristic of tinea capitis. Most cases today are caused by the nonfluorescent organism *Trichophyton tonsurans.*

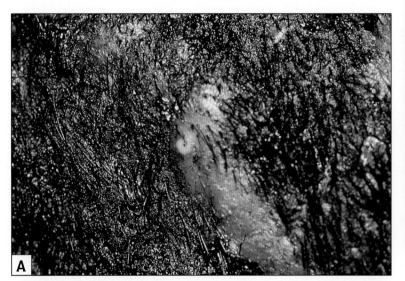

A

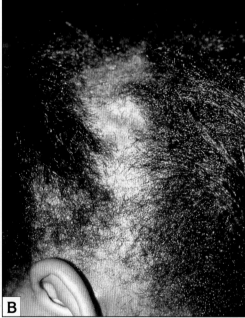

B

FIGURE 6-34 Kerion celsi. **A,** Kerion occurs when tinea capitis is accompanied by a vigorous cell-mediated immune response; the infected area may become edematous, boggy, and exudative. **B,** An exuberant inflammatory reaction to a dermatophyte infection of the hair may cause sufficient skin injury to produce a scar and permanent alopecia.

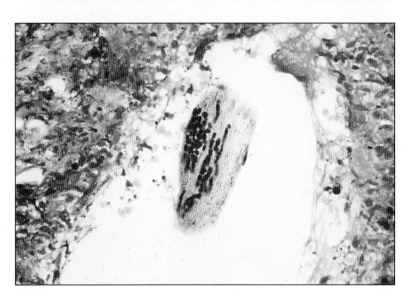

FIGURE 6-35 Histopathologic examination in tinea capitis. A hair follicle remnant contains a fragment of hair with periodic acid–Schiff–positive organisms on it. In a kerion, the immune response is so intense that demonstration of organisms by microscopic examination or culture is difficult. The diagnosis is made by biopsy of affected skin.

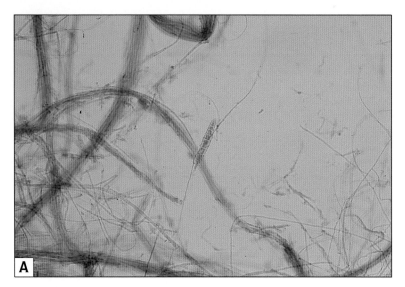

FIGURE 6-36 Etiologic organisms. Most cases of tinea capitis are caused by *Trichophyton tonsurans* or *Microsporum canis*. The clinical syndromes are indistinguishable, but each has a broad clinical spectrum depending on the host immune responses. **A**, *Microsporum canis* is readily identified in a lactophenol cotton blue preparation of cultured material by the presence of large macro- conidia with thick, echinulated walls. **B**, *Trichophyton tonsurans* is identified in a lactophenol cotton blue preparation by the presence of variably sized, teardrop-shaped to balloon-shaped microconidia attached to a conidiophore by a thin, short stalk. Smooth, elon- gated macroconidia, as shown in this micrograph, are rarely seen. (Panel 36B *courtesy of* K. Abson, MD.)

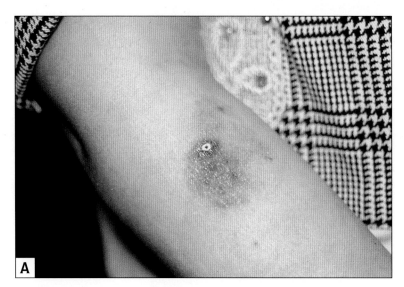

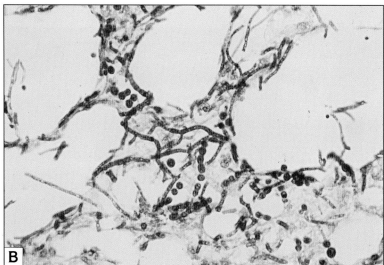

FIGURE 6-37 Majocchi's granuloma. **A**, The inflammatory, red to reddish-brown, grouped dermal papules of Majocchi's granuloma begin as a folliculitis caused by invasion of the hair follicle by der- matophytes. With rupture of the hair follicle, a neutrophilic inflammatory reaction occurs; this is superseded by a granuloma- tous reaction that may be due in part to the hair follicle contents. The evolution of the infection accounts for the spectrum of observed clinical lesions. (*Courtesy of* J. Francis, MD.) **B**, Periodic acid–Schiff–stained sections of skin show an abscess with abun- dant fungal elements. The organism, *Trichophyton rubrum*, is often easily seen in scrapings from infected surrounding skin but may be difficult to detect in scrapings from the lesion itself.

FUNGAL INFECTIONS OF THE NAILS

Types of onychomycoses		
Type	**Site of infection**	**Clinical appearance**
Distal subungual	Nailbed	Onycholysis
Superficial white	Dorsal surface of nail plate	Opaque white discoloration
Proximal subungual	Nail matrix	Dystrophic ridges in nail

FIGURE 6-38 Types of onychomycoses. There are three portals of entry for primary fungal infection of the nail unit. The most common is distal subungual onychomycosis, in which the infectious agent invades the nailbed, causing onycholysis (separation of the nail plate from the nailbed) as the cardinal physical finding. Next most common is superficial white onychomycosis, in which fungi invade the dorsal surface of the nail plate and produce an opaque white discoloration. Least common is proximal subungual onychomycosis. In this condition, fungi invade near or beneath the proximal nailfold and infect the nail matrix (the epithelium that makes the nail plate), causing the nail plate to grow out with dystrophic ridges and a clinically unaffected distal edge. Etiologic agents for primary dermatophyte infections of the nail unit include *Trichophyton rubrum*, *T. mentagrophytes*, *Epidermophyton floccosum*, and, occasionally, *T. tonsurans*. A number of saprophytic molds can also infect otherwise diseased nail plates and may obscure the cause of the primary nail problem.

Primary Dermatophyte Infections

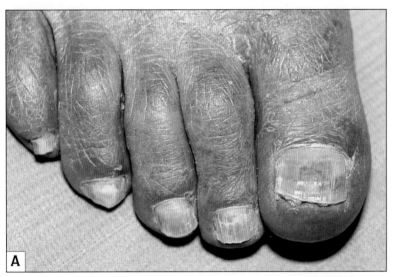

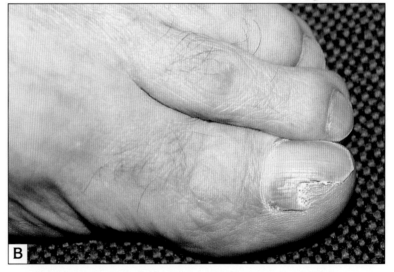

FIGURE 6-39 Distal subungual onychomycosis. **A**, Onycholysis, subungual debris, and yellowish thickening and dystrophic change of the nail plate occurring in the setting of a chronic dermatophyte infection of the feet characterize this challenging therapeutic problem. **B**, Early involvement of one nail demonstrates the proximal spread of disease nearly to the proximal nailfold. Differential diagnosis of this condition from early psoriasis requires trimming the nail plate as far proximally as possible and collecting subungual debris with a small curette for wet mount examination.

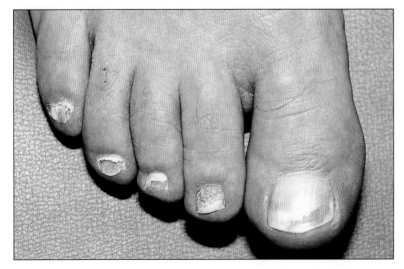

FIGURE 6-40 Superficial white onychomycosis and subungual onychomycosis. This patient demonstrates partial loss of the nail plates on three toes and opaque white discoloration of the remaining nail plate, pitting and ridging on one toe, and opaque white discoloration only on the great toenail. The simultaneous occurrence of superficial white onychomycosis and distal subungual onychomycosis is a common finding in HIV-1 infection.

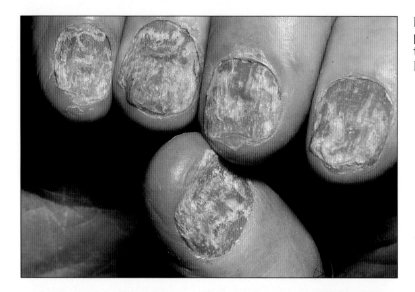

FIGURE 6-41 Proximal subungual onychomycosis. Note the dystrophy and ridging of all the nail plates. In this long-standing infection, the entire nail plate has become infected. (*Courtesy of* P. Fleckman, MD.)

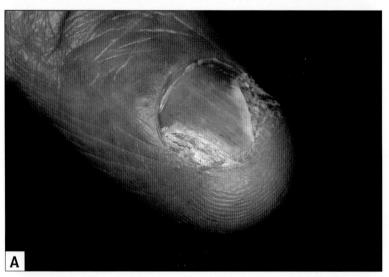

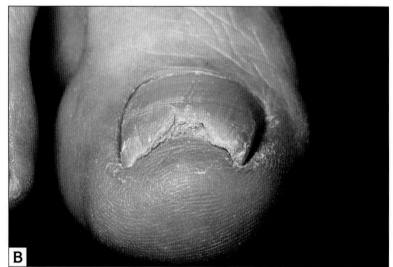

FIGURE 6-42 Candida infection of the nail plate. **A,** Onychomycosis is a prominent feature of candida infection of the nail plate with especially exuberant subungual debris. Culture is required to definitively establish *Candida* as the etiologic agent. **B,** The nail may become hyperconvex with the piled-up subungual debris. (*Courtesy of* P. Fleckman, MD.)

Other Fungal Infections

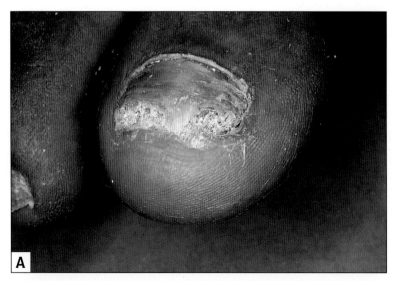

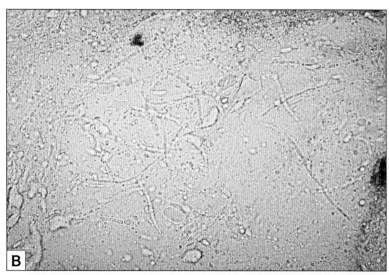

FIGURE 6-43 *Fusarium.* **A,** The yellow, thickened nail plate with abundant subungual debris has the appearance of a typical example of tinea unguium. **B,** The chartoconidium of *Fusarium* is evident on a KOH wet mount specimen. (*Courtesy of* D. Babel, MD.)

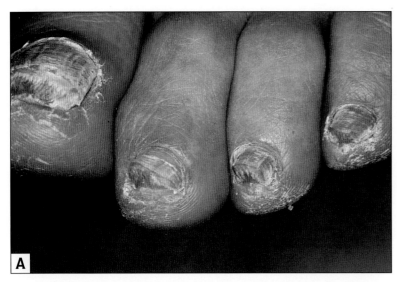

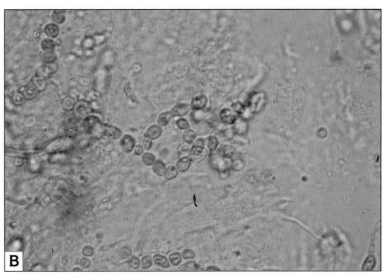

FIGURE 6-44 *Trichosporon.* **A,** The discolored, dystrophic, thickened, hyperconvex nails have the appearance of tinea unguium.

B, The toruloid hyphae and arthroconidia of *Trichosporon* are evident on the KOH wet mount. (*Courtesy of* D. Babel, MD.)

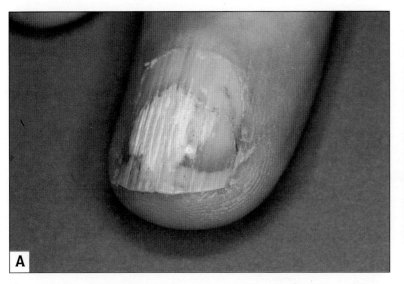

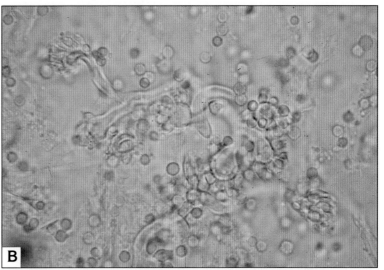

FIGURE 6-45 *Aspergillus.* **A,** The opaque white discoloration of the nail plate appears similar to superficial white onychomycosis. **B,** The

hyphae, fruiting head, and phialoconidia of *Aspergillus* are nicely seen in this KOH wet mount preparation. (*Courtesy of* D. Babel, MD.)

FUNGAL INFECTION IN COMPROMISED HOSTS

Alternariosis

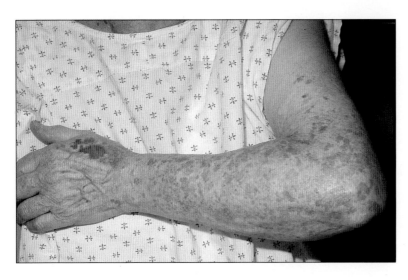

FIGURE 6-46 Cutaneous alternariosis. This confluent, inflammatory, papulonodular eruption occurred on the upper extremity of this woman with atopic dermatitis who had received extensive topical treatment with corticosteroids. *Alternaria* was cultured from the skin eruption. (*Courtesy of* J. Hanifin, MD.)

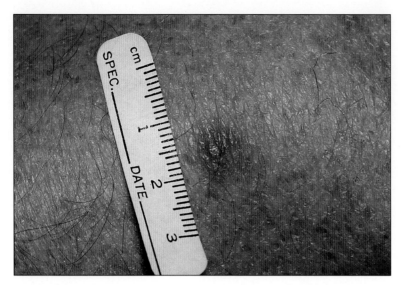

FIGURE 6-47 Cutaneous alternariosis. A solitary, minimally inflamed pustule occurred in this bone marrow transplant recipient.

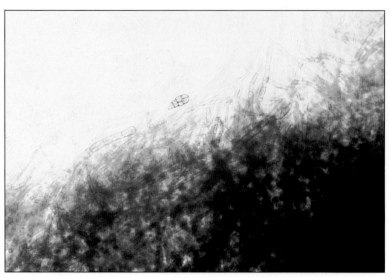

FIGURE 6-48 *Alternaria.* Lactophenol cotton blue preparation showing thick-walled septate hyphae and large pyriform conidia.

Trichophytosis

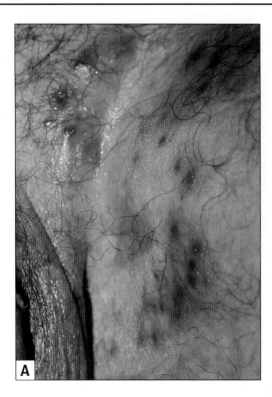

A

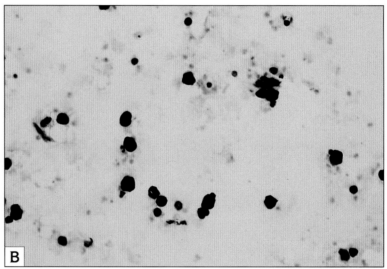

B

FIGURE 6-49 *Trichophyton rubrum* abscesses. **A,** Grouped dermal papules occurred symmetrically in the groin area and at one distant site in a bone marrow transplant recipient. *Trichophyton rubrum* was cultured from the skin lesions. **B,** A methenamine silver stain of abscess contents demonstrates the abundant fungal elements.

Fusarium Infection

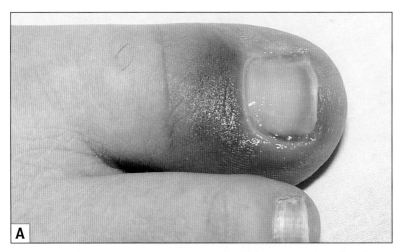

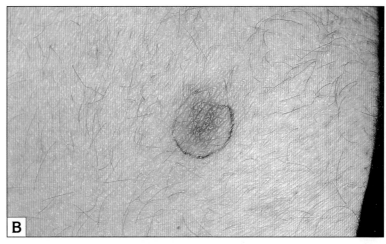

FIGURE 6-50 *Fusarium* paronychia. **A**, This paronychia developed 12 days after bone marrow transplantation. **B**, The paronychia was accompanied by eruption of papulonecrotic skin lesions.

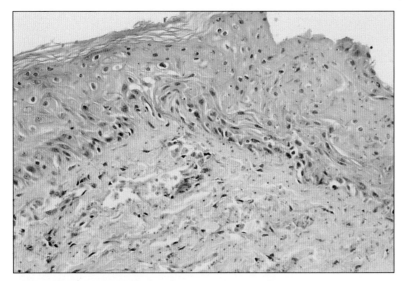

FIGURE 6-51 *Fusarium*. Hematoxylin-eosin–stained sections from a skin lesion demonstrate fungal organisms in the skin unaccompanied by an inflammatory infiltrate.

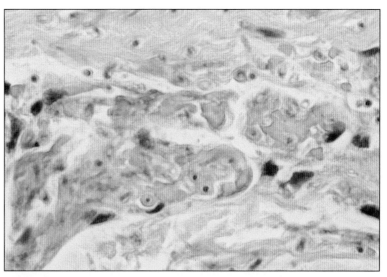

FIGURE 6-52 *Fusarium* infection. A micrograph shows abundant organisms in and around a vascular structure.

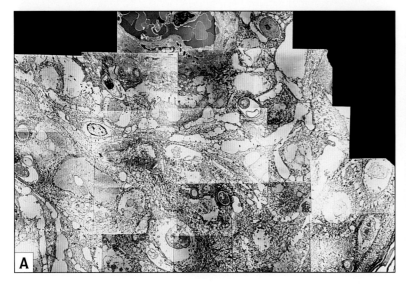

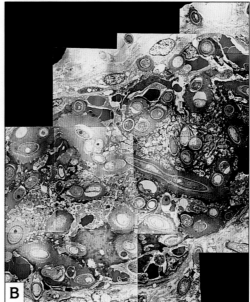

FIGURE 6-53 *Fusarium* infection. **A**, Electron micrograph photomontage of epidermis shows organisms within the epidermis and in a small dermal venule (*bottom left*). **B**, Electron micrograph photomontage of a dermal vessel shows abundant organisms within the vessel lumen. (*Courtesy of* D. Thorning, MD.)

Candidiasis

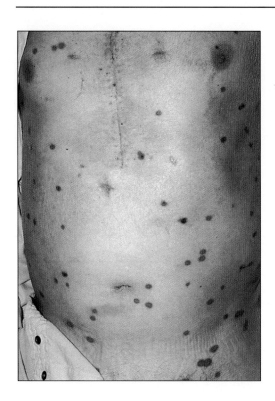

FIGURE 6-54
Disseminated candidiasis. A neutropenic chemotherapy patient developed fever, myalgias, and a purpuric rash. The source of this hematogenously disseminated infection is usually a contaminated vascular catheter. Biopsy of a skin lesion demonstrated clumps of organisms in the dermis without accompanying inflammation.

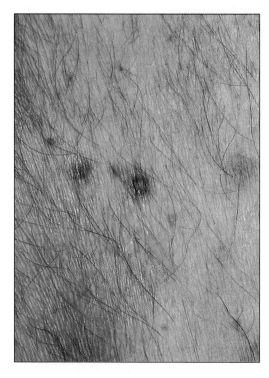

FIGURE 6-55
Disseminated candidiasis. A patient whose neutrophil count was recovering developed a rash with tiny central pustules, indicating an early neutrophilic response.

Coccidioidomycosis

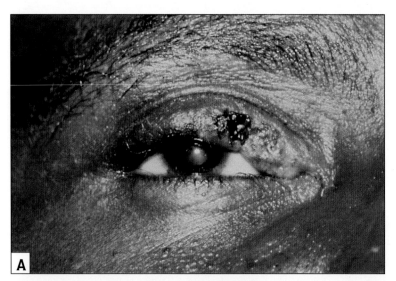

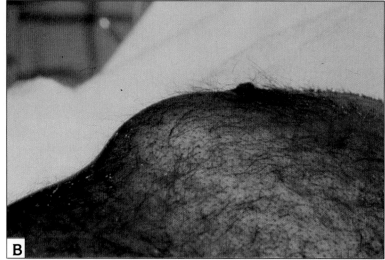

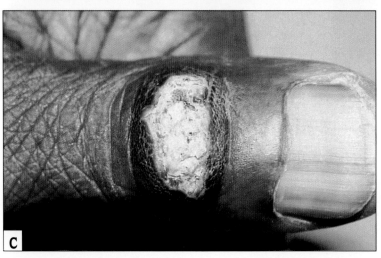

FIGURE 6-56 Disseminated coccidioidomycosis. Disseminated infection occurs in < 1% of cases of *Coccidioides* infection, but when it does occur, more than 50% of patients have skin lesions. The skin lesions are described as papulonodules, papulopustules, subcutaneous masses, or verrucous plaques. This 41-year-old man had an acute illness characterized by "total body pain," fever, headache, and nuchal rigidity. **A**, **B**, and **C**, The patient developed a warty whitish plaque over the right upper eyelid (*panel 56A*), a large subcutaneous mass on the chest wall (*panel 56B*), and a warty hyperkeratotic lesion on the thumb (*panel 56C*).

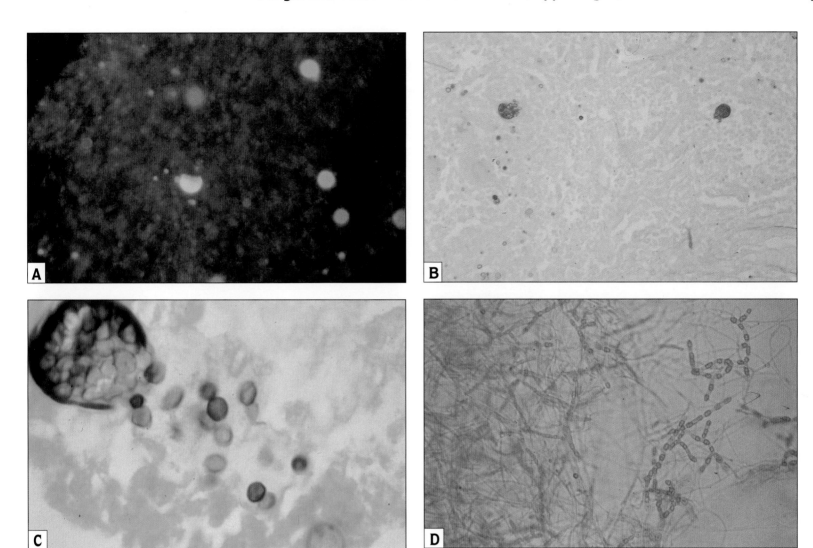

FIGURE 6-57 Histopathologic examination. **A,** Calcifluor stain of fluid aspirated from the chest wall lesion demonstrated the yeast forms. **B,** Periodic acid–Schiff staining of skin sections show yeast forms and spherules in the dermis. (*Courtesy of* K. Abson, MD.)

C, High-power micrograph of a spherule (silver stain). (*Courtesy of* D. Stevens, MD.) **D,** Lactophenol cotton blue preparation from cultured material shows typical barrel-shaped arthroconidia and 90° branching typical of *Coccidioides immitis.*

Cryptococcosis

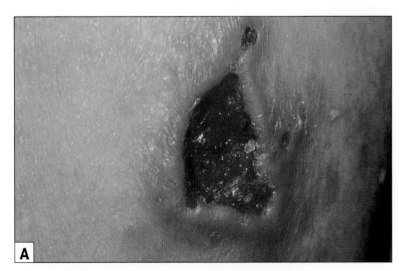

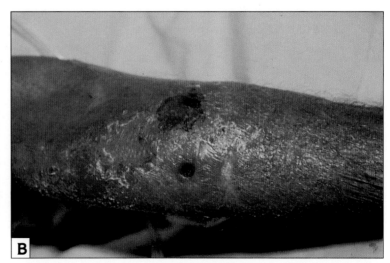

FIGURE 6-58 Cryptococcosis is caused by the yeast *Cryptococcosis neoformans.* Primary infection usually occurs in the lungs with dissemination in patients with leukemia, lymphoma, sarcoidosis, systemic lupus erythematosus, or HIV-1 infection. About 20% of patients with dissemination develop skin lesions. Skin lesions may be small translucent umbilicated papules resembling molluscum contágiosum, nodules, or ulcers, or infiltrated plaques resembling cellulitis. **A,** This punched-out irregular ulcer with the elevated border occurred in a patient with HIV-1 infection. (*Courtesy of* D. Spach, MD.) **B,** This indurated, erythematous plaque somewhat resembled a cellulitis. (*Courtesy of* K. Abson, MD.)

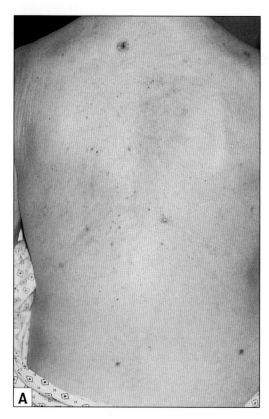
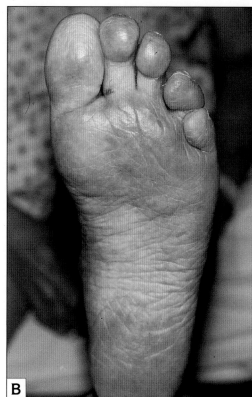
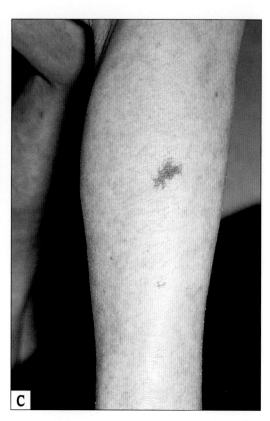

FIGURE 6-59 Cryptococcosis. **A**, **B**, and **C**, A patient undergoing chemotherapy developed a hemorrhagic nodule on the upper back (*panel 59A*) and other skin lesions, as well as a solitary papule at the base of the second toe (*panel 59B*) and a hemorrhagic area of superficial necrosis (*panel 59C*). (*Courtesy of* C. Bauman, MD.)

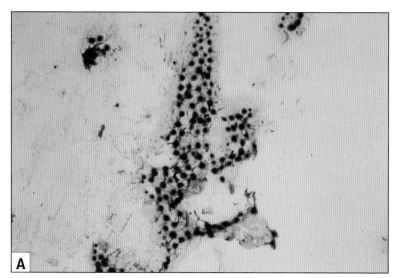
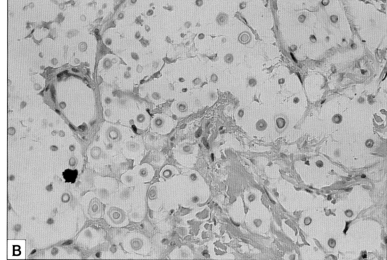

FIGURE 6-60 Histopathologic examination. **A**, Gram stain of fluid aspirated from one of the hemorrhagic areas from the patient in Fig. 6-59 shows many yeast forms. **B**, Hematoxylin-eosin–stained skin sections show abundant yeast forms surrounded by a thick mucinous capsule. (*Courtesy of* C. Bauman, MD.)

Aspergillosis

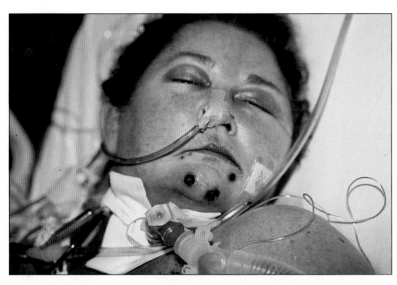

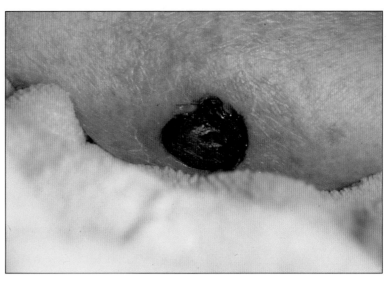

FIGURE 6-61 *Aspergillus* infection of the skin may occur by primary inoculation, as under an occlusive dressing, or by hematogenous dissemination. Necrosis of the skin is the result of angioinvasion and thrombosis. The characteristic lesion of cutaneous aspergillosis begins as an area of erythema and rapidly progresses to infarction and necrosis, somewhat resembling ecthyma gangrenosum. (*Courtesy of* K. Abson, MD.)

FIGURE 6-62 Aspergillosis. This rapidly progressing necrotic ulcer occurred in a patient receiving chemotherapy. (*Courtesy of* D. Thompson, MD.)

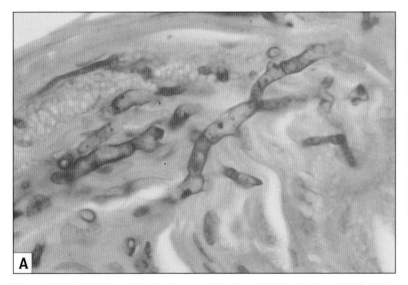

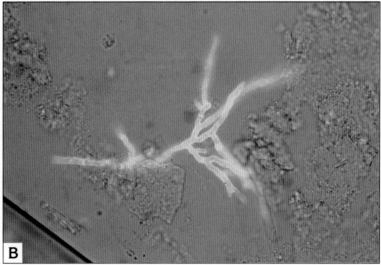

FIGURE 6-63 Histopathologic examination. **A**, Periodic acid–Schiff stain of a skin biopsy section readily demonstrates the thick, dichotomously branching hyphae. **B**, *Aspergillus* as visualized with calcifluor stain. (*Courtesy of* K. Abson, MD.)

Zygomycosis

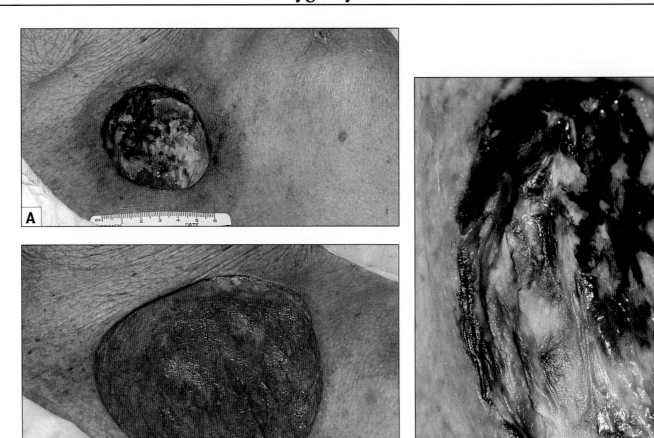

FIGURE 6-64 *Rhizopus* infection. Infection of the skin with the organisms *Rhizopus, Mucor*, or *Absidia* result in gangrenous cellulitis. Angioinvasion and thrombosis is a major component of the pathology of this lesion. The skin lesions resemble those seen in cutaneous aspergillosis, but progress more rapidly. This elderly patient developed an area of skin and subcutaneous fat necrosis at the site of an intravenous catheter. **A**, At 48 hours after surgical debridement, the lesion shows a raised dusky reddish border. **B**, A close-up view shows the grossly apparent colonies of mold growing on the subcutaneous fat and muscle. **C**, After additional surgical procedures, the wound is finally free of mold growth.

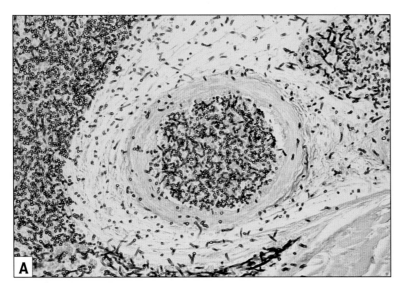

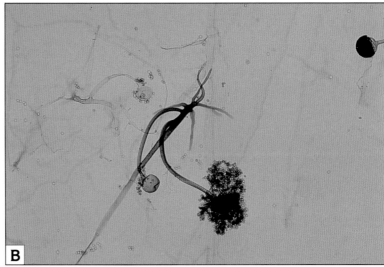

FIGURE 6-65 Histopathologic examination. **A**, Silver-stained sections of subcutaneous tissue show innumerable *Rhizopus* organisms in the subcutaneous fat and vascular lumen. **B**, Lactophenol cotton blue preparation shows sporangiophores arising directly from rhizoids. (*Courtesy of* K. Abson, MD.)

SUBCUTANEOUS AND DEEP MYCOSES

Actinomycosis

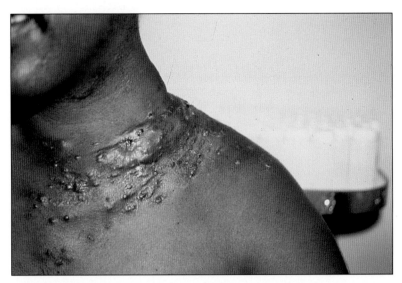

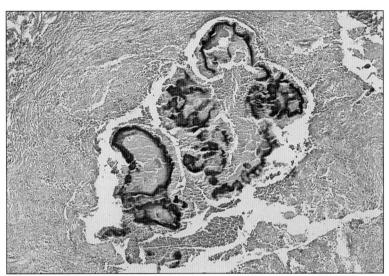

FIGURE 6-66 Actinomycosis. Actinomycosis is caused by the anaerobic gram-positive filamentous bacteria *Actinomyces israelii*. This organism has a strong tendency to cause chronic granulomatous inflammation and external sinuses. The organism normally lives in the mouth, and under conditions of reduced oxygen tension (*eg*, in the site of a dental extraction), it may proliferate, dissect along connective tissue planes, and exit to the skin. Hyperpigmented nodules on an indurated fibrotic base, seen here, are actually multiple draining sinuses. (*Courtesy of* K. Abson, MD.)

FIGURE 6-67 Actinomycosis. Micrograph of a "sulfur" granule of actinomycosis. (*Courtesy of* K. Abson, MD.)

Sporotrichosis

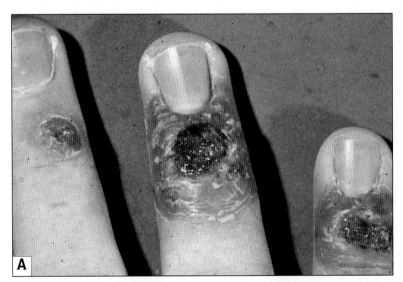

A

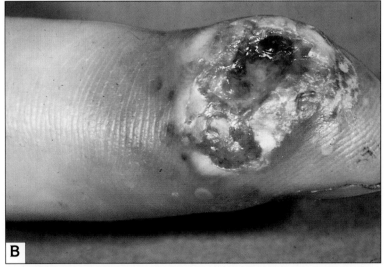

B

FIGURE 6-68 *Sporothrix* infection. Three weeks following accidental implantation of the fungus, a papule, papular-pustular lesion, or ulcer appears on the skin. Although this primary lesion may heal over a period of a few months, secondary dermal or subcutaneous nodules and ulcers, "nodular lymphangitis," develop along the distribution of the draining lymphatics. This constellation of findings is typical for infection with the causative agents for sporotrichosis, nocardiosis, tularemia, and atypical mycobacterial infection. Diagnosis is made on the basis of culture of *Sporothrix schenckii* from a skin biopsy specimen. In some patients proximal lesions do not develop (fixed cutaneous sporotrichosis); rarely, dissemination occurs with involvement of skin, bone, and synovium. **A,** Multiple sites of inoculation were observed in this young patient, who sustained many superficial skin wounds from handling holly packed in sphagnum moss. **B,** An ulcerated nodule with satellite pustules developed on the distal digit of this patient and was accompanied by nodular lymphangitis.

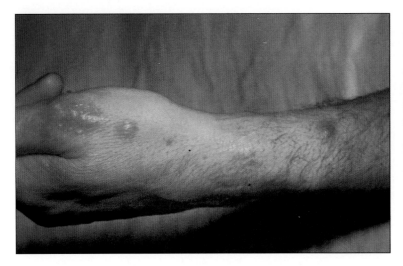

FIGURE 6-69 Nodular lymphangitis from sporotrichosis. Note the nearly linear distribution of dermal or subcutaneous papules and nodules on the forearm. (*Courtesy of* K. Abson, MD.)

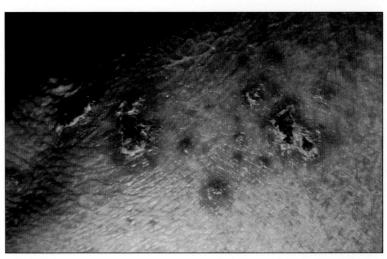

FIGURE 6-70 Fixed cutaneous sporotrichosis. Grouped reddish-brown dermal papules and ulcers consistent with granulomatous dermal inflammation were seen in a patient who never developed nodular lymphangitis. (*Courtesy of* K. Abson, MD.)

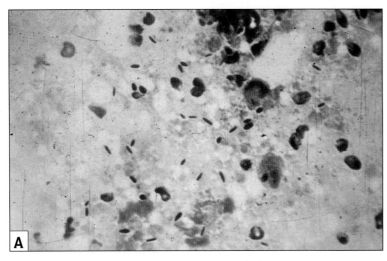

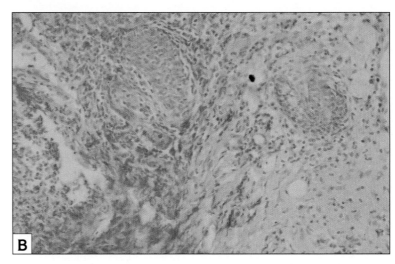

FIGURE 6-71 Histopathologic examination in sporotrichosis. **A**, Methenamine silver stain of wound exudate demonstrates abundant yeast forms. **B**, Periodic acid–Schiff–stained skin sec- tions show granulomatous inflammation and a single yeast form. (*Courtesy of* K. Abson, MD.)

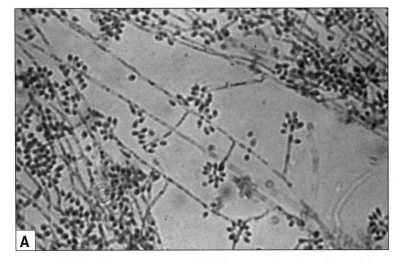

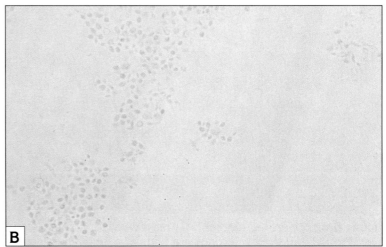

FIGURE 6-72 *Sporothrix schenckii.* The organism is a dimorphic fungus. **A**, At 26° C, the colony is composed of septate hyphae. Slender conidiophores branch off at right angles and bear clusters of oval conidia. **B**, At 37° C, the organism grows exclusively in the yeast form. *(continued)*

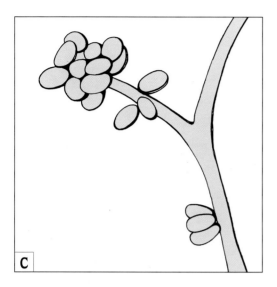

Figure 6-72 *(continued)* **C**, In the vegetative phase, bouquets of conidia are produced at the tips of the conidiophore.

Blastomycosis

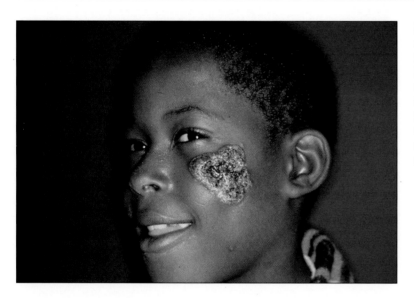

Figure 6-73 Blastomycosis. Skin lesions occur after systemic dissemination of *Blastomyces dermatitidis* from a primary pulmonary focus. Skin lesions occur in about 70% of patients with systemic blastomycosis and are usually vegetating plaques with slowly advancing, raised, hyperkeratotic, or verrucous borders with central healing and scarring. Small pustules are present in the verrucous border, and thrombosed dermal capillaries are present in the central scar. In this patient, *Blastomyces* was recovered from the darkly pigmented ulcerated plaque with verrucous indurated borders. (*Courtesy of* K. Abson, MD.)

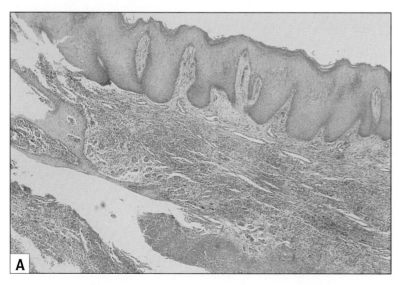

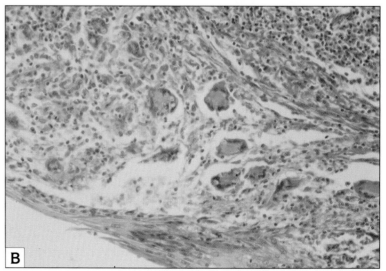

Figure 6-74 Blastomycosis. **A**, Microscopic examination shows prominent pseudoepitheliomatous hyperplasia, diffuse infiltration of the dermis with inflammatory cells, and many giant cells. **B**, This micrograph shows histiocytic infiltration of the dermis with multinucleated giant cells. Organisms are found in multinucleated giant cells in the dermis or free in the micropustules of the epidermis. (*Courtesy of* K. Abson, MD.)

Paracoccidioidomycosis

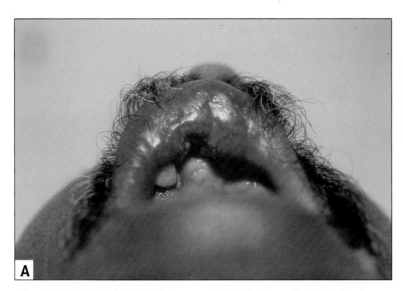

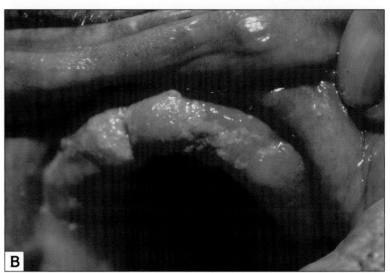

FIGURE 6-75 Mucocutaneous paracoccidioidomycosis. Infection with *Paracoccidioides* occurs by inhalation of spores. Typically, the patients are young adults living in tropical or subtropical forests in the endemic areas of Latin America between 23° N and 34° S latitude. Primary infection is usually self-limited; dissemination occurs most often in older men. Dissemination to the oropharynx is the most frequently involved extrapulmonary site.

The lesions vary from a painful stomatitis to deeply ulcerating granulomatous lesions of the lips, gingivae, tongue, or palate. Nonsuppurating cervical lymphadenopathy may accompany the oropharyngeal lesions. **A,** This view of the upper lip shows marked edema and dermal papules and nodules. **B,** The gingival ridge shows granulomatous infiltration and loss of all teeth. (*Courtesy of* K. Hansen, MD.)

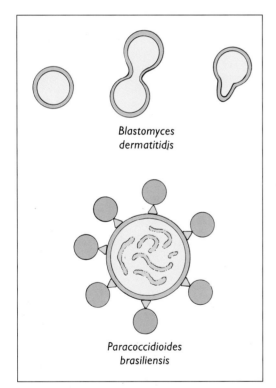

Blastomyces
dermatitidis

Paracoccidioides
brasiliensis

FIGURE 6-76 Differential diagnosis. *Blastomyces* has large, thick-walled yeast forms with single buds. In contrast, *Paracoccidioides* has multiply budding yeast forms. These are occasionally seen in sections as a "pilot's wheel," as shown here.

Histoplasmosis

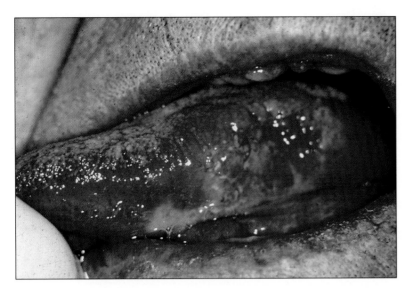

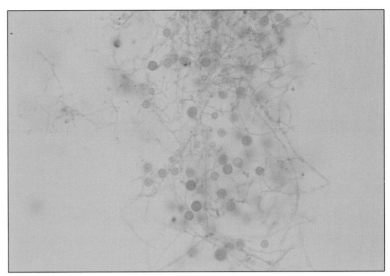

FIGURE 6-77 Histoplasmosis. Infection with *Histoplasma capsulatum* occurs when microconidia are inhaled into the lungs. Most cases go unrecognized or asymptomatic; the severity of illness depends on the size of the inoculum, whether the host had experienced previous infection, the presence of underlying chronic obstructive pulmonary disease, and the general immune status of the host. Dissemination from the primary pulmonary focus occurs only in about 1 in 2000 cases, but over half develop oropharyngeal ulcers. In this patient, the indurated ulcer on the tongue was shown to contain *Histoplasma* in stained sections and by culture. (*Courtesy of* E.D. Everett, MD.)

FIGURE 6-78 *Histoplasma capsulatum.* Lactophenol cotton blue preparation of a sporulating culture of *H. capsulatum* demonstrates the characteristic mycelia, microconidia, and tuberculate macroconidia. (*Courtesy of* K. Abson, MD.)

Mycetoma

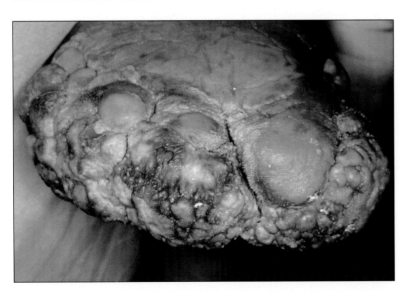

FIGURE 6-79 Mycetoma (Madura foot). This indolent and usually painless local infection is characterized by induration and tumefaction, with sinus tract formation and drainage of granule-containing pus. Late in the course of the disease, the bones may become involved. Two groups of organisms may cause this clinical presentation. Actinomycetoma is caused by filamentous bacteria, including *Nocardia* and *Actinomyces* species. Eumycetoma is caused by a group of true fungi, including *Petriellidium* and *Madurella* species. Gram stain is useful in distinguishing those cases caused by filamentous bacteria (gram positive) from those caused by the true fungi (not stained), whereas periodic acid–Schiff and methenamine silver reagents stain both. This view of a patient's foot shows the grotesque deformity (maduramycosis) that accompanies long-standing infection. (*Courtesy of* K. Abson, MD.)

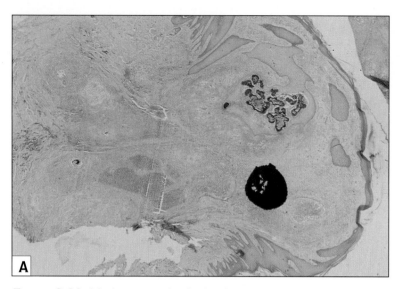

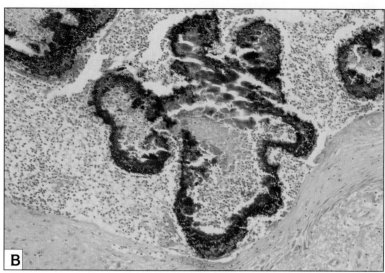

FIGURE 6-80 Maduramycosis. **A**, A micrograph shows a large dark granule in the dermis. **B**, A high-power view shows a black "sulfur granule" with dark fungal material at the periphery of the granule. (*Courtesy of* K. Abson, MD.)

ACKNOWLEDGMENTS

The author is grateful to Dale Tilly and the staff of Medical Media Production Services at the Seattle VA Medical Center and to the many individuals who contributed images for this chapter.

SELECTED BIBLIOGRAPHY

Braun-Falco O, Plewig G, Wolff HH, Winkelmann RK: *Dermatology*. New York: Springer-Verlag; 1991.

Kwon-Chung KJ, Bennett JE: *Medical Mycology*. Philadelphia: Lea & Febiger; 1992.

Lever WF, Schaumberg-Lever G: *Histopathology of the Skin*, 7th ed. Philadelphia: J.B. Lippincott; 1990.

Scher RK, Daniel CR (eds.): *Nails: Therapy, Diagnosis, Surgery*. Philadelphia: W.B. Saunders; 1990.

CHAPTER 7

Viral Infections of the Skin and Soft Tissues

Julie S. Francis
John Neff

MOLLUSCUM CONTAGIOSUM

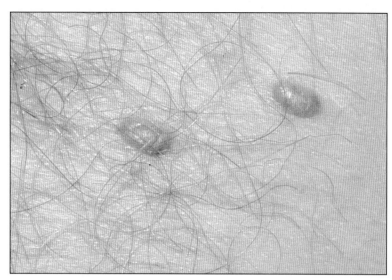

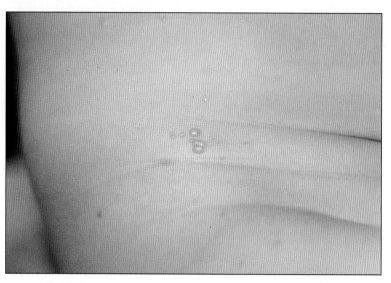

FIGURE 7-1 Molluscum contagiosum. Molluscum is a common, benign viral infection of the skin and mucous membranes, which can occur at any age but is most common in children. It is characterized by distinct single or multiple, dome-shaped papules, which are flesh or pink-colored. Lesions generally range in size from 1–5 mm, although larger papules measuring 10–15 mm are occasionally seen. With time, central umbilication of the papules can occur. (*Courtesy of* G. Raugi, MD.)

FIGURE 7-2 Molluscum contagiosum. Molluscum can occur anywhere on the skin but has a predilection to the central body, particularly the trunk, axillae, medial thighs, and groin as seen in this figure. An eczematous reaction can sometimes be seen near molluscum papules and may represent the beginnings of a cell-mediated immune response against the virus.

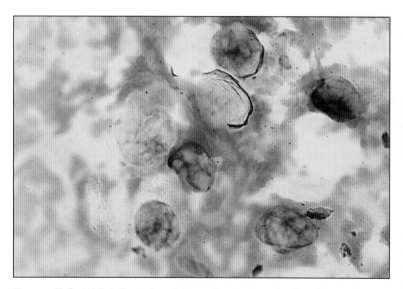

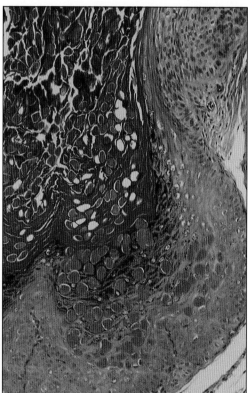

FIGURE 7-3 Wright's stain of the extruded contents of a molluscum papule. Note the blue-stained viral inclusions (known as molluscum bodies) within the cytoplasm of epidermal cells. Molluscum contagiosum is caused by a DNA pox virus, the largest virus to infect humans. The infection is limited to the skin and mucous membranes; there are no systemic manifestations. Considered moderately contagious, molluscum is spread via autoinoculation and direct contact. (*Courtesy of* G. Raugi, MD.)

FIGURE 7-4 Histopathology of molluscum contagiosum. Viral infection induces proliferation of epidermal cells, which project downward into the dermis. Infected cells are filled with intracytoplasmic round-to-oval inclusion bodies, which represent the molluscum virus. (Hematoxylin-eosin stain, × 100.) (*Courtesy of* D. Benjamin, MD.)

WARTS

Main clinical presentations of warts

Verruca vulgaris (common warts)
Verruca plana (flat warts)
Verruca plantaris (plantar warts)
Condylomata acuminata
  (anogenital warts)

FIGURE 7-5 Main clinical presentations of warts. Warts are caused by localized infection of the skin and/or mucous membranes with one of over 60 types of DNA-containing human papillomavirus (HPV). Specific HPV types can cause specific clinical infections. Common, flat, and plantar warts can occur in any age group but are most common in children and adolescents.

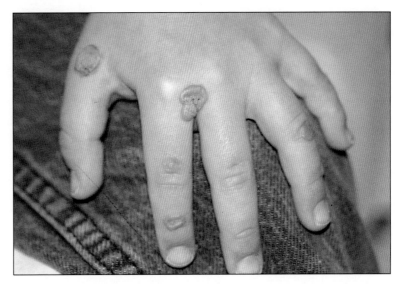

FIGURE 7-6 Verruca vulgaris. A number of human papillomavirus (HPV) types, including types 1, 2, and 4, cause common warts. Common warts are typically single or multiple, flesh-colored, dome-shaped papules with a rough, verrucous surface. They can occur anywhere on the skin but are most common on exposed surfaces, such as the fingers, hands, feet, and face. The boy in this figure had his warts frozen with liquid nitrogen and then developed blisters and enlargement of his warts. This isomorphic phenomenon, known as Koebner's phenomenon, in which trauma induces autoinoculation of the wart virus, is a common method of HPV spread and can sometimes be seen as a side effect of various treatments.

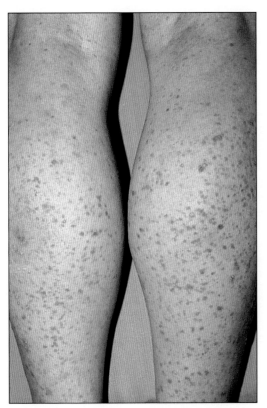

FIGURE 7-7 Verruca plana. Flat warts, commonly caused by human papillomavirus types 3 and 10, occur primarily on the face and extremities. They are generally small, flesh or brown-colored, broad-based papules and can vary in number from a few to several hundred. Autoinoculation from trauma, such as shaving, is a common means of viral spread. (*Courtesy of* G. Raugi, MD.)

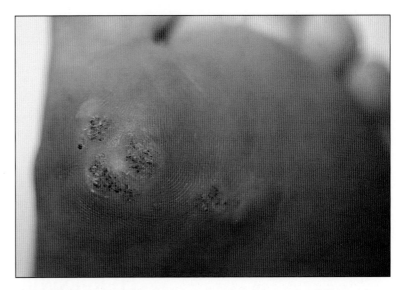

FIGURE 7-8 Verruca plantaris. A number of human papillomavirus (HPV) types, including types 1, 2, and 4, cause plantar warts. These occur on weight-bearing areas of the feet and commonly exhibit overlying hyperkeratosis. This figure illustrates the discontinuation of normal skin lines, classically seen in areas of HPV infection; in contrast, in a callus, the skin lines are preserved. Note the punctate dark-brown dots, which represent vessel thrombosis in the superficial dermis and can be a helpful diagnostic clue in differentiating plantar warts from calluses.

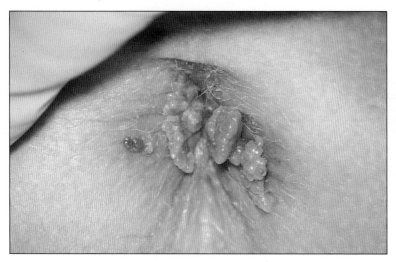

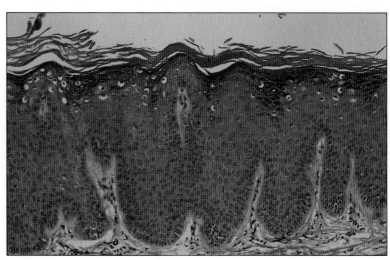

FIGURE 7-9 Condylomata acuminata. Condylomata acuminata is the clinical term given to the soft, flesh-colored polypoid or acuminate warts that occur in the anogenital region. In some patients, viral infection can be extensive and cause pain, itching, and bleeding. Most anogenital warts are caused by infections with human papillomavirus (HPV) types 6 and 11; however, other HPV types can also cause infections in the anogenital region, including HPV types 16 and 18, both of which can cause cellular atypia and induce malignant transformation. (*Courtesy of* A. Giesel, MD.)

FIGURE 7-10 Histopathology of verruca vulgaris. Human papillomavirus infection of the skin causes acanthosis with downward growth of the rete ridges. The stratum corneum is thickened with scattered columns of retained nuclei. (Hematoxylin-eosin stain, × 100.) (*Courtesy of* D. Benjamin, MD.)

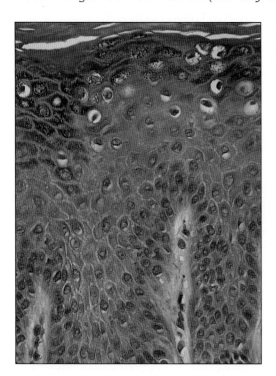

FIGURE 7-11 Histopathology of verruca vulgaris. The characteristic histologic feature is the presence of large vacuolated cells in the upper layers of the epidermis. These cells have dark basophilic nuclei surrounded by a clear zone. (Hematoxylin-eosin stain, × 400.) (*Courtesy of* D. Benjamin, MD.)

HERPESVIRUS INFECTIONS

Herpesvirus group
Herpes simplex virus
Varicella-zoster virus
Cytomegalovirus
Epstein-Barr virus
Human herpesvirus-6

FIGURE 7-12 Herpesvirus group. Five DNA viruses are members of the herpesvirus family. They cause a variety of diseases and respond quite differently to antiviral therapy.

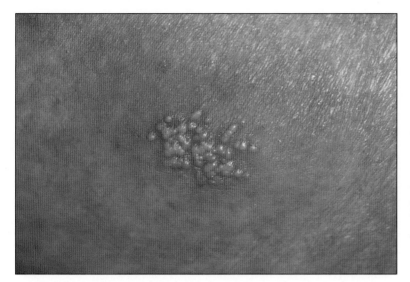

FIGURE 7-13 Herpes simplex virus (HSV). *Herpesvirus hominis* is the causative agent in herpes simplex infections and is characterized by two major serologic types. Type I HSV (HSV-1) usually causes infections on the head, neck, and upper torso. Type 2 HSV (HSV-2) usually causes recurrent genital herpes infections and is primarily responsible for neonatal herpes. Both types of HSV cause primary and recurrent infections. This figure illustrates a classic example of recurrent HSV-1 infection. Note the grouped vesicles and pustules on an erythematous base. (*Courtesy of* M. Welch, MD.)

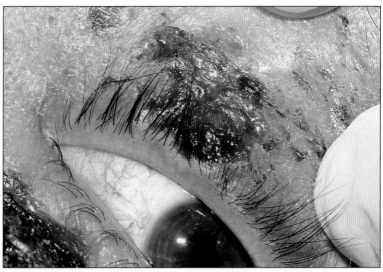

FIGURE 7-14 Chronic cutaneous herpes simplex infection. In immunocompromised hosts, recurrent herpes simplex virus (HSV) infections can be more severe. This patient with AIDS has chronic HSV-1 infection of the skin around the eye, with ulceration, crusting, and pain. (*Courtesy of* G. Raugi, MD.)

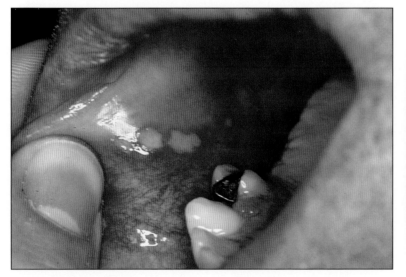

FIGURE 7-15 Herpetic gingivostomatitis. Gingivostomatitis is the most common presentation of herpes simplex virus-1 infection in children. After an incubation period of a few days, vesicles, erythema, and swelling occur in the oral cavity and on the lips. The vesicles soon erode, leaving small shallow ulcers on an erythematous base. The mucocutaneous infection is frequently associated with fever, malaise, irritability, pain, and adenopathy. (*Courtesy of* B. Myall, MD.)

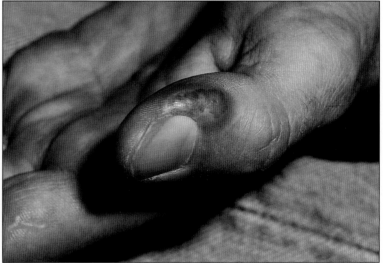

FIGURE 7-16 Herpetic whitlow. Herpetic whitlow is a specific clinical type of herpes simplex virus (HSV) infection characterized by inoculation of the HSV virus into the skin of one or more fingers. It can cause painful superficial or deep vesicles or bullae with a whitish-blue hue. It is most commonly seen in health-care personnel. (*Courtesy of* P. Kirby, MD.)

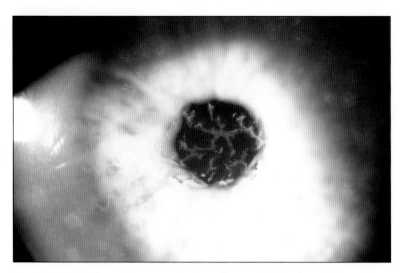

FIGURE 7-17 Herpetic corneal ulcer. Corneal infection is just one presentation of herpes simplex virus (HSV) infections of the eye and is best seen by slit-lamp examination using topical fluorescein or rose bengal dye. The infection is characterized by dendritic ulcers, a term that refers to the branching morphologic appearance of these corneal lesions. Recurrent corneal HSV infection can lead to scarring and impairment of vision. (*Courtesy of* T. Lindquist, MD.)

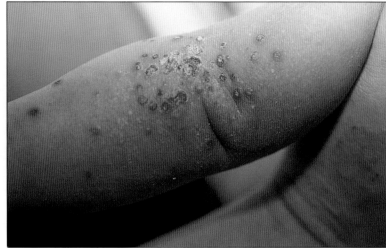

FIGURE 7-18 Eczema herpeticum. Also known as Kaposi's varicelliform eruption, eczema herpeticum refers to widespread herpes simplex virus (HSV) infection in patients with underlying skin disorders, most commonly atopic dermatitis. It can occur with both primary and recurrent HSV infections. Note the vesicles, superficial ulcers, and crusts in the antecubital fossa of this toddler with atopic dermatitis. Her infection began as primary herpetic gingivostomatitis and soon spread to areas of skin involved with atopic dermatitis.

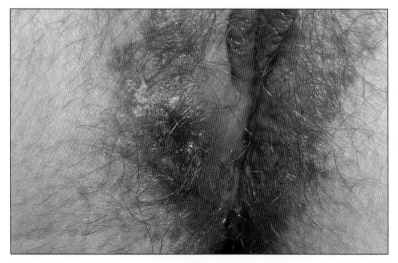

FIGURE 7-19 Genital herpes. Herpes simplex virus (HSV) infections in the genital area begin as vesicles or pustules, which progress to erosions and ulcers, generally lasting 1–3 weeks. Associated local symptoms for both primary and recurrent genital HSV infections include severe pain, itching, dysuria, inguinal adenopathy, and urethral or vaginal discharge. Constitutional symptoms occur mainly with primary genital infection and can include fever, myalgias, malaise, and headache. (*Courtesy of* P. Kirby, MD.)

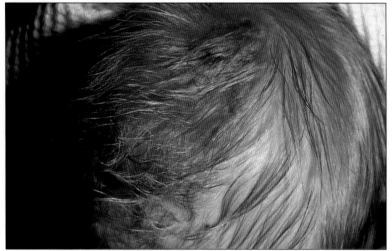

FIGURE 7-20 Neonatal herpes. Newborns may acquire primary herpes simplex virus (HSV) infection *in utero*, during delivery, or postnatally. Most neonatal HSV infections are caused by HSV-2, but 15% to 20% are caused by HSV-1. Cutaneous involvement may be minimal or extensive and is not necessarily indicative of the severity of concurrent systemic disease. (*From* Frieden IJ: Blisters and pustules in the newborn. *Curr Probl Pediatr* 1989, 19:578; with permission.)

FIGURE 7-21 Tzanck stain of a herpetic vesicle. Note the large multinucleated giant cell. The preparation is obtained by scraping the base of a new, freshly opened vesicle and staining with Giemsa stain or toluidine blue. (*Courtesy of* D. Benjamin, MD.)

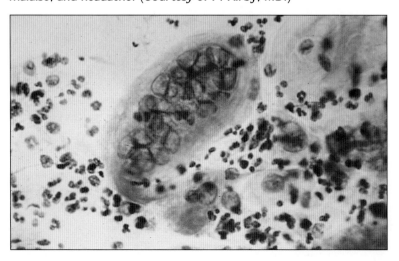

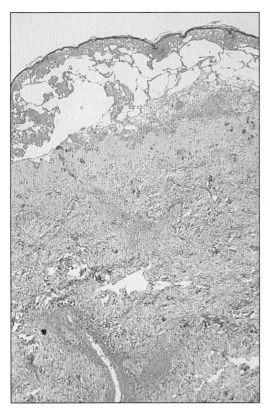

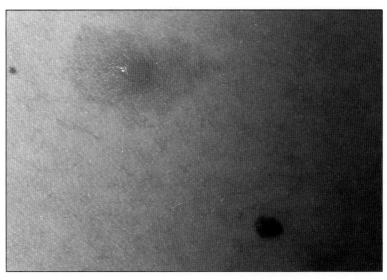

FIGURE 7-22 Histopathology of herpes simplex virus (HSV) infection of the skin. The characteristic lesion of HSV infection is an intraepidermal vesicle with marked degeneration of the epidermal cells. The infected cells may become swollen and lose their attachment to surrounding cells, a process known as ballooning degeneration. The infected cells may become so distended that they burst, leaving a loculated vesicle, as seen in this figure, a process known as reticular degeneration. (Hematoxylin-eosin stain, × 50.) (*Courtesy of* D. Benjamin, MD.)

FIGURE 7-23 Varicella. Chickenpox is caused by a primary infection with varicella-zoster virus. After an incubation period of approximately 14–16 days, the disease begins with low-grade fever, malaise, and the appearance of a characteristic generalized pruritic vesicular eruption. The early morphology of the vesicles has been likened to a "dewdrop on a rose petal," a comparison that can be appreciated in this figure. (*Courtesy of* G. Raugi, MD.)

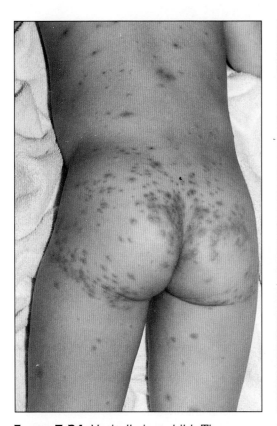

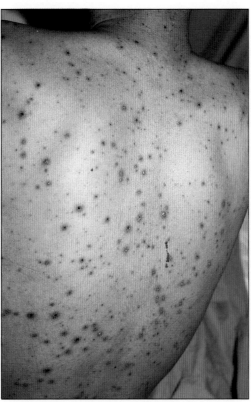

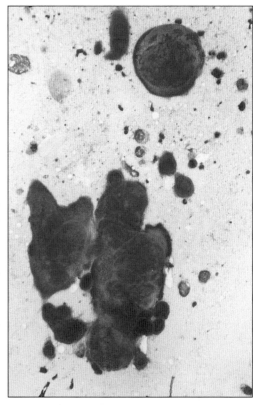

FIGURE 7-24 Varicella in a child. The eruption generally begins on the trunk or head and spreads centrifugally. New lesions generally begin to crust within 1–2 days. It is common to find various-sized papules, vesicles, pustules, and crusts all present on the skin at the same time. (*Courtesy of* D. Stevens, MD.)

FIGURE 7-25 Varicella in an adult. Over 90% of primary varicella infections occur in children. In adolescents, adults, and immunocompromised patients, the disease can be more severe. Secondary bacterial skin infections, otitis media, pneumonia, encephalitis, hepatitis, and Reye's syndrome are well-known complications of varicella infection. (*Courtesy of* D. Stevens, MD.)

FIGURE 7-26 Tzanck stain of the contents of a varicella vesicle. Note the multinucleated giant cells. These represent swollen epidermal cells containing intracytoplasmic viral inclusions. (*Courtesy of* D. Benjamin, MD.)

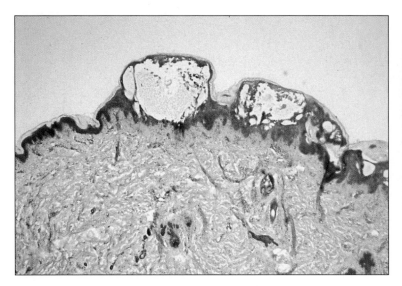

FIGURE 7-27 Histopathology of varicella. Note the intraepidermal vesicles. The skin lesions of varicella are histologically indistinguishable from those seen in herpes simplex virus infections. (*Courtesy of* D. Benjamin, MD.)

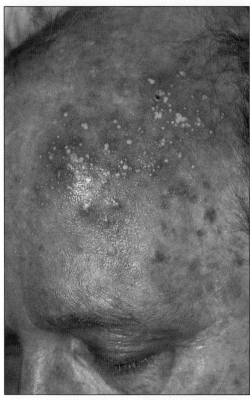

FIGURE 7-28 Acute herpes zoster. After primary varicella-zoster virus infection, the virus persists in a latent form and can be reactivated, resulting in herpes zoster or "shingles." Herpes zoster is characterized by papules, vesicles, and pustules on an inflammatory base in a dermatomal distribution, frequently associated with burning pain and tenderness. (*Courtesy of* G. Raugi, MD.)

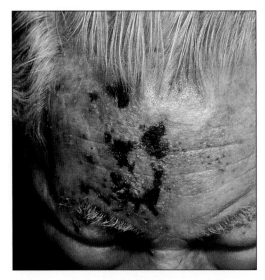

FIGURE 7-29 Resolving herpes zoster. Crops of vesicles appear for about 1 week and then dry out and crust over. The infection usually lasts 1–3 weeks. Other than mild fever, systemic symptoms are usually absent. (*Courtesy of* G. Raugi, MD.)

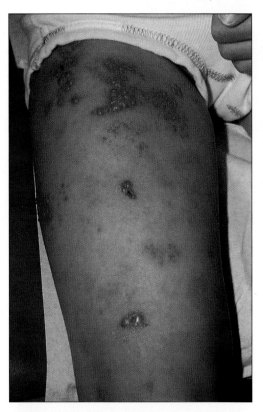

FIGURE 7-30 Disseminated herpes zoster in a child. Herpes zoster usually involves one or a few dermatomes. Occasionally, patients may develop disseminated infection with herpes zoster that can be associated with severe systemic symptoms, including fever, malaise, pneumonia, hepatitis, and meningoencephalitis. Dissemination can occur in immunocompetent as well as immunocompromised adults; however, disseminated zoster in children is seen almost always in immunocompromised individuals. (*Courtesy of* G. Raugi, MD.)

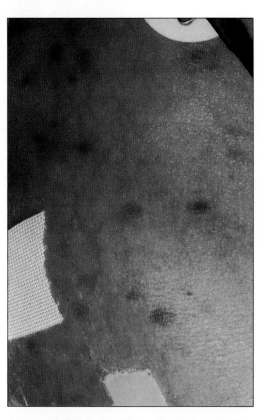

FIGURE 7-31 Congenital cytomegalovirus (CMV) infection. Cutaneous rash is unusual in acquired CMV infections but is common in congenital CMV infections. Congenital CMV infection can present in a variety of ways, ranging from asymptomatic to profound, with systemic manifestations including intrauterine growth retardation, hepatosplenomegaly, pneumonia, neonatal jaundice, thrombocytopenia, central nervous system involvement, and chorioretinitis. Skin findings include purpuric papules and nodules, as seen in this ill infant with congenital CMV infection.

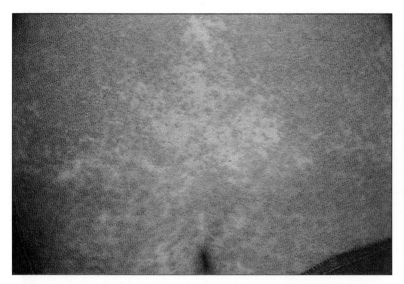

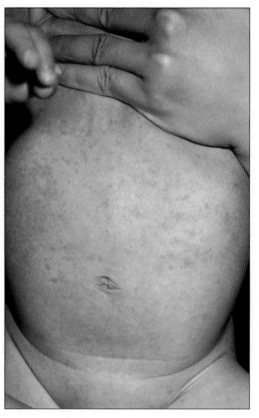

FIGURE 7-33 Roseola. Roseola infantum, also known as exanthem subitem, is a common exanthem of childhood caused by infection with human herpesvirus-6. Similar "roseola-like" illnesses occur and have been linked to other viruses. Roseola is characterized by a febrile illness with mild constitutional symptoms lasting 3–5 days. After rapid defervescence, a pink macular or maculopapular rash appears, primarily on the trunk and lasting hours to days. (*From* Frieden IJ: Childhood exanthems. *Curr Opin Dermatol* 1994, 1:285–289; with permission.)

FIGURE 7-32 Ampicillin rash in a patient with infectious mononucleosis. Infectious mononucleosis is caused by an acute infection with Epstein-Barr virus (EBV). Primary EBV infection in children is usually asymptomatic, but some children, adolescents, and young adults may develop infectious mononucleosis. When antibiotics (usually ampicillin) are administered during primary EBV infection, a red or copper-colored morbilliform eruption may appear. The rash begins on the trunk and gradually spreads over the entire body. (*Courtesy of* A. Smith, MD.)

OTHER VIRAL INFECTIONS

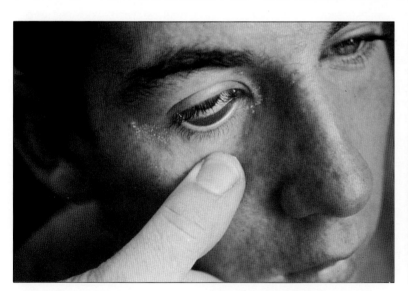

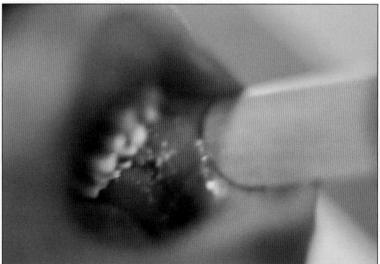

FIGURE 7-34 Conjunctivitis in a patient with measles. Rubeola, or measles, is a systemic disease caused by infection with a large RNA virus of the paramyxovirus family. Following an incubation period of 10–12 days, typical measles is characterized by fever, chills, headache, coryza, persistent cough, photophobia, and conjunctivitis. Palpebral conjunctivitis is seen in this ill-appearing patient. (*Courtesy of* D. Stevens, MD.)

FIGURE 7-35 Koplik's spots in a patient with measles. Approximately 2 days before the onset of the morbilliform exanthem, these highly characteristic Koplik's spots appear on the buccal mucosa. They are small, 1–2-mm, white or gray-blue papules, dotted on a bright red background. They usually disappear once the rash begins. (*Courtesy of* D. Stevens, MD.)

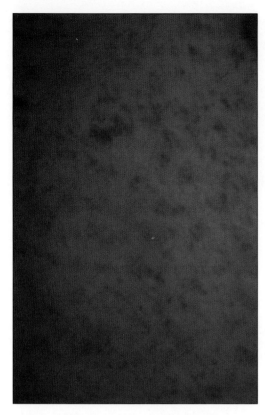

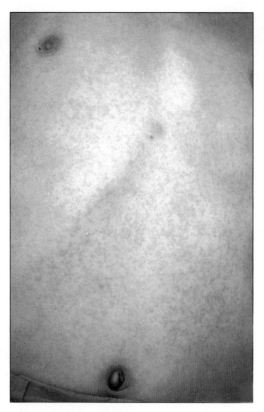

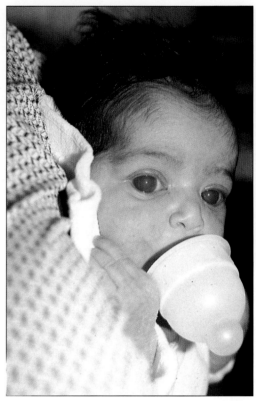

FIGURE 7-36 Measles exanthem. The measles exanthem begins 3–4 days into the illness as discrete erythematous papules that can coalesce with time. The exanthem starts first on the forehead, hairline, and behind the ears and then spreads down the body to involve the face, neck, trunk, upper extremities, and finally the lower extremities and feet. As the rash begins to fade, it turns brown, as seen in this figure, and can resolve with fine desquamation. (*Courtesy of* D. Stevens, MD.)

FIGURE 7-37 Rubella exanthem. The rubella virus, a member of the togaviridae family, causes a relatively mild illness usually in the winter and spring. The exanthem begins after a usual 14–16-day incubation period and consists of a myriad of small, discrete, rose-colored macules and papules that first appear on the face and rapidly spread downward to involve the rest of the body. Lymphadenopathy is the most notable clinical manifestation of rubella; the most prominent enlargement occurs in the sub-occipital and posterior auricular nodes generally several days before the rash appears. (*Courtesy of* D. Stevens, MD.)

FIGURE 7-38 Congenital rubella. Congenital rubella is the result of fetal infection with the virus, usually during the first trimester. There are a host of clinical findings in congenital rubella infection; the most frequent include intrauterine growth retardation, auditory nerve deafness, structural heart defects, congenital cataracts, and "salt and pepper" retinopathy. This infant demonstrates some of the eye findings of congenital rubella infection—congenital cataracts and corneal cloudiness due to congenital glaucoma. (*Courtesy of* D. Stevens, MD.)

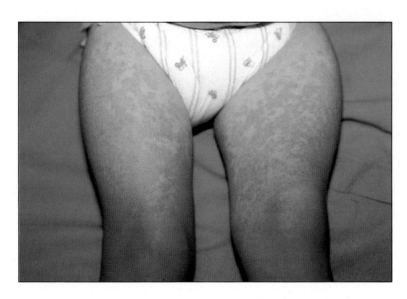

FIGURE 7-39 Erythema infectiosum. Fifth's disease, or erythema infectiosum, is caused by human parvovirus B19. The exanthem occurs in three stages and is usually not associated with constitutional symptoms. The first stage is characterized by a bright red malar rash that looks like a sunburn. The second stage occurs 1–4 days later as an erythematous maculopapular eruption primarily involving the extensor surfaces of the extremities. The eruption may become confluent in areas as seen in this figure.

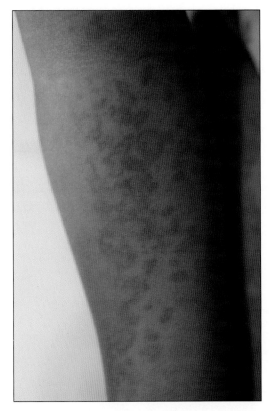

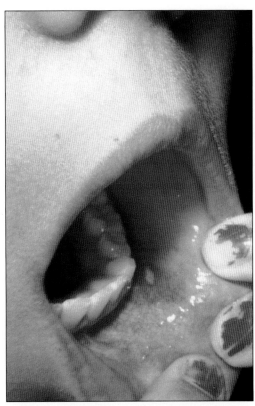

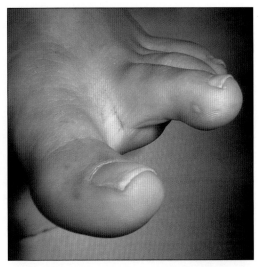

FIGURE 7-42 Hand, foot, and mouth disease. The exanthem characteristically involves the hands and feet but may involve the buttocks as well. The lesions on the hands and feet consist of 3–7-mm gray-white vesicles on an erythematous base. They frequently have an elliptical or "football-shaped" appearance. (*Courtesy of* G. Raugi, MD.)

FIGURE 7-40 Erythema infectiosum. The third stage of Fifth's disease begins as the rash starts to fade with areas of central clearing. This leaves a reticulated or lacy pattern of erythema, as seen in this figure, which can last several weeks. The most common complication of erythema infectiosum is joint involvement, ranging from mild arthralgias to overt arthritis, findings which are common in adults but relatively rare in children.

FIGURE 7-41 Hand, foot, and mouth disease. Coxsackievirus A16 is the most common cause of hand, foot, and mouth disease. The illness begins with a prodrome of fever, malaise, anorexia, and sore mouth. The enanthem occurs 1–2 days after the onset of fever, and the exanthem appears shortly after. The oral lesions appear as various-sized erosions and ulcerations on an erythematous base. The tongue and buccal mucosa are the areas most frequently affected.

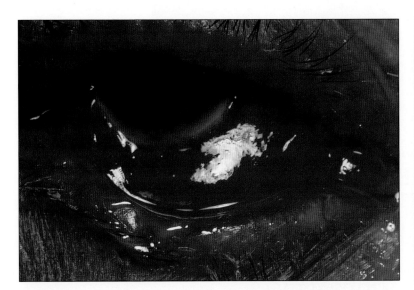

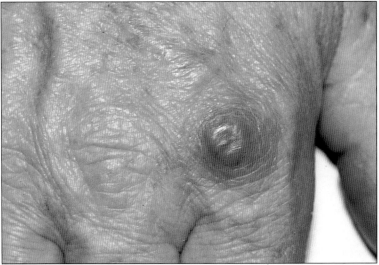

FIGURE 7-43 Adenovirus conjunctivitis. Adenoviruses cause an array of symptoms and clinical findings. Adenoviral exanthems are frequently generalized and nonspecific in appearance. Other associated findings include fever, rhinitis, pharyngitis, adenopathy, and conjunctivitis. (*Courtesy of* D. Stevens, MD.)

FIGURE 7-44 Orf. Ecthyma contagiosum, or orf, is caused by a parapox virus that causes endemic infection in sheep and goats. In humans, after an incubation period of 3–6 days, the infection is characterized by single or multiple papules or nodules, generally located on the dorsum of the hand, fingers, or thumb, which resolve spontaneously within 7–10 weeks. The individual pictured here was a sheep farmer when he acquired his infection. (*Courtesy of* G. Raugi, MD.)

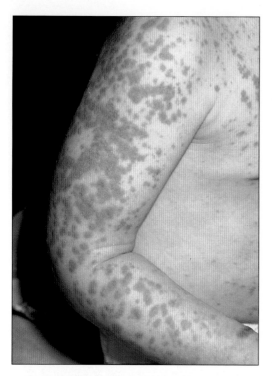

FIGURE 7-45 Papular acrodermatitis of childhood (Gianotti-Crosti disease). This is the term used to describe a distinctive erythematous, discrete papular eruption that is acrally located with relative sparing of the trunk. Associated findings may include lymphadenopathy, hepatomegaly, and evidence of hepatitis. The disease may be caused by a number of different viruses including hepatitis B, hepatitis A, Epstein-Barr virus (EBV), cytomegalovirus, coxsackievirus A16, and parainfluenza virus. The child in this figure has papular acrodermatitis of childhood due to an infection with EBV. (*Courtesy of* I.J. Frieden, MD.)

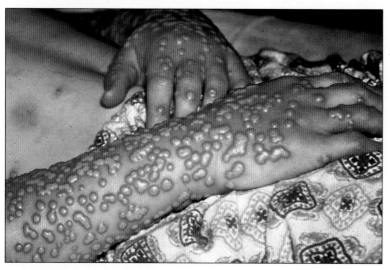

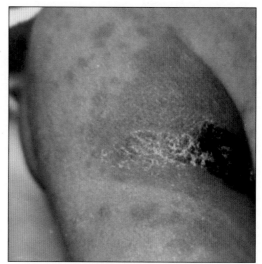

FIGURE 7-47 Vaccinia. Now that smallpox apparently has been eradicated, the need for vaccinia vaccinations is exceedingly rare. Three to 5 days after primary inoculation with vaccinia virus, a vesicle forms, followed by a pustule, which increases in size for 9–10 days and then heals leaving a scar. Severe localized erythema may occur at the injection site as seen in the figure.

FIGURE 7-46 Discrete vesiculopustular stage of smallpox. Smallpox (variola) is a highly contagious disease caused by poxvirus variolae, which apparently has been eradicated from the world. The last naturally occurring case of smallpox was in Somalia in 1977.

ACKNOWLEDGMENTS

The authors thank Cathy Moore-Daugherty for her assistance in preparing the chapter.

SELECTED BIBLIOGRAPHY

Peter G, Halsey NA, Marcuse EK, Pickering LK (eds.): *1994 Red Book: Report of the Committee on Infectious Diseases*, 23rd ed. Elk Grove Village, IL: American Academy of Pediatrics; 1994.

Feigin RD, Cherry JD (eds.): *Textbook of Pediatric Infectious Diseases*, 3rd ed. Philadelphia: W.B. Saunders Co; 1992.

Hurwitz S: *Clinical Pediatric Dermatology*, 2nd ed. Philadelphia: W.B. Saunders Co; 1993.

Lever WF, Schaumburg-Lever G: *Histopathology of the Skin*, 7th ed. Philadelphia: J.B. Lippincott Co; 1990.

Schachner LA, Hansen RC (eds.): *Pediatric Dermatology*. New York: Churchill Livingstone, Inc.; 1988.

CHAPTER 8

Ectoparasitic Diseases of the Skin

Milan Trpis

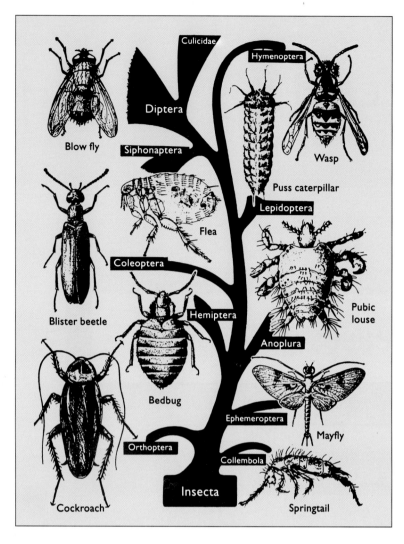

FIGURE 8-1 Evolutionary tree of some medically important insects. Cockroaches (Orthoptera) are mechanical vectors of pathogenic viruses and bacteria and biologic vectors of parasitic helminths. Mayflies (Ephemeroptera) may cause seasonal allergic reactions to exuviae. Bedbugs (Hemiptera) are unpleasant blood-suckers but are seldom vectors of any pathogens. Beetles (Coleoptera) of the family Cantharidae, when disturbed, release hemolymph, which causes blisters upon contact with human skin. Some butterflies (Lepidoptera), in their caterpillar stage, may cause skin irritation by releasing toxins from fragments of urticarial hairs. Fleas (Siphonaptera) are vectors of plague-causing bacteria (*Yersinia pestis*) and murine typhus (*Rickettsia typhi*). Flies (Diptera) cause various forms of myiasis, which is invasion of human tissue by fly maggots. Bees, wasps, hornets, and bumblebees (Hymenoptera) introduce venom to the human body by stings. (*From* Patton WS, Evans AM: *Insects, Ticks, Mites, and Venomous Animals of Medical and Veterinary Importance.* Croydon: H.R. Grubb, Ltd.; 1929; with permission.)

SKIN PATHOLOGY RELATED TO CERATOPOGONIDS AND PHLEBOTOMIDS

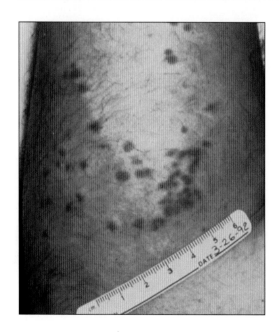

FIGURE 8-2 Severe reaction to bites of the sand fly *Phlebotomus longipalpis*. The rash may persist for several weeks. Phlebotomids are also vectors of cutaneous or visceral leishmaniasis. (*Courtesy* of F. Neva, MD.)

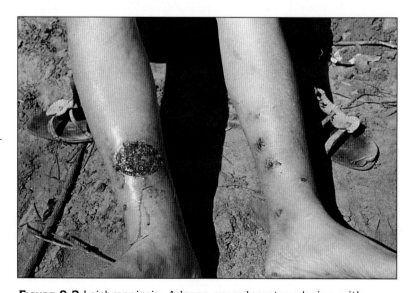

FIGURE 8-3 Leishmaniasis. A large granulomatous lesion with rolled or rigid borders, typical of cutaneous leishmaniasis caused by *Leishmania braziliensis* in high and dry western slopes of the Andes Mountains. Dogs are the reservoir animals for *L. braziliensis*. (*From* Murdoch WP, Hayneman D: Epidemiology of Leishmaniasis. *In* Tipton VJ (ed.): *Medical Entomology.* Salt Lake City: Entomological Society of America and Brigham Young University; 1970:215–230; with permission.)

TRUE BUGS AND SKIN INJURY

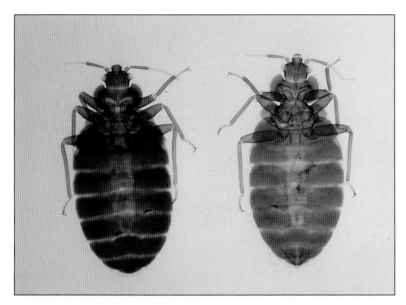

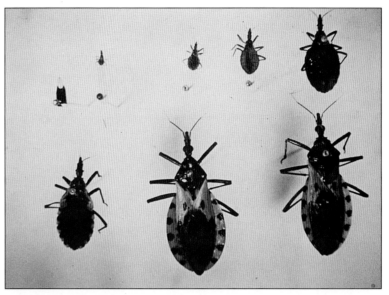

FIGURE 8-4 Bedbugs. *Cimex lectularius* are distributed in the temperate zone and *Cimex heteropterus* in the tropics. Bedbugs are vicious biters that feed on people during the night. Despite frequent feeding on people, they are not known to be vectors of human pathogens. However, some pathogens, such as hepatitis virus, have been transmitted experimentally in the laboratory.

FIGURE 8-5 Developmental stages of triatomid bugs. This type of development, called hemimetabolous, consists of gradual metamorphosis (from egg, to nymph, to adult). Insects of all developmental stages are parasitic and voracious, ingesting large amounts of blood. Feeding usually occurs during the night. When a vertebrate host is not available, triatomid bugs can endure starvation for several months. (*From* Zeledon R: American Trypanosomiasis. *In* Tipton VJ (ed.): *Medical Entomology.* Salt Lake City: Entomological Society of America and Brigham Young University; 1970: 193–200; with permission.)

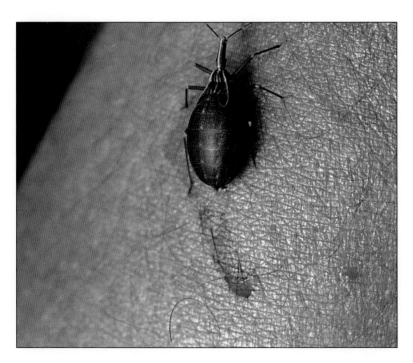

FIGURE 8-6 Triatomid bugs are the vectors of *Trypanosoma cruzi*, the etiologic agent of Chagas' disease in humans. The crithidial forms of this pathogen are transmitted when the insect defecates during feeding, as shown here. The pathogens are introduced into the human body in bug feces rubbed into excoriated skin, mucosa of the eye, or injured skin after feeding. (*Courtesy of* The Pan American Health Organization.)

INSECT VENOMS

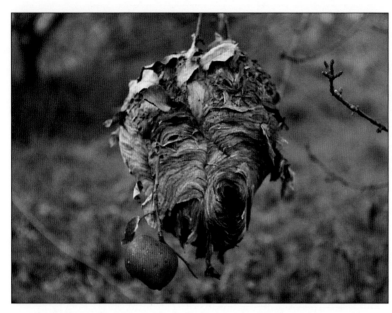

FIGURE 8-7 Hornets' nest of *Vespa crabro*. Hornets are capable of multiple attacks by the same individual without loosing the stinger. Hornets' venom may trigger anaphylactic shock and often death in people oversensitive to venoms of Hymenoptera.

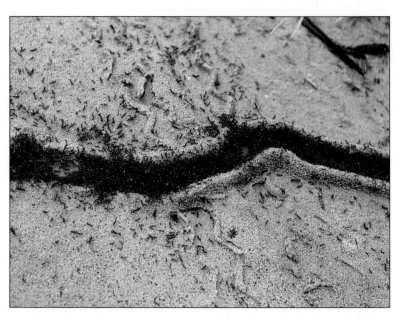

FIGURE 8-8 Safari ants. A trail of "safari ants" across a busy road during the night in western Africa. These ants do not build typical ant hills, but are always on the move, carrying their developing offspring, attacking prey, and feeding on the move. Most safari ants stay in the grooved trail, but up to 1 m from the trail are soldiers with large mandibles, which protect the moving colony. Soldier ants are very aggressive. When they attack intruders, they cut the skin with their large, strong jaws and spray the wound with myrmic acid, causing a painful burning sensation and rash that lasts several hours.

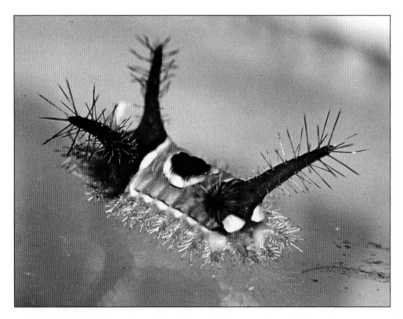

FIGURE 8-9 A bizarre caterpillar with hollow urticarial bristles filled with venom. Urticarial hairs and bristles are brittle and often break when they penetrate human skin, releasing venom from the fragments. These structures do not exist in adult butterflies. (*From* Scott HG: Envenomization. *In* Tipton VJ (ed.): *Medical Entomology*. Salt Lake City: Entomological Society of America and Brigham Young University; 1970:257–269; with permission.)

MITES AND TICKS

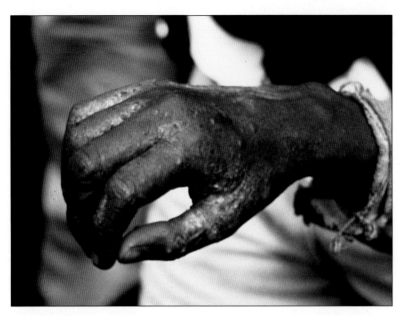

FIGURE 8-10 The hand of a person infested with the scab mite *Sarcoptes scabiei*. Female mites burrow in the skin, make corridors in the upper layer of the skin, and feed on dermal tissue and oozing lymph. Mating takes place on the skin. Inseminated females make new corridors as they burrow into the skin and lay their eggs there. Lymph oozing from injured skin forms scabs that grow progressively thicker. To remove the scabies condition, mites must be removed from infested areas by treatment with acaricides.

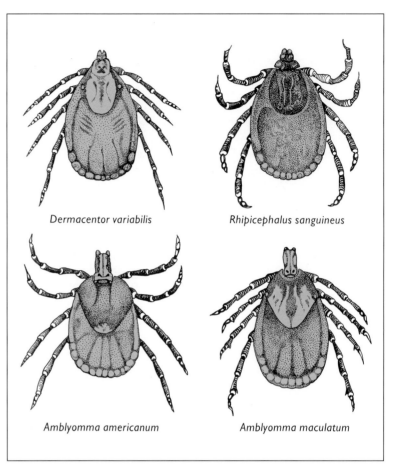

Dermacentor variabilis

Rhipicephalus sanguineus

Amblyomma americanum

Amblyomma maculatum

FIGURE 8-11 Hard ticks of three genera: *Dermacentor*, *Rhipicephalus*, and *Amblyomma*. Attachment and feeding by ticks takes several hours. Depending on a developmental stage (larva, nymph, adult) and the species, ticks may molt several times within larval or nymph developmental stages. Ticks may transmit to humans rickettsial pathogens such as *Rickettsia rickettsii*, the etiologic agent of Rocky Mountain spotted fever, and *Borrelia burgdorferi*, the causative agent of Lyme disease transmitted by the *Ixodes scapularis* tick. Ticks may cause conditions called "tick paralysis," a reaction to tick saliva released into the body during feeding. To relieve the condition, ticks must be removed from attachment to human skin. (*From* Tipton VJ: Scrub Typhus. *In* Tipton VJ (ed.): *Medical Entomology*. Salt Lake City: Entomological Society of America and Brigham Young University; 1970:133–140; with permission.)

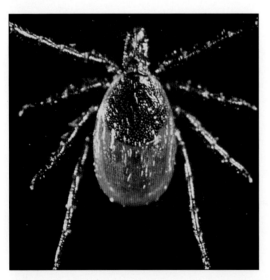

FIGURE 8-12 *Ixodes scapularis*, a hard tick that feeds on wild animals and humans. *I. scapularis* is the principal vector of *Borrelia burgdorferi*, the pathogen that is responsible for a complex disease condition called Lyme disease. (*Courtesy of* Northwest Infectious Diseases Consultants.)

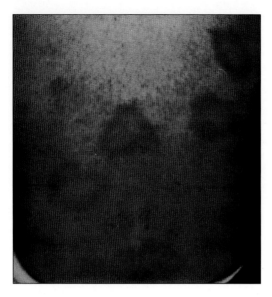

FIGURE 8-13 Lyme disease erythema migrans. Several organs and conditions may be involved in manifestations of Lyme disease: neurologic, ocular, cardiovascular, respiratory, liver, spleen, gastrointestinal, urinary, skin, and muscles. Single or multiple erythema migrans may occur and last for weeks to months. Symptoms vary greatly. Other vectors of Lyme disease are dog ticks *Dermacentor andersoni* (both males and females) and the lone star tick *Amblyomma americanum* (nymphs, females, and males). (*Courtesy of* B. Berger, MD.)

SPIDERS AND SKIN NECROSES

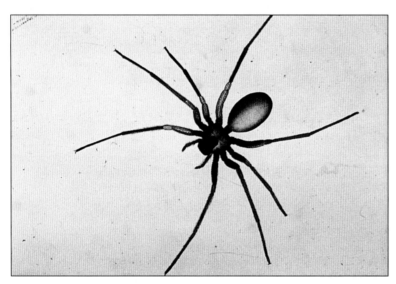

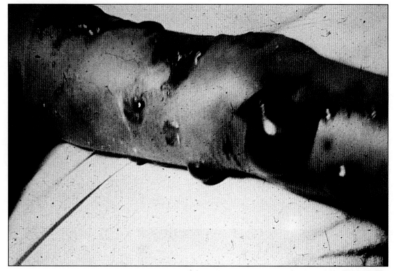

FIGURE 8-14 Brown recluse spider *Loxosceles reclusa*. Also known as the violin spider due to the dark violin-shaped spot on its cephalothorax, the brown recluse spider is a nocturnal spider and bites people when it is disturbed. It can be found both outdoors and indoors. The brown recluse spider introduces venom into the human body, which then remains local or spreads systemically. The reaction to spider venom is a small blister (2–6 hrs after the bite), which grows in size and may spread to the surrounding skin tissue. The endothelial damage results in necrosis by formation of microthrombic aggregates of leukocytes and platelets in small vessels. (*From* Scott HG: Envenomization. *In* Tipton VJ (ed.): *Medical Entomology*. Salt Lake City: Entomological Society of America and Brigham Young University; 1970:257–269; with permission.)

FIGURE 8-15 Multiple necroses on the arm caused by bites of the recluse spider, *L. reclusa*. The bites are not painful and usually unnoticeable. However, after 2–6 hrs, a blue-white circle is formed at the site of the bite, which changes into a blister that becomes red and later black. The affected area becomes necrotic, and dermal and subdermal tissue are destroyed. Regeneration of the necrotic tissue is limited and often needs surgical repair by skin grafting. (*From* Scott HG: Envenomization. *In* Tipton VJ (ed.): *Medical Entomology*. Salt Lake City: Entomological Society of America and Brigham Young University; 1970:257–269; with permission.)

DERMAL MYIASIS

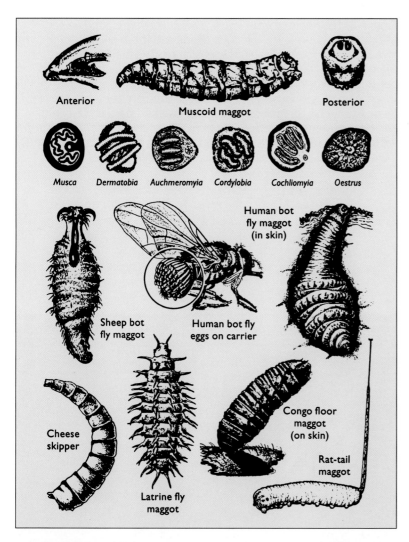

FIGURE 8-16 Maggots of different fly species causing myiasis. Myiasis is invasion of human tissue by larvae of the higher flies, such as Muscidae, Calliphoridae, Gastrophillidae, and other families. The *top row* shows the morphology of the anterior and posterior ends of a fly maggot. The *second row* shows the types of stigmal plates used in species identification. The *third row* illustrates the sheep bot fly maggot, *Oestrus ovis*, that affects the nasal cavity. Eggs of the human bot fly, *Dermatobia hominis*, attached by a female *D. hominis* to a nonbiting fly carrier. When the carrier fly or mosquito lands on a human or animal, the larvae hatch and penetrate the victim's skin. The *bottom row* shows the cheese skipper, *Piophila casei*, an agent of enteric myiasis; latrine fly maggot; Congo floor maggot, *Auchmeromyia luteola*; and rat-tail maggot *Eristalis tenax*. (*From* Patton WS, Evans AM: *Insects, Ticks, Mites, and Venomous Animals of Medical and Veterinary Importance*. Croydon: H.R. Grubb, Ltd.; 1929; with permission.)

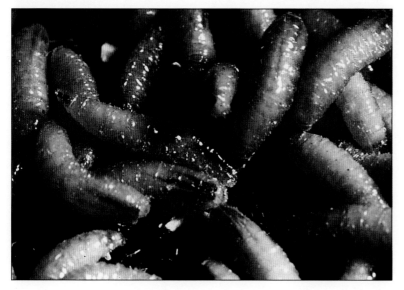

FIGURE 8-17 Screw worm maggots. Maggots of the screw worm fly, *Cochliomyia hominivorax*, which can produce myiasis in humans, are here produced in the laboratory for a genetic control. Males are irradiated to induce sterility and then released in the field into the natural population of *C. hominivorax*. Females are inseminated by sterile males but produce no offspring. (*From* Crystal MM: Veterinary entomology: Screwworms, blowflies, and myiasis. *In* Tipton VJ (ed.): *Medical Entomology*. Salt Lake City: Entomological Society of America and Brigham Young University; 1970:319–324; with permission.)

HUMAN LICE AND SKIN PATHOLOGY

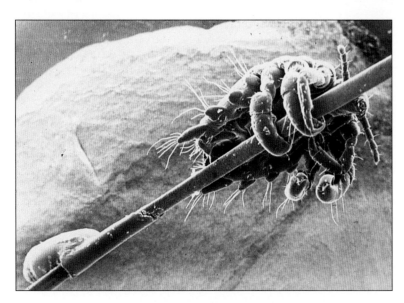

FIGURE 8-18 Pubic or crab louse, *Phthirus pubis* L., and an egg (nit) attached to a hair. The body shape and its strong grasping legs give the pubic louse a crablike appearance. The public louse prefers the pubic area, where it finds suitable temperature and humidity, but it may occasionally be found on a moustache or eyebrows. Infestation of new hosts occurs through intimate contacts. Development from a nit to an adult takes 2–3 weeks, and the lifespan of adult lice averages 3 weeks. The pubic louse is not an important vector of any louse-borne diseases transmitted by the human body louse or head louse. The pubic louse feeds several times a day.

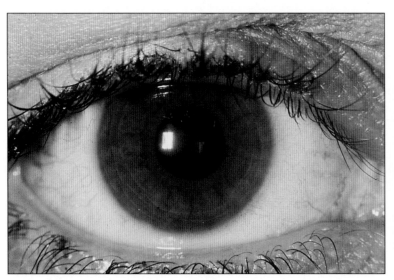

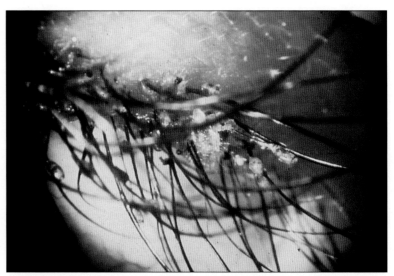

FIGURE 8-19 Heavy infestation of a woman's eye lashes with pubic lice, acquired most probably during sexual activity. Redness of the eyelids results from lice feeding. Infestation occasionally spreads to eyebrows.

FIGURE 8-20 A detail of an eye infestation with pubic lice. *Phthirus pubis* lice are attached near the base of eye lashes.

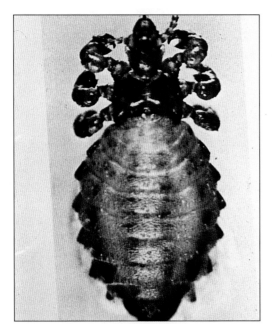

FIGURE 8-21 Human body louse, *Pediculus humanus*. The human body louse is morphologically indistinguishable from the head louse *Pediculus capitis* De Geer. However, these two species are separated on the human body by different niche selection. Only the body louse causes a skin crust (impetigo) resulting in the vagabond's disease. The body louse is also an efficient vector of louse-borne (epidemic) typhus caused by *Rickettsia prowazekii*, trench fever caused by *Rochalimaea quintana*, and epidemic relapsing fever caused by *Borrelia recurrentis*. (*From* Felsenfeld O: Relapsing Fever. *In* Tipton VJ (ed.): *Medical Entomology*. Salt Lake City: Entomological Society of America and Brigham Young University; 1970:167–174; with permission.)

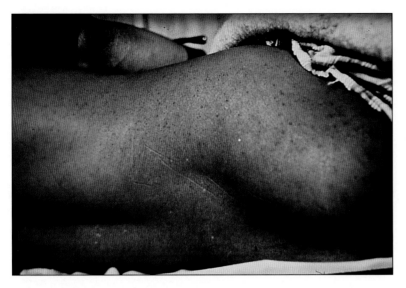

FIGURE 8-22 Skin rash of louse-borne typhus. A typical macular skin rash results from infection with *R. prowazekii*, the etiologic agent of epidemic louse-borne typhus. The rash becomes apparent first on the trunk and later spreads over the whole body. (*Courtesy of* L.L. Shold, MD.)

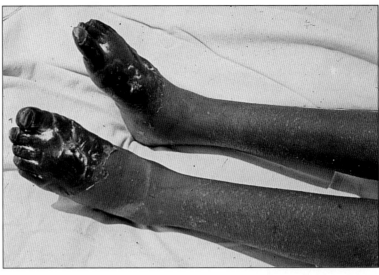

FIGURE 8-23 Gangrene of the toes after infection with epidemic louse-borne typhus. Similar gangrene manifestations may occur on the feet, fingertips, ear lobes, nose, penis, scrotum, or vulva. (*Courtesy of* L.L. Shold, MD.)

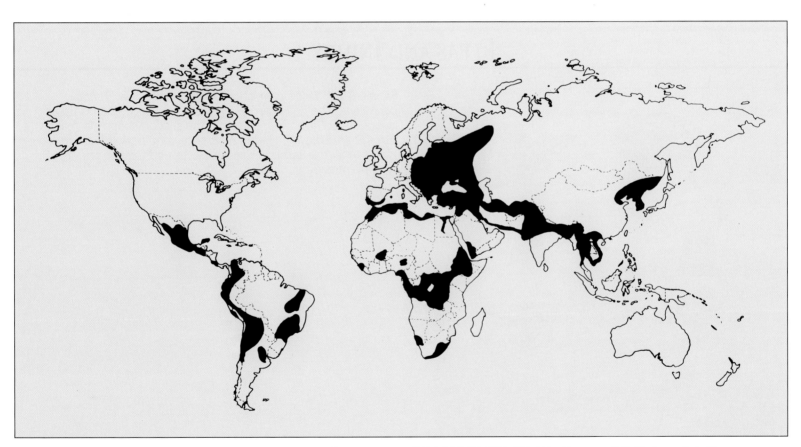

FIGURE 8-24 World distribution of louse-borne typhus fever. (*From Handbook of Diseases of Military Importance*. Publ no. DST-1810H-001-82. Washington, DC: Defense Intelligence Agency; 1982; with permission.)

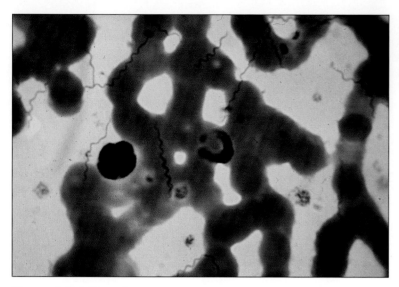

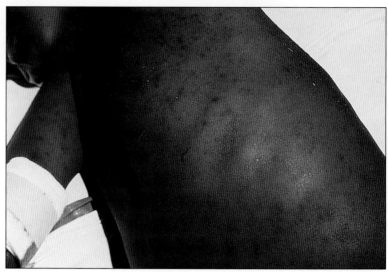

FIGURE 8-25 *Borrelia recurrentis* in a blood smear. Relapsing fever spirochetes of the genus *Borrelia* are transmitted by lice to humans worldwide, with the exception of New Zealand, Australia, and Oceania. Outbreaks are sporadic.

FIGURE 8-26 Rash from infection with louse-borne *B. recurrentis.* Epidemic relapsing fever transmitted by lice has a clinical picture similar to endemic relapsing fever transmitted by ticks. The fever, which may reach 41° C, may alter with chills, vertigo, cephalgia, myalgia, excessive sweating, and vomiting. Erythema and jaundice of varying degrees may be observed.

FLEAS AND INJURY

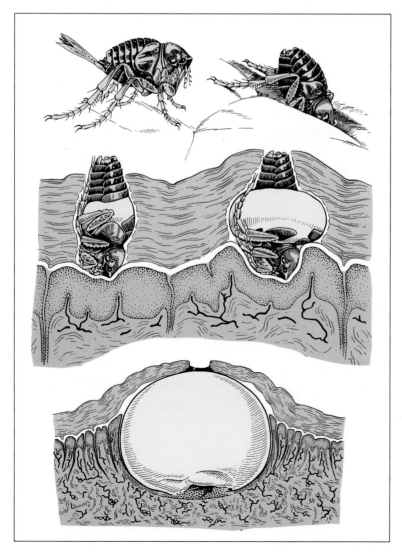

FIGURE 8-27 Skin penetration by the chigoe flea, *Tunga penetrans.* The flea burrows to reach the subcutaneous tissue layers, where it positions itself in the subcutaneous, dermal tissue. (*From* Geigy R, Herbig A: *Erreger und Überträger tropischer Krankenheiten.* Basel: Verlag für Recht und Geselschaft; 1955; with permission.)

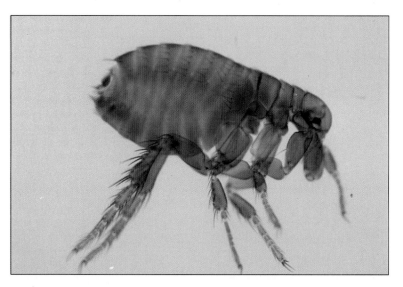

FIGURE 8-28 The Oriental rat flea, *Xenopsylla cheopis* (female). This is a cosmopolitan flea, occurring everywhere *Rattus norvegicus* is found except in northern latitudes, where the flea is scarce or absent. It has been responsible for spreading plague from harbor rats to ground squirrels in San Francisco, California. It has been a vector of endemic or murine typhus caused by *Rickettsia typhi*.

BLACK FLIES AND ONCHOCERCIASIS

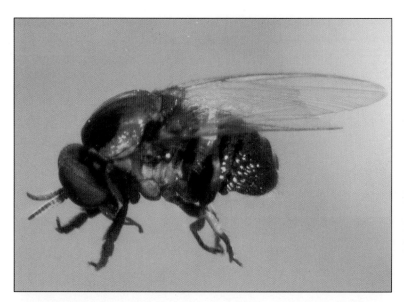

FIGURE 8-29 Black flies *Simulium yahense*, the vector for human onchocerciasis. These flies are vicious biters and blood suckers in West African countries. Black fly larvae and pupae live in fast-flowing African and Central American rivers, from which adult fly males and females emerge. *Simulium* flies are intermediate hosts of *Onchocerca volvulus*. They support the development of *O. volvulus* through three larval stages and then transmit the third larval stage (infective larvae) to humans.

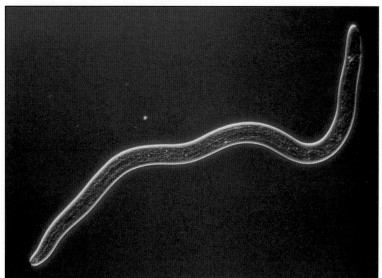

FIGURE 8-30 Infective larvae of *Onchocerca volvulus*. The third larval stage (L_3), infective larvae, are transmitted to humans by black fly bites. The disease caused by *O. volvulus* is called "onchocerciasis" or "river blindness."

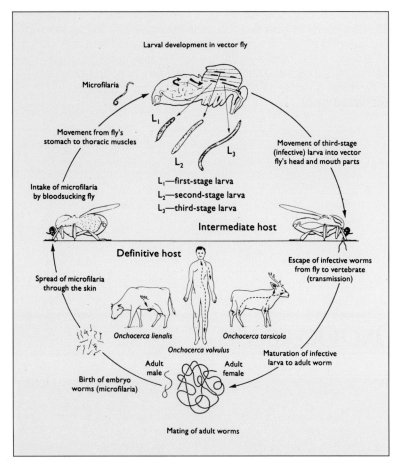

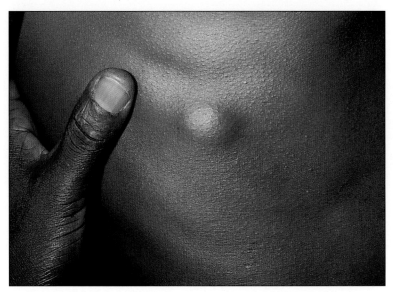

FIGURE 8-32 Onchocerciasis nodule. *Onchocerca* nodule on the trunk of a male from Sierra Leone. Several males and females of *O. volvulus* live in one nodule. Females produce hundreds of embryos daily. The embryos free themselves from shells and penetrate the ectodermal tissue, and many may remain trapped in the eye, where they eventually die.

FIGURE 8-31 Developmental cycle of *Onchocerca* species in black fly vectors and transmitted to human or animal hosts. Different *Onchocerca* species are highly host-specific in both simulids (larval stages) and mammalian hosts (adult male and females). (*Courtesy of* the World Health Organization.)

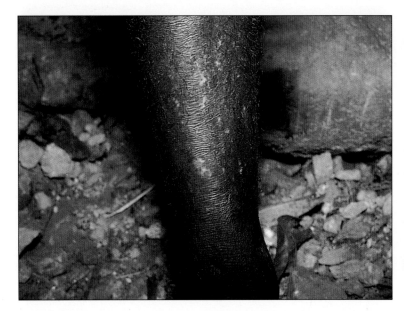

FIGURE 8-33 Onchoceriasis skin depigmentation. Depigmentation of skin (leopard skin) on an onchocercal patient. The skin loses its elasticity and has a scaly appearance. The dead filarial bodies cause itching.

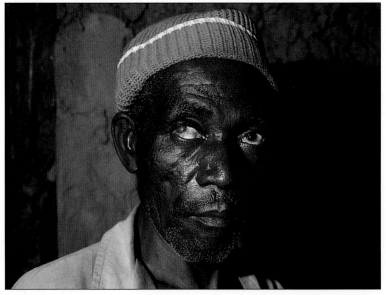

FIGURE 8-34 Onchocerciasis. This man is completely blind in the right eye and has blurry vision in the left eye. River blindness is a progressive chronic disease. The eye damage is irreversible even after removal of adult worms and microfilariae from the tissues.

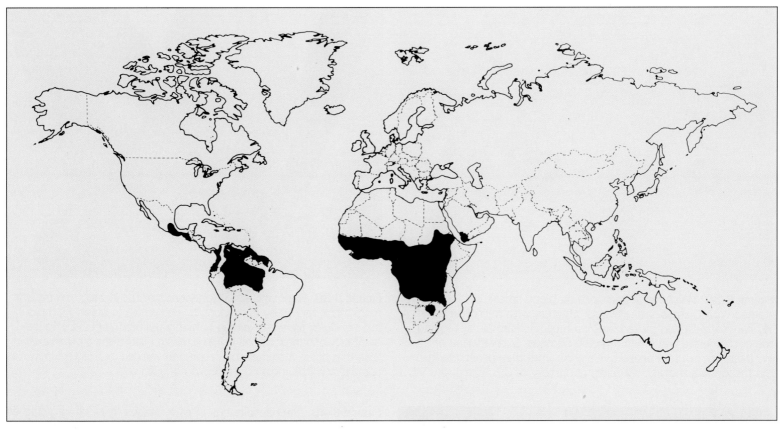

FIGURE 8-35 Worldwide distribution of onchocerciasis. (*From Handbook of Diseases of Military Importance.* Publ no. DST- 1810H-001-82. Washington, DC: Defense Intelligence Agency; 1982; with permission.)

MOSQUITOES: ALLERGY TO BITES AND TRANSMISSION OF FILARIASIS

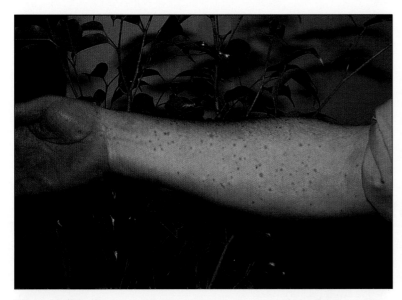

FIGURE 8-36 Rash on the forearm developed within 24 hrs after multiple bites by *Culex pipiens* mosquitoes. This condition is caused by saliva from the female insect introduced into the human tissues in the process of feeding.

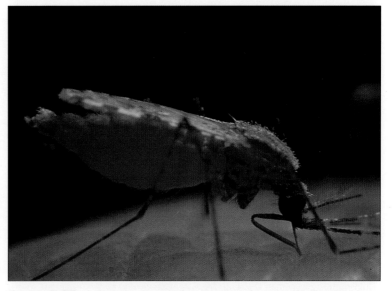

FIGURE 8-37 A female *Anopheles stephensi* mosquito feeding on a human host. *Anopheles*, *Culex*, and *Mansonia* mosquito females may transmit lymphatic filariasis, a disease caused by filarial worms *Wuchereria bancrofti* and *Brugia malayi* in humans, *Brugia pahangi* in cats, and *Dirofilaria immitis* (heartworm) in dogs. (*Courtesy of* R. Noonan, MD.)

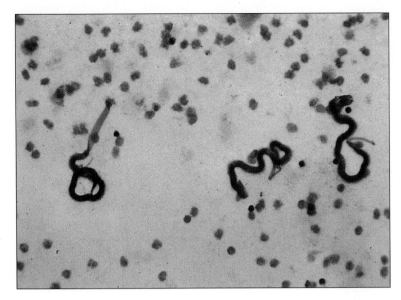

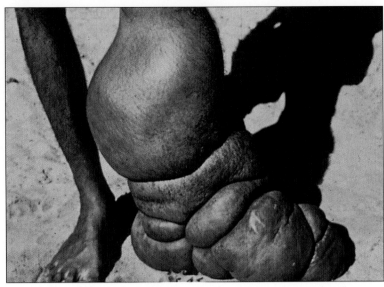

FIGURE 8-38 *Wuchereria bancrofti* on blood smear. A blood smear stained with Giemsa stain reveals infection with microfilariae of *W. bancrofti*. Unless picked up by a mosquito female at feeding, the microfilariae will die in infected humans. Microfilariae of *W. bancrofti* are in a protective sheath until they penetrate into the mosquito's thoracic muscles. (*Courtesy of* G.B. Craig, Jr, MD.)

FIGURE 8-39 Elephantiasis. Elephantiasis of the left leg of a patient from India, caused by *W. bancrofti*. The vector in urban filariasis in India is *Culex pipiens* breeding in highly polluted water. Disfigurement of elephantoid limbs is irreversible. Filariasis is a chronic disease that poses a tremendous economic burden in affected countries. (*Courtesy of* the Indian Commission on Filariasis.)

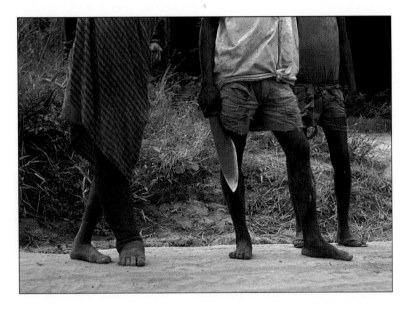

FIGURE 8-40 Elephantoid legs in early stages. A random group of men infected with human *W. bancrofti* in southern coastal area of Tanzania. There, the primary vector is *Culex pipiens* breeding in pit latrines.

SELECTED BIBLIOGRAPHY

Acha PN, Szyfres B: *Zoonoses and Communicable Diseases Common to Man and Animals*, 2nd ed. Scientific Publ no. 503. Washington, DC: Pan American Health Organization; 1987.

Goldsmith R, Heyneman D (eds.): *Tropical Medicine and Parasitology*. Norwalk, CT: Appleton & Lange; 1989.

Hoeprich PD, Hordan MC (eds.): *Infectious Diseases*, 4th ed. Philadelphia: J.B. Lippincott Co.; 1992.

Woods GL, Gutierrez Y: *Diagnostic Pathology of Infectious Diseases*. Malvern, PA: Lea & Febiger; 1993.

CHAPTER 9

Cutaneous Manifestations of Rickettsial Infections

Theodore E. Woodward
Daniel J. Sexton
David H. Walker

SPOTTED FEVER GROUP RICKETTSIOSES

Rocky Mountain Spotted Fever

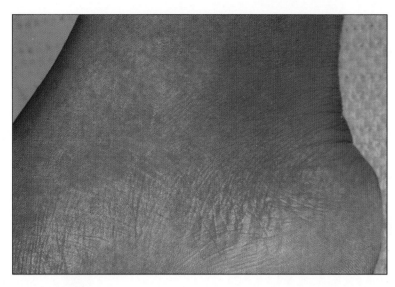

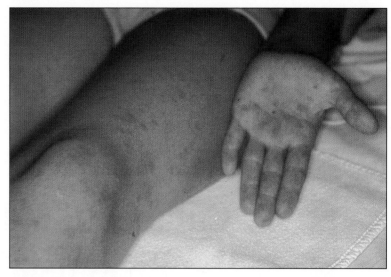

FIGURE 9-1 Rocky Mountain spotted fever, the prototype and most severe rickettsiosis, usually manifests a rash, which appears first as blanchable macules on the wrists and ankles on day 3–5 of illness. This patient developed severe Rocky Mountain spotted fever with long-term neurologic sequelae, yet his skin rash was confined to a small patch on one ankle. A biopsy specimen of this rash disclosed *Rickettsia rickettsii* in blood vessels, and his illness was confirmed serologically. Occasionally, patients with severe Rocky Mountain spotted fever will develop a skin rash late in their illness or, in 10% of cases, not at all. (Kaplowitz LG, Fischer JJ, Sparling PF: Rocky Mountain spotted fever: A clinical dilemma. *Curr Clin Top Infect Dis* 1981, 2:89–108.) These cases of "Rocky Mountain *spotless* fever" may be extremely difficult to diagnose unless a high index of clinical suspicion is present.

FIGURE 9-2 The characteristic pink macular rash of Rocky Mountain spotted fever on the palm and leg as seen in this 5-year-old girl fades on pressure and is accentuated by a warm compress. Her illness was associated with headache, muscle pains, and elevated temperature for 3 days. The patient's illness responded rapidly to specific antirickettsial therapy. The diagnosis was confirmed by identification of *R. rickettsii* in a biopsy sample of a cutaneous lesion by immunofluorescent examination (Woodward TE, Pedersen CE Jr, Oster CN, *et al.*: Prompt confirmation of Rocky Mountain spotted fever identification of rickettsiae in skin tissues. *J Infect Dis* 1976, 134:297.) (*From* Woodward TE: Rocky Mountain spotted fever: Diagnosis and treatment. *Resid Staff Physician* 1978, 24(May):56–61; with permission.)

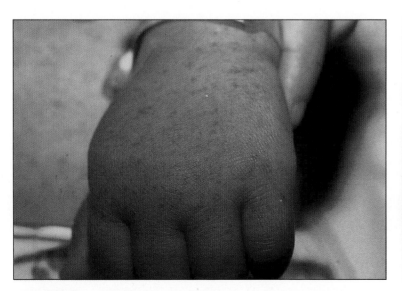

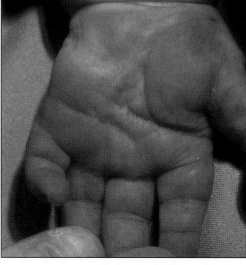

FIGURE 9-4 Palmar rash in Rocky Mountain spotted fever. The rash in Rocky Mountain spotted fever involves the palms and soles in approximately half of patients, usually appearing relatively late in the course of illness. Thus, this sign is not a reliable early diagnostic clue.

FIGURE 9-3 In addition to rash, which is petechial in this patient but may be maculopapular or purpuric, children with Rocky Mountain spotted fever frequently have edema of the face and extremities, as seen in this hand.

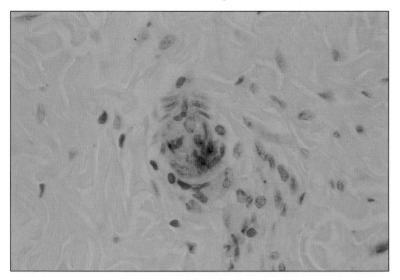

FIGURE 9-5 Immunoperoxidase stain of *R. rickettsii* in a dermal blood vessel. Early in the course of Rocky Mountain spotted fever, there is little or no host cellular response to the infection. (Dumler JS, Gage WR, Pettis GL, *et al.*: Rapid immunoperoxidase demonstration of *Rickettsia rickettsii* in fixed cutaneous specimens from patients with Rocky Mountain spotted fever. *Am J Clin Pathol* 1990, 93:410–414.)

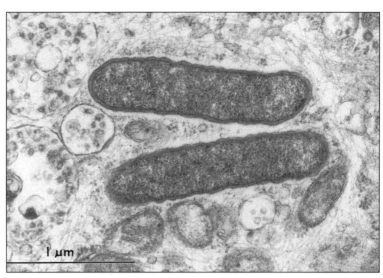

FIGURE 9-6 Electron photomicrograph of two rickettsiae in the host cell cytosol shows a thin (0.4 × 1.6 μm) bacillus with a gram-negative bacterial cell wall.

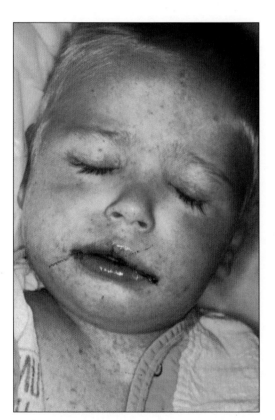

FIGURE 9-7 A 4-year-old boy with Rocky Mountain spotted fever in semicoma on the 9th day of illness. Note the swollen face, rash on the face, neck, and upper chest, and encrusted oral blood. (*Courtesy of* T.E. Woodward, MD.)

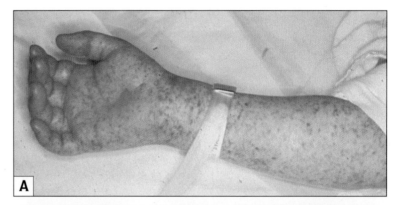

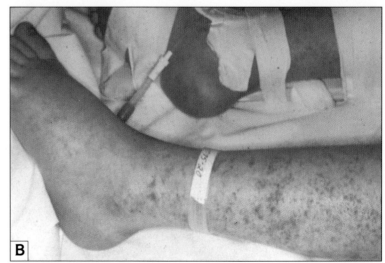

FIGURE 9-8 **A**, Small cutaneous petechiae are present on the swollen forearm and hand of this semicomatose boy. The edema resulted from increased vascular permeability and escape of fluid, electrolytes, and albumin into the extravascular space. **B**, In the same patient, late petechial lesions are seen on the leg and edematous feet. *(continued)*

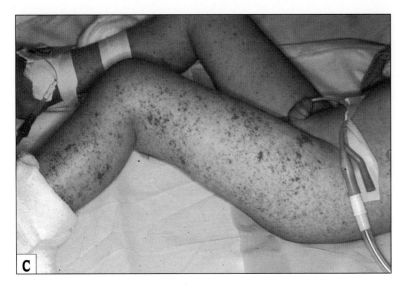

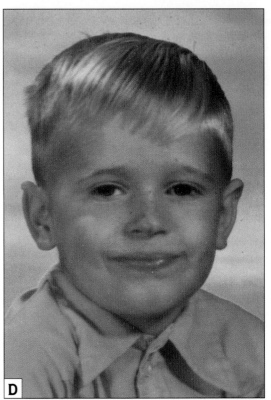

FIGURE 9-8 *(continued)* **C**, In the same patient, small and large hemorrhagic lesions are present on the legs. **D**, The same patient after recovery has resolved the edema. He suffered mild deafness for about 6 months after his recovery.

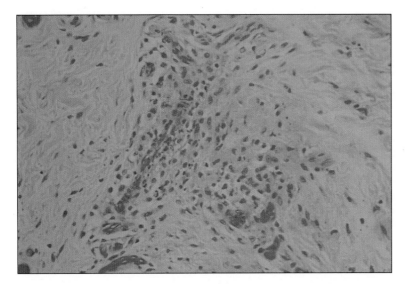

FIGURE 9-9 Vasculitis in the skin rash of Rocky Mountain spotted fever results from rickettsial infection of and injury to endothelium of dermal blood vessels, stimulating a lymphohistiocytic immune response later in the course of the infection.

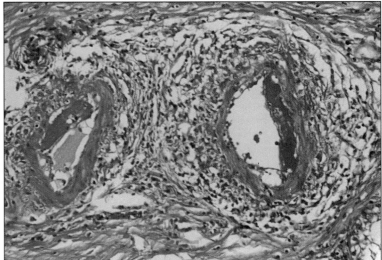

FIGURE 9-10 Late in the course of severe cases of Rocky Mountain spotted fever, there is marked vascular injury, as observed in these two blood vessels of the scrotal skin on the 10th day of illness. Fibrinoid necrosis and thrombus formation are present, and marked perivascular mononuclear infiltration typifies the late host response. (*From* Woodward TE: Clues to better understanding of the nature of certain infectious diseases. *Am J Med Sci* 1956, 231:3761; with permission.)

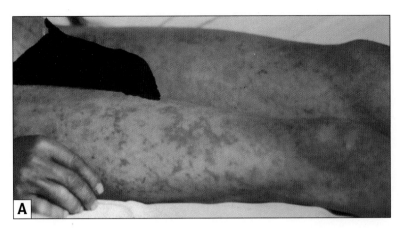

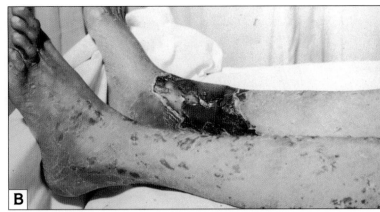

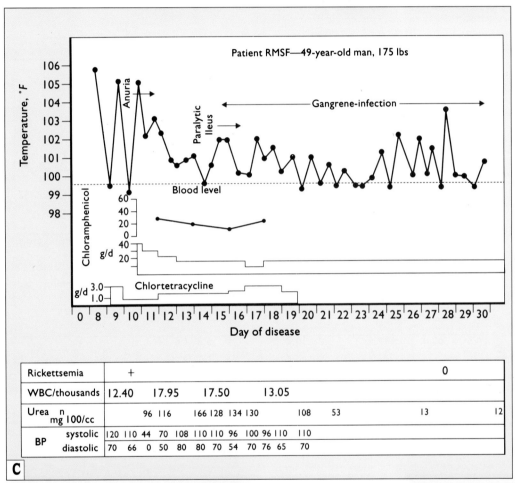

FIGURE 9-11 A, This adult male patient with an extensive cutaneous ecchymoses on the 10th day of illness was unresponsive and had muttering delirium. This type of rash is often confused with fulminant meningococcemia. **B,** The same patient at a later stage showing a large gangrenous lesion of the right ankle. He recovered fully after an extensive course of antibiotic treatment and supportive care. **C,** The temperature graph and clinical course of this patient, who walked out of the hospital. This patient suffered acute renal failure (blood urea nitrogen, 166 mg/dL) and hypotensive shock (blood pressure, 44/0 mm Hg). (Walker DH, Mattern WD: Acute renal failure in Rocky Mountain spotted fever. *Arch Intern Med* 1979, 139:443–448.)

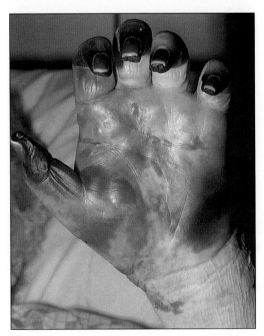

FIGURE 9-12 Digital gangrene in a patient who survived severe Rocky Mountain spotted fever. Most patients have a maculopapular skin rash with or without petechiae. However, some develop gangrene of the extremities eventually resulting in the need for amputation. (Kirkland KB, Marcom PK, Sexton DJ, *et al.*: Rocky Mountain spotted fever complicated by gangrene: Report of six cases and review. *Clin Infect Dis* 1993, 16:629–634.)

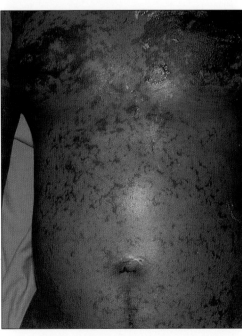

FIGURE 9-13 Cutaneous purpurea and necrosis of the late rash in a fatal case of Rocky Mountain spotted fever.

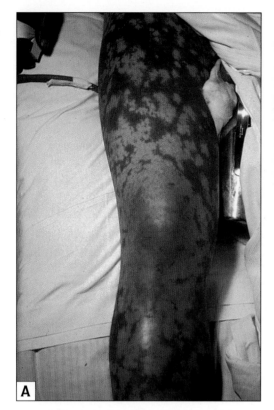

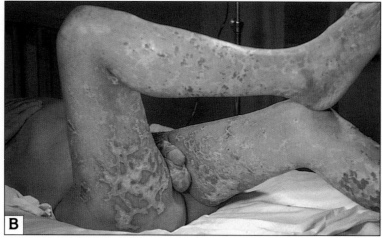

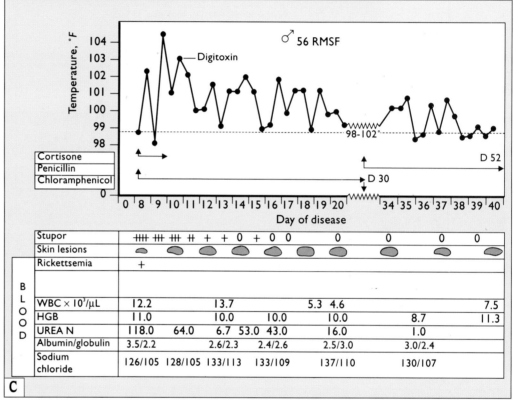

FIGURE 9-14 A, A severe ecchymotic rash was observed in a comatose patient with Rocky Mountain spotted fever on the 8th day of illness. The patient was discharged after 33 days of hospitalization. (*Courtesy of* T.E. Woodward, MD.) **B**, The same patient is shown with extensive early scars consequent to the hemorrhagic, necrotic skin lesions. **C**, Temperature graph and clinical course of the above patient with progressive large necrotic skin lesions and acute renal failure (blood urea nitrogen, 118 mg/dL). The diagnosis was confirmed by rickettsial isolation and increased specific antibody titer.

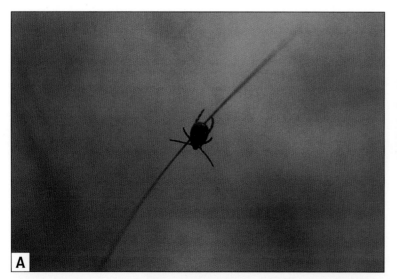

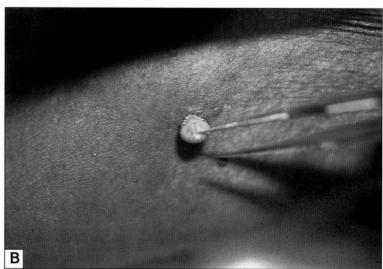

FIGURE 9-15 *Dermacentor variabilis*, the principal reservoir and vector of *R. rickettsii* in the eastern United States. The vectors of spotted fever group rickettsioses maintain rickettsiae by transo- varial transmission and transmit the infection to humans during feeding. **A**, The tick awaiting a host to provide a blood meal. **B**, An engorged female *D. variabilis* in the axilla.

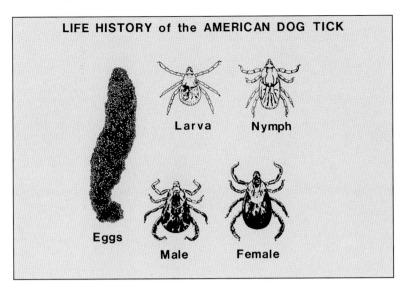

LIFE HISTORY of the AMERICAN DOG TICK

Larva Nymph

Eggs

Male Female

FIGURE 9-16 Life history of the American dog tick, *D. variabilis*. Eggs hatch into larvae, which molt into nymphs, which in turn molt into either male or female adults. Infection is maintained from stage to stage (*transstadial transmission*). Vertical transmission of infected ova from infected adult female ticks is known as *transovarial* transmission. If infected larvae, nymphs, or adult ticks take a blood meal from a rickettsemic animal, the ticks will remain infected throughout this life cycle. (Burgdorfer W: Ecological and epidemiological considerations of Rocky Mountain spotted fever and scrub typhus. *In* Walker DH (ed.): *Biology of Rickettsial Diseases*. Boca Raton, FL: CRC Press; 1988:33–50.)

Primary Lesions at Portal of Infection

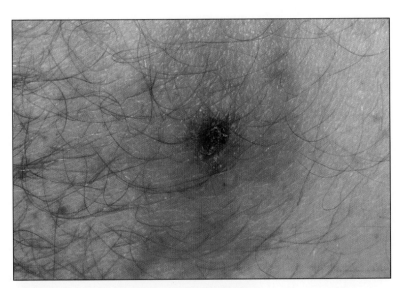

FIGURE 9-17 Many rickettsial diseases, including boutonneuse fever, rickettsialpox, North Asian tick typhus, Oriental spotted fever, Queensland tick typhus, and scrub typhus, frequently have an *eschar*, focal necrosis of the epidermis and dermis, at the site of inoculation of rickettsiae by the tick or mite bite. This eschar, or tâche noire of boutonneuse fever, is surrounded by an erythematous halo owing to vasodilation. (Walker DH, Occhino C, Tringali GR, *et al.*: Pathogenesis of rickettsial eschars: The tâche noire of boutonneuse fever. *Hum Pathol* 1988, 19:1449–1454.)

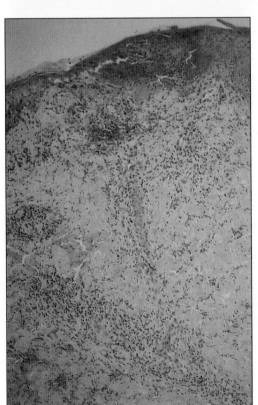

FIGURE 9-18 The microscopic appearance of an eschar in boutonneuse fever consists of epidermal necrosis accompanied by a prominent perivascular lymphohistiocytic infiltrate. Cytokines from these cells, particularly interferon-γ and tumor necrosis factor-α, stimulate intraendothelial synthesis of rickettsicidal nitric oxide. (Feng H-M, Walker DH: Interferon-γ and tumor necrosis factor-α exert their antirickettsial effect via induction of synthesis of nitric oxide. *Am J Pathol* 1993, 143:1016–1023.)

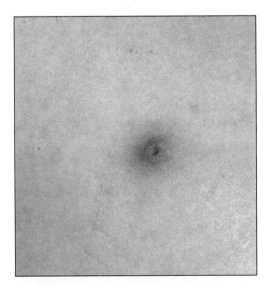

FIGURE 9-19 Small primary lesions develop at the site of tick attachment in a small proportion of patients with Rocky Mountain spotted fever, and rarely a fully developed eschar occurs.

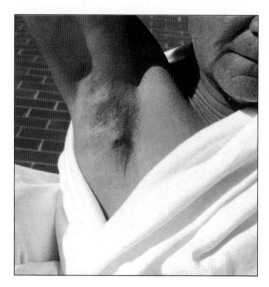

FIGURE 9-20 The primary lesion in a patient with boutonneuse fever is an encrusted lesion that developed at the site of tick attachment. Axillary lymphadenopathy presumably represents the response to the initial regional lymphatic spread of rickettsiae.

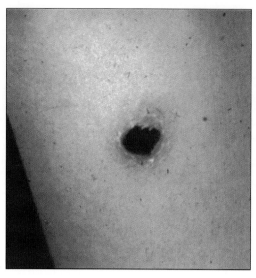

FIGURE 9-21 A typical encrusted primary lesion was seen at site of mite attachment in a patient with rickettsialpox. (*Courtesy of* H. Rose, MD.) (Brettman LR, Lewin S, Holzman RS, *et al.*: Rickettsialpox: Report of an outbreak and a contemporary review. *Medicine* 1981, 60:363–372.)

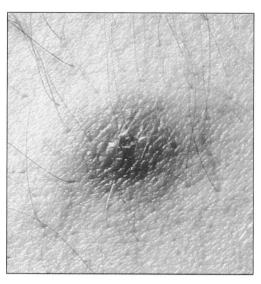

FIGURE 9-22 This typical early lesion develops into the eschar of scrub typhus. This lesion was present at the onset of illness prior to the appearance of a rash. (*Courtesy of* USA Typhus Mission to Kuala Lumpur Malaysia, 1948.)

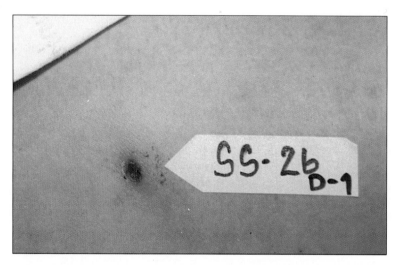

FIGURE 9-23 A fully developed eschar seen in a patient with scrub typhus. (Brown G: Scrub typhus: Pathogenesis and clinical syndrome. *In* Walker DH (ed.): *Biology of Rickettsial Diseases*. Boca Raton, FL: CRC Press; 1988:93–100.) (*Courtesy of* G. Watt, MD.)

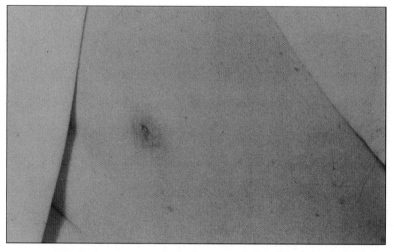

FIGURE 9-24 Several other infectious diseases have a lesion at the portal of entry resembling a rickettsial disease eschar. This primary lesion (eschar) was present on the abdominal wall of a patient with tick-transmitted tularemia. The eschar developed at the site of tick attachment. Inguinal lymphadenopathy was present. There was no rash. The patient recovered fully with chloramphenicol treatment.

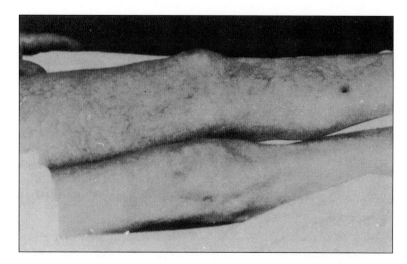

FIGURE 9-25 A small primary lesion was present on the leg at the site of an infected flea attachment in a patient with bubonic plague. (*From* Pollitzer R: *Plague*. Geneva: World Health Organization; 1954; with permission.)

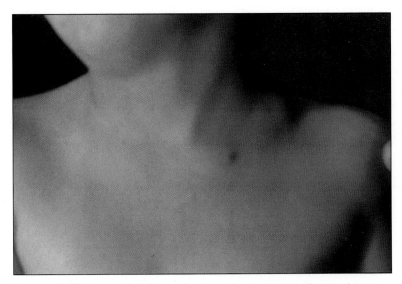

FIGURE 9-26 A small primary lesion of cat scratch disease is present at the site of a kitten scratch and is accompanied by lymphadenitis in the shoulder and neck region. There was no rash.

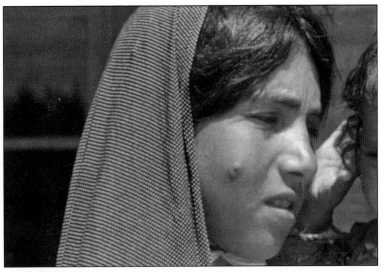

FIGURE 9-27 A cutaneous anthrax lesion on the cheek of a young Iranian woman who tended sheep, some of which died of anthrax. Large gram-positive bacilli were detected by aspiration from the periphery of the lesion.

Rash and Vectors of Other Spotted Fever Group Rickettsioses

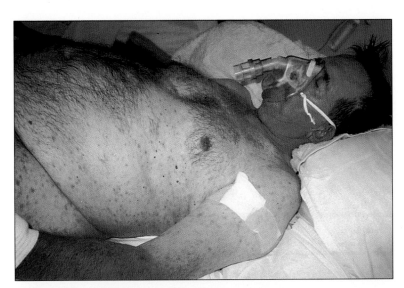

FIGURE 9-28 After the appearance of an eschar, a rash develops in most patients diagnosed with rickettsial infection. The rash of boutonneuse fever may be maculopapular with or without petechiae. Although most patients with boutonneuse fever have a relatively mild illness, severe disease resulting in multiple organ failure occasionally occurs. (*Courtesy of* M. Drancourt, MD.)

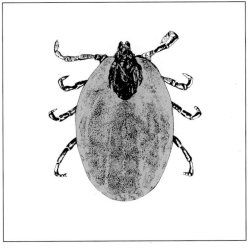

FIGURE 9-29 Female *Rhipicephalus sanguineus* (brown dog tick) is the vector of *Rickettsia conorii* (boutonneuse fever) in the Eastern Hemisphere and of *Rickettsia rickettsii* (Rocky Mountain spotted fever) in Mexico.

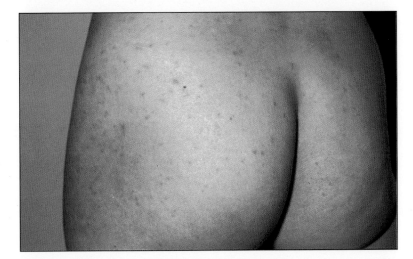

FIGURE 9-30 Maculopapules, some of which are petechial, are characteristic of rickettsial infection, as in this patient with Flinders Island spotted fever. Queensland tick typhus (QTT) and Flinders Island spotted fever are two illnesses due to the spotted fever group rickettsiae occurring in Australia. Patients with Flinders Island spotted fever and QTT typically have mild illnesses, often with an eschar at the site of tick attachment. In addition to fever and localized lymphadenopathy, maculopapular rash is seen on the trunk and extremities. (Sexton DJ, Dwyer B, Kemp R, Graves S: Spotted fever group rickettsial infections in Australia. *Rev Infect Dis* 1991, 13:876–886.)

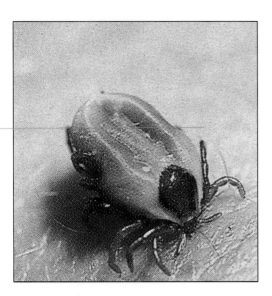

FIGURE 9-31 Mating female and male *Ixodes holocyclus*, which is a principal vector of *Rickettsia australis*, the agent of Queensland tick typhus.

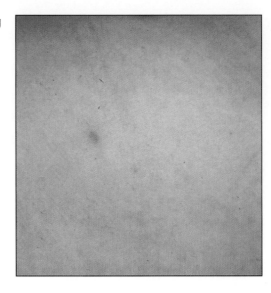

FIGURE 9-32 A maculopapular rash is seen in some patients with rickettsialpox and at some stages of the illness.

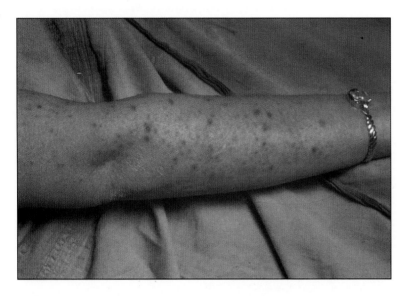

FIGURE 9-33 The rickettsialpox rash is typically vesicular but may be maculopapular. Most patients have mild illness. Rickettsialpox is caused by *Rickettsia akari*, a member of the spotted fever group that is transmitted by the gamasid mite, *Liponyssoides sanguineus*. These mites maintain the rickettsia by transovarian transmission and by horizontal transmission through mice.

TYPHUS FEVERS

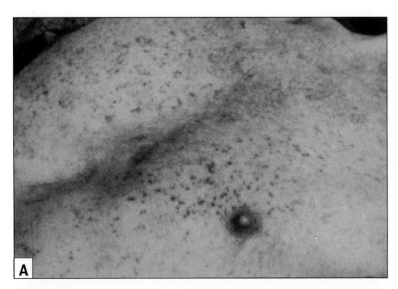

A

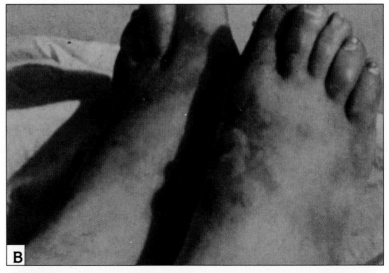

B

FIGURE 9-34 A, Typical petechial skin lesions are seen in a patient with epidemic typhus fever on the 10th day of illness. The patient died of his infection during World War II when specific antirickettsial treatment was not available. (Wolbach SB, Todd JL, Palfrey FW: Pathology of typhus in man. *In* Wolbach SB, Todd JL, Palfrey FW (eds.): *The Etiology and Pathology of Typhus.* Cambridge: League Red Cross Society, Harvard University; 1922:152–221.) **B,** The same patient with epidemic typhus fever a few days later had symmetric early gangrene of the medial aspect of the feet caused by the severe vascular injury by *Rickettsia prowazekii*.

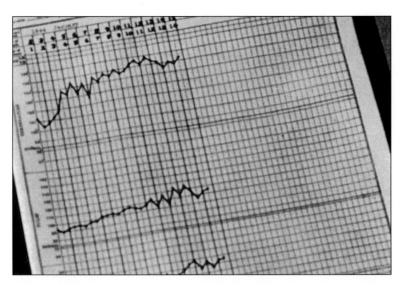

FIGURE 9-35 The characteristic temperature, heart rate, and respiratory rate curves (*top* to *bottom*) of fatal louse-borne epidemic typhus show a continuous febrile course typical of most severe rickettsioses and accelerated rates of pulse and respiration. (*Courtesy of* USA Typhus Fever Commission.)

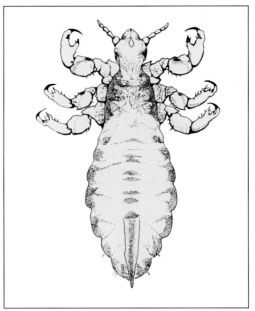

FIGURE 9-36 The human body louse, *Pediculus humanus corporis*, is the vector of classic epidemic typhus (*R. prowazekii*). The feces of infected lice contain large quantities of infectious *R. prowazekii*.

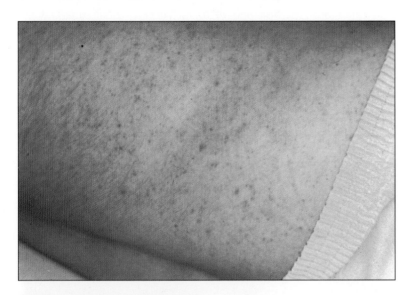

FIGURE 9-37 The typical faint, pink, macular rash of recrudescent typhus fever (Brill-Zinsser disease) was observed in a patient who was moderately ill with fever and headache. Twenty-five years earlier, he had experienced louse-borne typhus fever in Poland. The diagnosis was confirmed serologically by demonstration of IgG antibody to *R. prowazekii*.

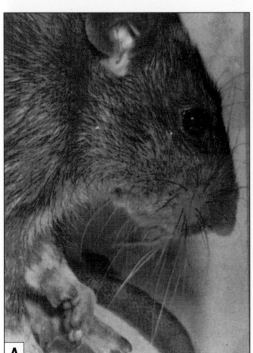

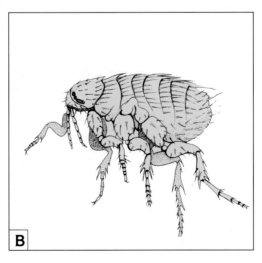

FIGURE 9-38 A similar illness is seen in patients with murine typhus. **A** and **B**, The classic natural cycle of *Rickettsia typhi* includes rats (*Rattus rattus* and *R. norvegicus*) (*panel 38A*) and the Oriental rat flea (*Xenopsylla cheopis*) (*panel 38B*).

SCRUB TYPHUS

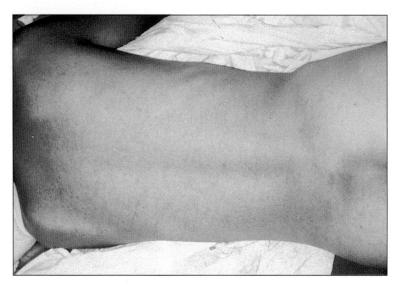

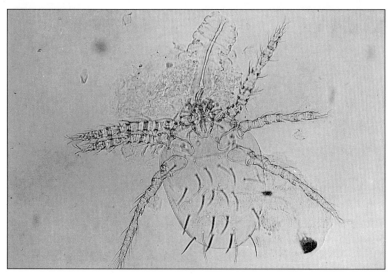

FIGURE 9-39 This patient with scrub typhus has a rash. Fewer than half of patients with scrub typhus develop a cutaneous eruption.

FIGURE 9-40 The trombiculid mite, *Leptotrombidium deliensis*, is an important reservoir and vector of *Rickettsia tsutsugamushi*, which causes scrub typhus. (Audy JR: *Red Mites and Typhus*. New York: Oxford University Press; 1968:153–160.)

EHRLICHIOSIS

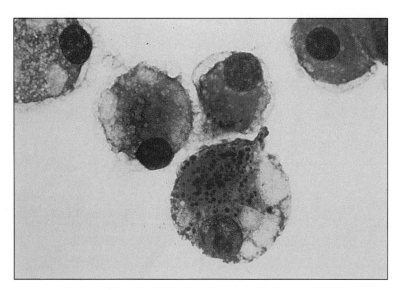

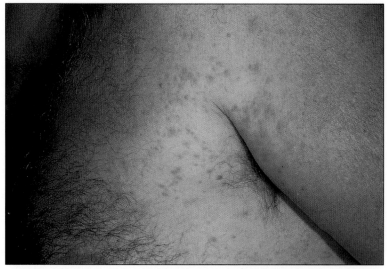

FIGURE 9-41 *Ehrlichia chaffeensis*, an obligate intracellular bacterium that parasitizes phagosomes of mononuclear phagocytes, is the cause of a newly recognized disease, ehrlichiosis. Ehrlichiae are extremely difficult to propagate *in vitro*. They have been successfully isolated in the continuous canine cell line DH-82. (Dawson JE, Anderson BE, Fishbein DB, *et al.*: Isolation and characterization of an *Ehrlichia* sp. from a patient diagnosed with human ehrlichiosis. *J Clin Microbiol* 1991, 29:2741–2745.) (*Courtesy of* J.E. Dawson, MD.)

FIGURE 9-42 Skin rash in a patient with human ehrlichiosis. Only a small percentage of patients with human ehrlichiosis have a skin rash. However, most patients have thrombocytopenia, leukopenia, elevated hepatic transaminases, fever, and a history of tick exposure. Diagnosis of a human illness due to *E. chaffeensis* is best obtained by serology or polymerase chain reaction. (Eng TR, Harkess JR, Fishbein DB, *et al.*: Epidemiologic, clinical, and laboratory findings of human ehrlichiosis in the United States, 1988. *JAMA* 1990, 264:2251–2258.) (*Courtesy of* C. Van Stecker, MD, and E.D. Everett, MD.)

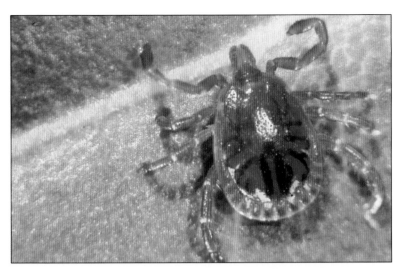

FIGURE 9-43 Lone star tick, *Amblyomma americanum*, is a vector of *E. chaffeensis* (Anderson BE, Sims KG, Olson JG, *et al.*: *Amblyomma americanum*: A potential vector of human ehrlichiosis. *Am J Trop Med Hyg* 1993, 49:239–244.)

Rickettsial diseases of humans

Disease	Etiologic agent	Transmission	Geographic distribution
Spotted fever group			
Rocky Mountain spotted fever	R. rickettsii	Tick bite	North and South America
Rickettsialpox	R. akari	Mite bite	United States, Europe, Korea
Boutonneuse fever	R. conorii	Tick bite	Mediterranean, Black Sea basin, Africa, India
North Asian tick typhus	R. sibirica	Tick bite	Asiatic Russia, China, Mongolia
Queensland tick typhus	R. australis	Tick bite	Australia
Oriental spotted fever	R. japonica	Tick bite	Japan
Typhus group			
Epidemic typhus	R. prowazekii	Louse feces	Potentially worldwide, recently in Africa, South America, Central America, Mexico, Asia
Brill-Zinsser disease	R. prowazekii	Reactivation of latent infection	Potentially worldwide, including the United States, Canada, and Eastern Europe
Flying squirrel typhus	R. prowazekii	Ectoparasite of flying squirrel	United States
Murine typhus	R. typhi	Flea feces	Worldwide
Cat flea typhus	Unnamed *Rickettsia* sp.	Flea	Texas and California
Scrub typhus group	R. tsutsugamushi	Chigger bite	Southern Asia, Japan, Western Pacific, Indonesia, Australia, Korea, Asiatic Russia, India, Sri Lanka, China
Ehrlichioses			
Human monocytic ehrlichiosis	*Ehrlichia chaffeensis*	Tick bite	United States, Europe, Africa, possibly worldwide
Human granulocyte ehrlichiosis	*Ehrlichia* sp. closely related to *E. phagocytophila*	Probable tick bite	United States
Sennetsu ehrlichiosis	*E. sennetsu*	Unknown	

FIGURE 9-44 Rickettsial disease in humans. A summary table lists key information on the etiology and distribution of the rickettsioses.

SELECTED BIBLIOGRAPHY

Walker DH (ed.): *Biology of Rickettsial Diseases*. Boca Raton, FL: CRC Press; 1988.

Hechemy KE, Paretsky D, Walker DH, Mallavia LP (eds.): Rickettsiology: Current Issues and Perspectives. *Ann N Y Acad Sci* 1990:590.

CHAPTER 10

Parasitic Diseases of the Skin and Soft Tissue

Herman Zaiman
Elaine C. Jong

LESIONS LOCALIZED TO THE SKIN AND SOFT TISSUE

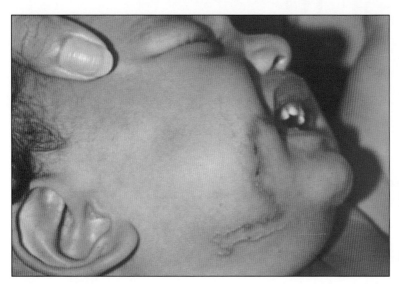

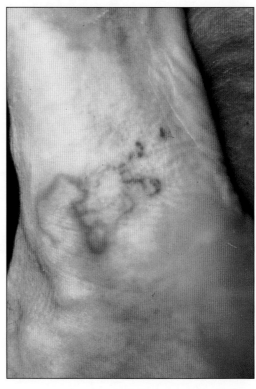

FIGURE 10-2 Cutaneous larva migrans. A typical serpiginous lesion is present on the foot of a traveler returned from the Caribbean.

FIGURE 10-1 Cutaneous larva migrans. The face of a 2-year-old boy from Venezuela is shown. This infection is acquired from direct skin contact with soil contaminated by dog or cat feces containing hookworm eggs. These develop into infective larvae that penetrate skin they contact. Such larvae are usually limited to the skin because they are in an inappropriate host. (*Courtesy of* F. Battistini, MD.)

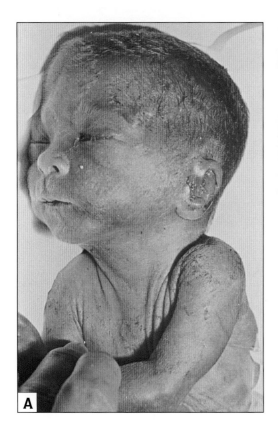

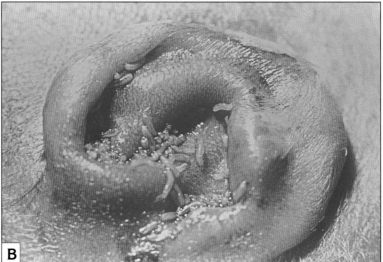

FIGURE 10-3 Cutaneous myiasis. **A**, Fly larvae are present in the ear and orbits of a newborn child in West Virginia. These were acquired during passage through the birth canal of the mother who had genital myiasis. **B**, A close-up view shows maggots in the child's ear. (*Courtesy of* J.E. Hall, PhD, and M.B. Ayoubi, MD.)

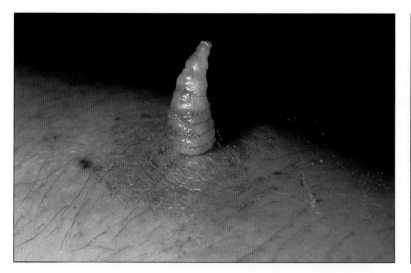

FIGURE 10-4 Cutaneous myiasis. A larva of *Dermatobia hominis* is shown emerging from the skin. Female flies of the genus *Dermatobia* use mosquitoes to transport their eggs. When such a mosquito bites, the fly eggs are deposited on the victim's skin. The larvae hatch and rapidly penetrate the skin, inciting the development of small nodule around each larva. (*Courtesy of* J. Keystone, MD.)

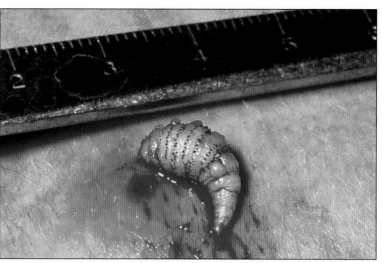

FIGURE 10-5 Cutaneous myiasis. A *D. hominis* larva is removed from a boillike lesion with a central punctum by incision and drainage. The central punctum serves as an air vent. The lesion was on a traveler who returned from Central America. (*Courtesy of* H. Rosen, MD.)

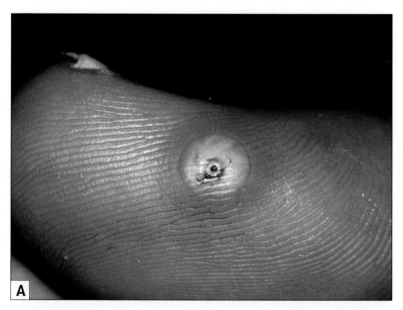

FIGURE 10-6 Tungiasis. **A,** A female sand flea or jigger (*Tunga penetrans*) is present on the medial aspect of the great toe, the typical attack site. The jigger is found in Central America, South America, West and East Africa, and the Indian subcontinent.

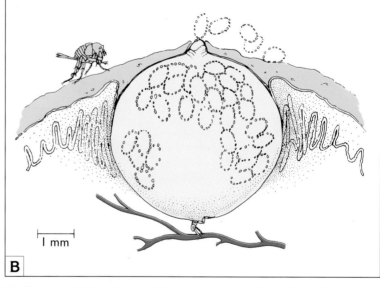

B, The gravid female sand flea burrows into the skin and extrudes her eggs through the skin, where they fall to the ground. (*From* Zalar GL, Walther RR: Infestation by *Tunga penetrans. Arch Dermatol* 1980, 116:80–81; with permission.)

FIGURE 10-7 Leeches. *Haemadipsa ornata* (terrestrial leeches) from North Borneo are shown feeding on a man. Leeches still have medical usage, *eg,* to evacuate fluid blebs under skin transplants. (*Courtesy of* B.C. Walton, PhD.)

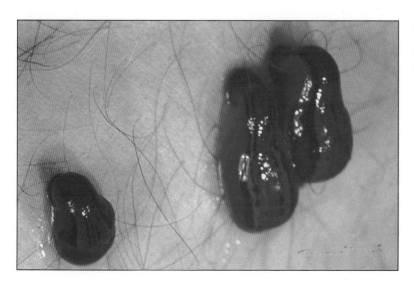

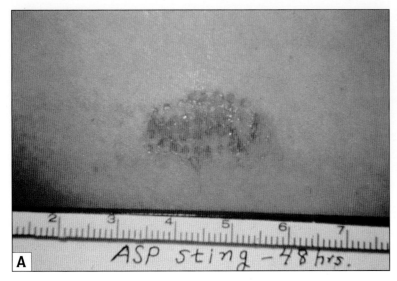

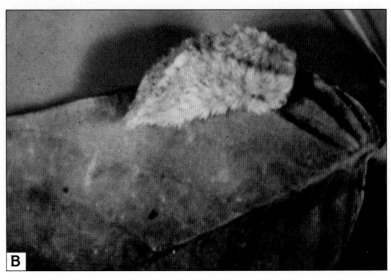

FIGURE 10-8 *Megalopyge opercularis.* **A**, A dermatitis is shown at 48 hours following contact with the puss caterpillar (also known as the tree asp) in Africa. **B**, A puss caterpillar is seen on a leaf. Severe local pain often follows contact with these caterpillars, which are the larval stage of a small moth. Clusters of venomous spines are hidden among the fine hairs on the back of the caterpillar. (*Courtesy of* A. Ewert, PhD.)

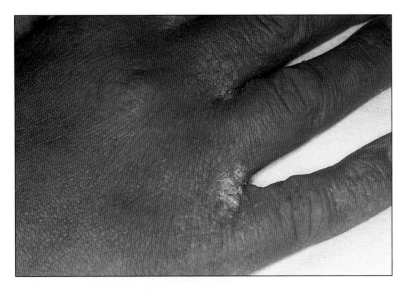

FIGURE 10-9 Scabies. A severe keratotic interdigital skin lesion due to *Sarcoptes scabiei* mites is present. (*Courtesy of* S.D. Glazer, MD.)

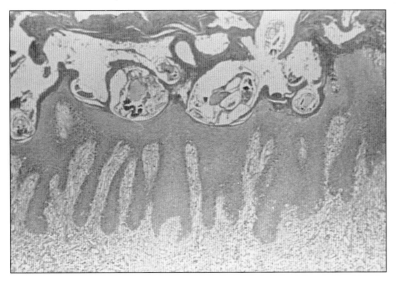

FIGURE 10-10 Scabies. A microscopic section of a scabies lesion shows multiple sections of the mites in the epidermis. (Hematoxylin-eosin stain.) (*Courtesy of* S.D. Glazer, MD.)

PARASITIC INFECTIONS TRANSMITTED BY INSECT BITES

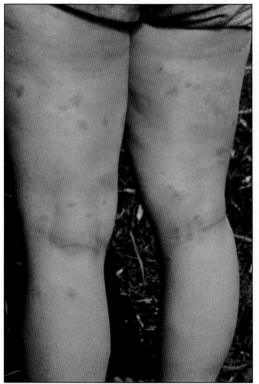

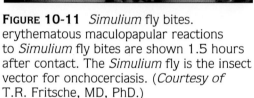

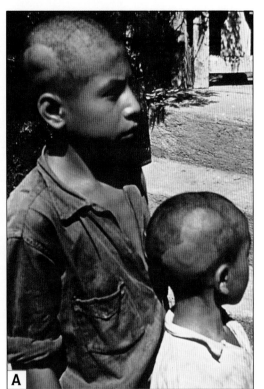

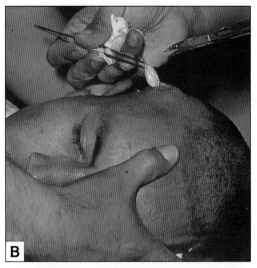

FIGURE 10-11 *Simulium* fly bites. erythematous maculopapular reactions to *Simulium* fly bites are shown 1.5 hours after contact. The *Simulium* fly is the insect vector for onchocerciasis. (*Courtesy of* T.R. Fritsche, MD, PhD.)

FIGURE 10-12 Onchocerciasis. **A**, Two boys in Central America show skin nodules (onchocercoma) typical of infection with *Onchocerca volvulus*. The nodules contain adult onchocerca, usually surrounded by a fibrous reaction. (*Courtesy of* D. Price, PhD.) **B**, Excision of a subcutaneous nodule is shown. (*Courtesy of* A.M. Fallis, PhD.)

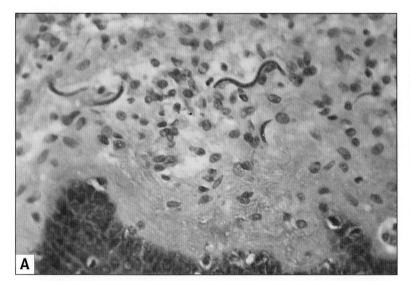

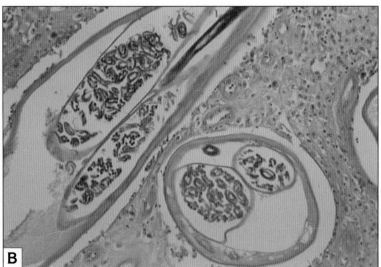

FIGURE 10-13 *Onchocerca* microfilariae. **A**, Subcutaneous micro-filariae of *O. volvulus* are demonstrated. Blindness may result from migration of larvae into the eye. **B**, Microscopic section through an onchocercoma shows microfilariae, which appear as circuitous lines within the adult female worm. The worm gut is seen as a cross-section in the lower parasite and longitudinally in the upper parasite. (Hematoxylin-eosin stain.)(*Courtesy of* M. Wittner, MD, PhD.)

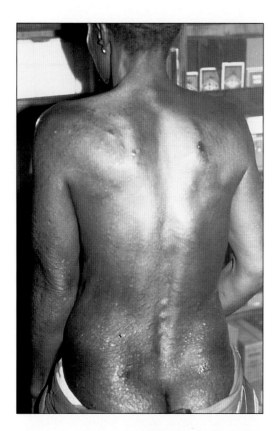

FIGURE 10-14
Onchocerciasis. The patient shows atrophic dermatitis, connective tissue loss, glossy wrinkled skin, and multiple small nodules plus excoriations due to scratching. There is an intense pruritic reaction to the migrating larvae over a long period of time. (*Courtesy of* S.E. Maddison, MD.)

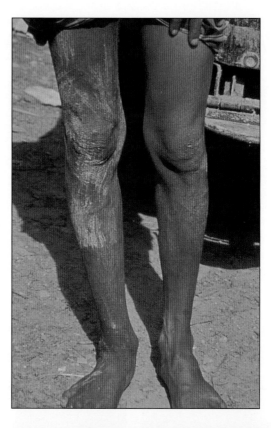

FIGURE 10-15
Sowdah. An adult man from the Yeman Arab Republic shows typical sowdah of the right leg. Many lesions result from scratching due to the intense pruritus caused by migrating *Onchocerca* larvae. (*Courtesy of* D.W. Buttner, MD.)

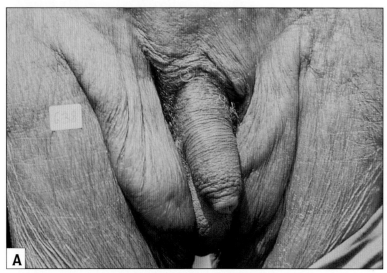

FIGURE 10-16   Hanging groin due to onchocerciasis. **A** and **B**, Bilateral hanging groin is shown in a blind man of about 52 years of age (*panel 16A*) and in a woman of about 45 years of age

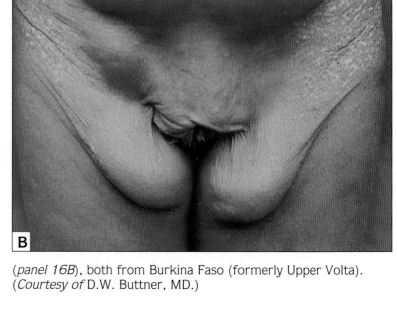

(*panel 16B*), both from Burkina Faso (formerly Upper Volta). (*Courtesy of* D.W. Buttner, MD.)

FIGURE 10-17   Filariasis. Early inguinal lymphadenopathy due to infection with *Wuchereria bancrofti* is present in this patient. (*Courtesy of* D. Price, PhD.)

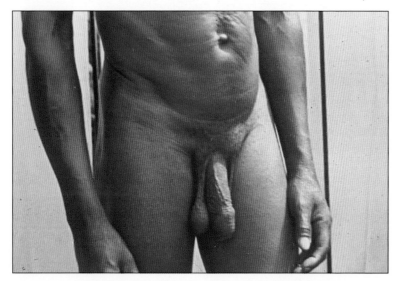

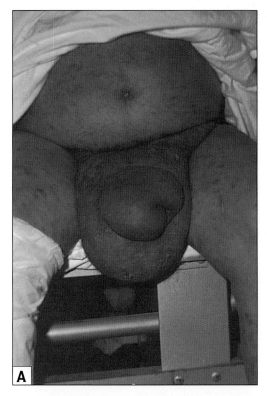 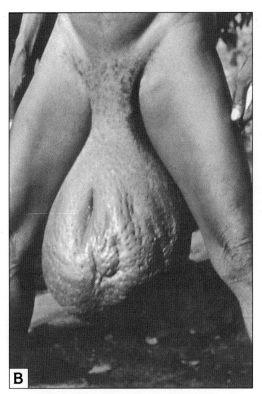

FIGURE 10-18 Genital enlargement of filariasis. **A** and **B**, Moderate (*panel 18A*) and marked genital enlargement (*panel 18B*) due to infection with *W. bancrofti* is shown. (Panel 18A *courtesy of* M. Wittner, MD, PhD; and panel 18B *courtesy of* B. Kean, MD.)

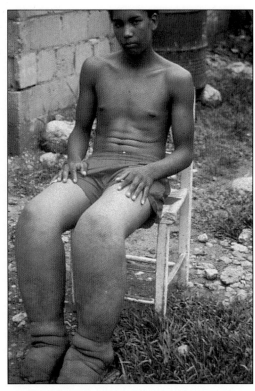

FIGURE 10-19 Lymphadenopathy in filariasis. Lymphedema involving both lower extremities is present in a young man from the Dominican Republic. (*Courtesy of* A.L. Vincent, PhD.)

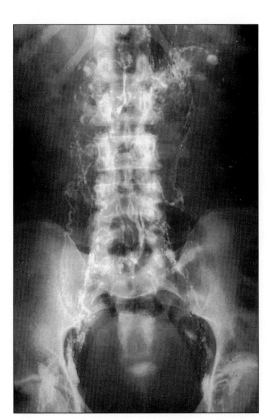

FIGURE 10-20 Lymphadenopathy in filariasis. A bilateral lymphangiogram shows dilated tortuous lymph channels caused by obstruction to centripetal lymph flow due to the presence of adult *W. bancrofti*. This obstruction causes backflow to the pericalyceal lymph channels in the kidney. Contrast flows into and fills some of the calyces, then flows distally to the urinary bladder, which becomes relatively opaque. (*Courtesy of* N. Katz, MD.)

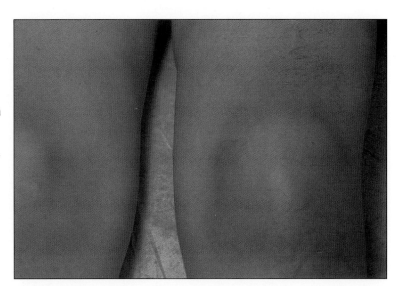

FIGURE 10-21 Calabar swelling due to *Loa loa*. An acute inflammatory reaction of the left knee is present secondary to migration of the filarid nematode *L. loa*. This patient was a 38-year-old geologist who worked in Zaire for 3 years. (*Courtesy of* F. Ciferri, MD, MPh.)

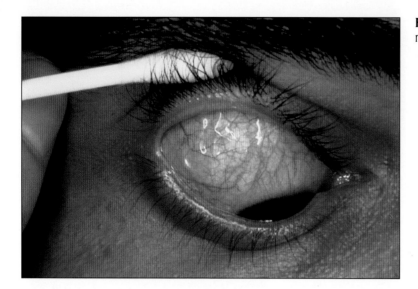

FIGURE 10-22 *Loa Loa.* Subconjunctival migration of the filarid nematode *L. loa* is demonstrated. (*Courtesy of* D. Gendelman, MD.)

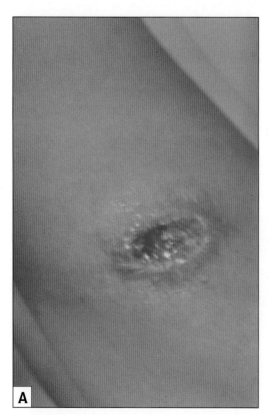

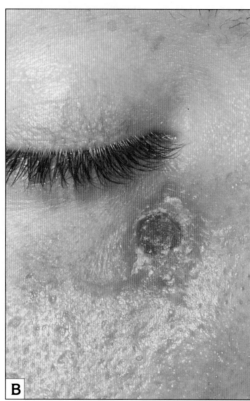

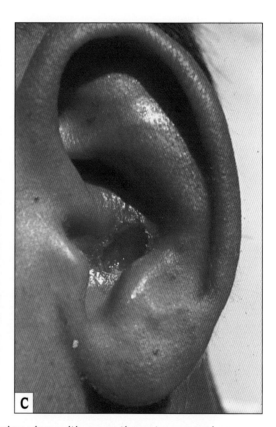

FIGURE 10-23 Leishmaniasis ulcers. **A**, An ulcer is present at the site of a *Phlebotomus* fly bite from 3 weeks previously. Note the sharply defined, rolled, elevated edges of the ulcer. (*Courtesy of* F. Etges, PhD.) **B**, Slowly enlarging ulcer with an erythematous margin on the face of an American student who studied in Guatemala. **C**, Leishmanial ulceration on the pinna. (*Courtesy of* F. Beltran, MD.)

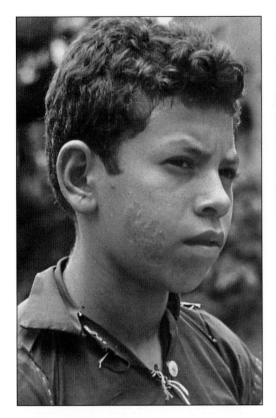

FIGURE 10-24 Healed facial scar due to multiple leishmanial ulcers. Such scarring is known as "seal of the forest" in Costa Rica. (*Courtesy of* D. Reifsnyder, PhD.)

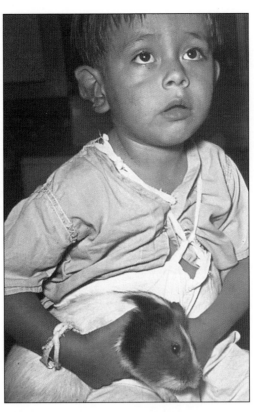

FIGURE 10-25 Ear notching secondary to leishmanial ulceration. The boy is holding a guinea pig, which is one of the reservoir hosts. (*Courtesy of* E.C. Nelson, PhD.)

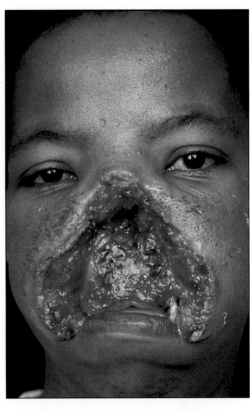

FIGURE 10-26 Mucocutaneous leishmaniasis destruction of the nose and mouth due to leishmaniasis in a patient from Colombia, South America. (*Courtesy of* F. Etges, PhD.)

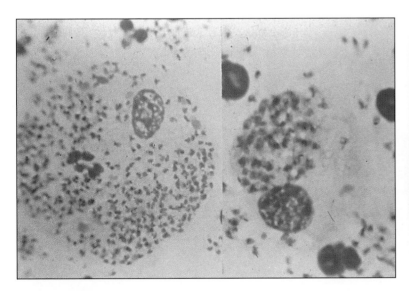

FIGURE 10-27 Leishmania amastigotes. A touch preparation of biopsied tissue shows multiple leishmania amastigotes. (*Courtesy of* B.H. Kean, MD.)

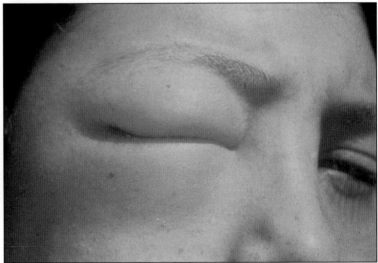

FIGURE 10-28 Chagas' disease. A woman from Argentina shows Romaña's sign, a unilateral swelling about the eye, which is a typical early finding in Chagas' disease. The causative parasite *Trypanosoma cruzi* is transmitted in the feces of a reduviid bug. (*Courtesy of* E. Kuschnir, MD.)

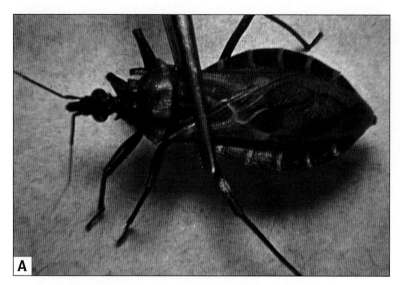

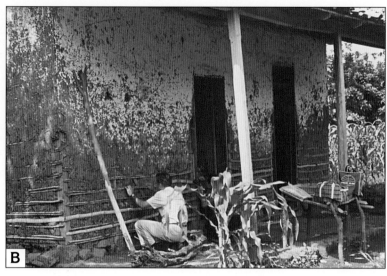

FIGURE 10-29 Reduviid bug. **A**, Many closely-related species may transmit *T. cruzi*, and multiple mammals may serve as reservoir hosts (they, too, may be infected). (*Courtesy of* D. Kaye, MD.)

B, Reduviid bugs hide in the cracks and crevices of this typical mud and wooden house, coming out at night to bite the sleeping inhabitants. (*Courtesy of* D. Reifsnyder, MD.)

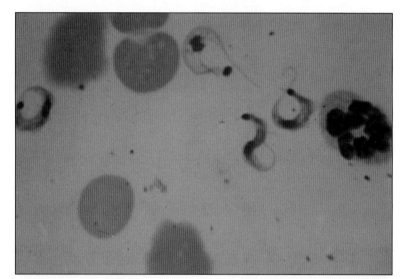

FIGURE 10-30 *Trypanosoma cruzi* trypanosomes. A thin smear of human blood shows multiple trypanosomes typical of *T. cruzi*. These often take C- or U-shapes and have large kinetoplasts posteriorly. The kinetoplasts are primitive mitochondria. A free visible flagellum and an undulating membrane (not visible on this slide) are present. The nucleus is placed centrally. (*Courtesy of* R.E. Kuntz, PhD.)

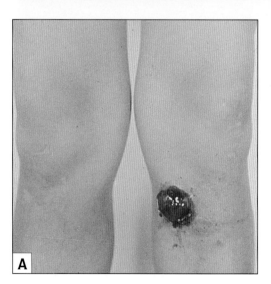

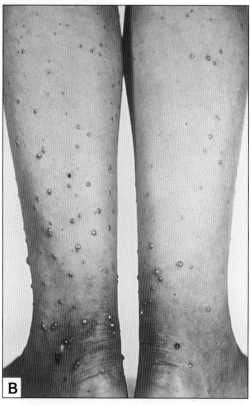

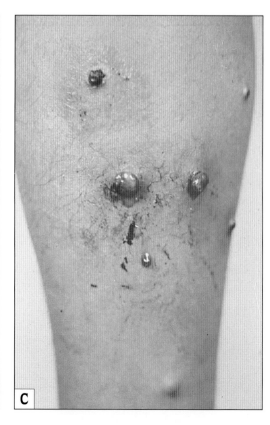

FIGURE 10-31 Verruca peruana. **A**, Gigantic verrucous lesions are present on the legs. This disease, caused by *Bartonella*, is transmitted by the bite of the *Phlebotomus* fly. The lesions may be misinterpreted as Kaposi's sarcoma. **B** and **C**, Nodular (*panel 31B*) and hematogenous nodular types (*panel 31C*) of verrucous eruption can also occur. (*Courtesy of* B.H. Kean, MD.)

GASTROINTESTINAL PARASITES WITH CUTANEOUS MANIFESTATIONS

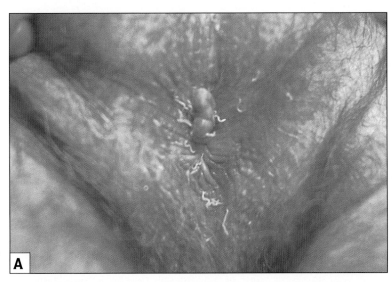

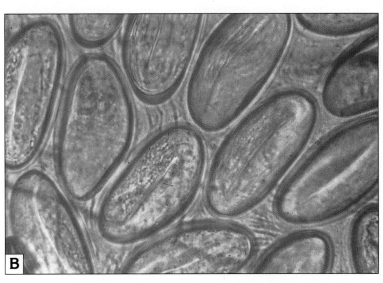

FIGURE 10-32 Pinworm. **A**, Multiple adult worms (*Enterobius vermicularis*) are present on the perianal skin. (*Courtesy of* F. Ciferri, MD, MPh.) **B**, Multiple pinworm eggs containing embryo worms are present on this perianal sample taken with clear adhesive tape.

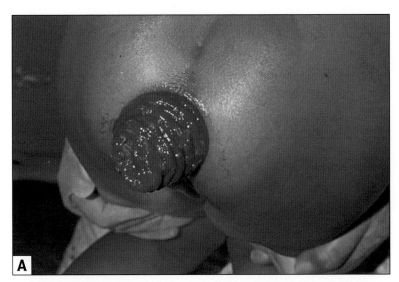

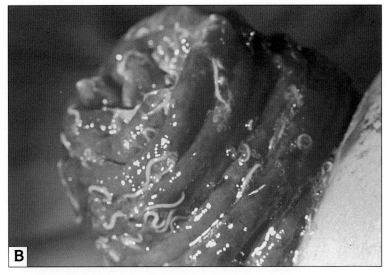

FIGURE 10-33 Whipworm. **A**, A prolapsed rectum in a child is due to presence of the whipworm (*Trichuris trichiura*). **B**, Close-up view of the adult whipworms on the prolapsed rectal mucosa. Only the posterior half of the worm projects into the lumen.

The anterior half, which is much thinner in cross-section, is woven into the mucosa and is not visible. This combination of a thick posterior (handle) and a thin anterior (lash) suggests the whipworm name. (*Courtesy of* F. Beltran, MD.)

FIGURE 10-34 Trichinosis. The patient shows mild periorbital edema due to infection with *Trichinella spiralis*. (*Courtesy of* I.G. Kagan, PhD.)

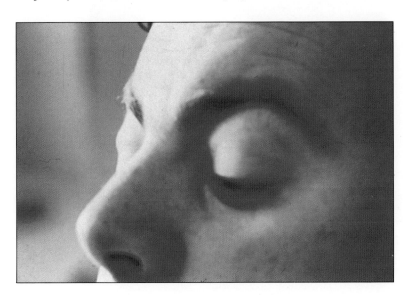

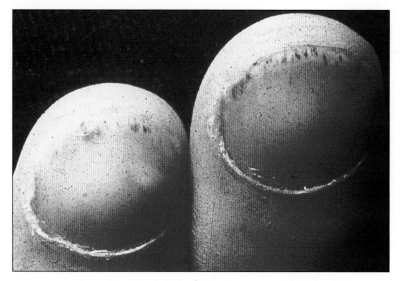

FIGURE 10-35 Subungual hemorrhages in trichinosis. Fingernails show subungual hemorrhages suggestive of subacute bacterial endocarditis, but they are actually due to trichinosis. Such patients often have a bleeding diathesis and a normal sedimentation rate despite a highly toxic presentation. A marked peripheral blood eosinophilia is often present. A precipitous fall of the eosinophilia is a grave prognostic sign. (*Courtesy of* I.G. Kagan, PhD.)

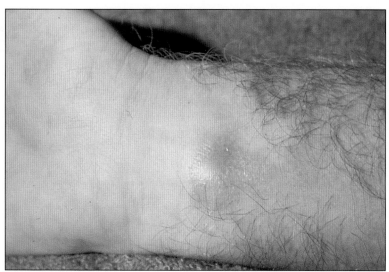

FIGURE 10-36 Gnathostomiasis. A swollen erythematous lesion on the volar aspect of the wrist is caused by the larval nematode, *Gnathostoma spinigerum*, which may be acquired by eating raw snakes, amphibians, fish, or undercooked chicken or duck. This infection occurs with frequency in the Far East. (*Courtesy of* K.G. Brand, MD.)

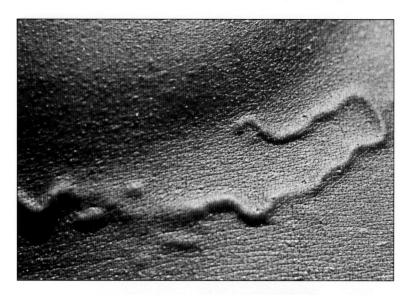

FIGURE 10-37 Dracunculiasis. A migrating adult female nematode, *Dracunculus medinensis*, is present in the subcutaneous tissues inferior to the breast of this African patient. (*Courtesy of* J. Donges, MD.)

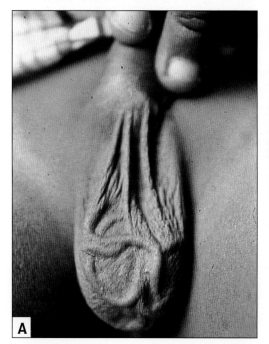

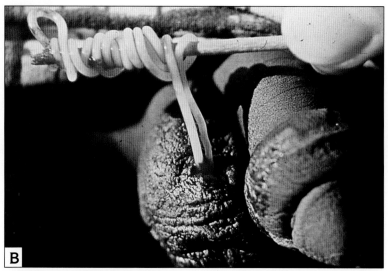

FIGURE 10-38 Dracunculiasis. **A**, A migrating adult female nematode, *D. medinensis*, is present in the scrotum. **B**, The classical matchstick recovery technique used in extracting the adult female worm is demonstrated. (*Courtesy of* J. Donges, MD.)

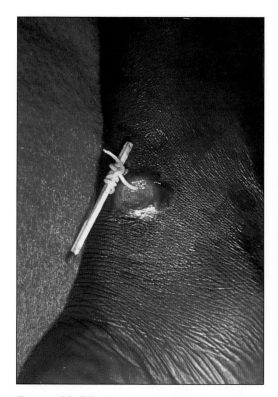

FIGURE 10-39 Cutaneous ulcer dracunculiasis. The adult female worms often induce cutaneous ulcer formation. When the ulcerated area is immersed in water, the female deposits many larvae into the water that eventually develop in microscopic copepods. When these are subsequently ingested by people drinking the contaminated water, the parasites are digested free of the copepods and migrate throughout the body, over a long period of time (months to years). The female worm can achieve lengths approximating 1 m. Note the atrophic circular scars present as the result of previous infection. (*Courtesy of* J. Donges, MD.)

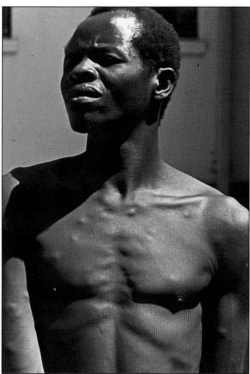

FIGURE 10-40 Cysticercosis. An adult African man shows numerous subcutaneous nodules of larval *Taenia solium* (*Cysticercus cellulosae*). (*Courtesy of* M. King, MD.)

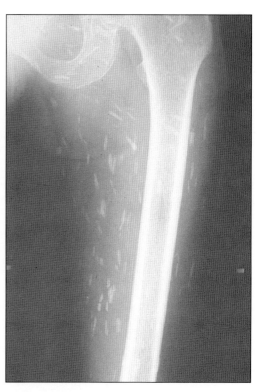

FIGURE 10-41 Cysticercosis. This radiograph shows soft-tissue calcifications resembling rice grains, which are characteristic of chronic cysticercosis. This patient was a refugee from Southeast Asia.

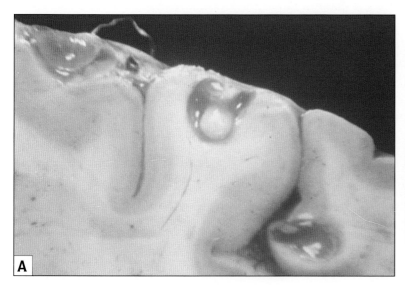

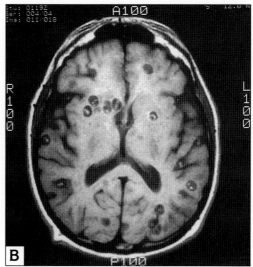

FIGURE 10-42 Neurocysticercosis. **A,** A gross section of a human brain shows three pearllike cysticerci. Such patients often present with seizures. (*Courtesy of* B. Kean, MD.) **B,** A CT scan of the brain shows multiple small circular densities. Within many of these, a calcified dot is present that represents calcification of the scolex within the cysticerci.

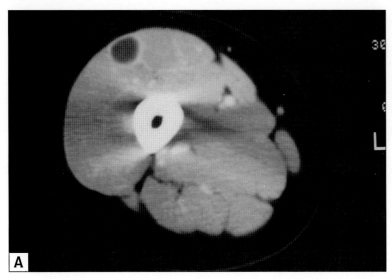

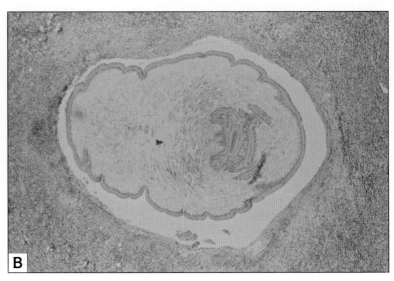

FIGURE 10-43 Sparganosis (tapeworm). **A,** A young adult man in the Air Force with a history of considerable Far East travel presented in California with a fluctuant migrating thigh mass. A computed tomography scan of the thigh showed a 1-cm hypodense lesion with peripheral soft-tissue inflammation. A larval tapeworm was removed. (*Courtesy of* Travis Air Force Base, Department of Radiology.) **B,** Microscopic cross-section through a sparganum larva is presented. Note the intense inflammatory response. (Hematoxylin-eosin stain.)

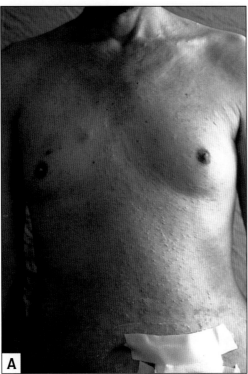

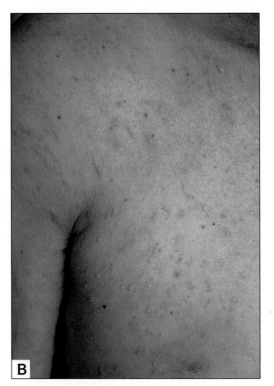

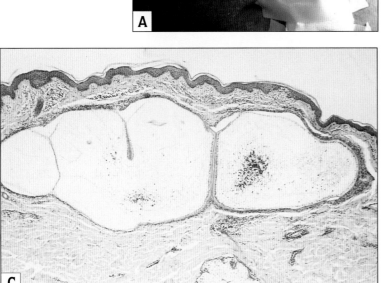

FIGURE 10-44 *Sparganum proliferum.* **A,** Multiple skin lesions and gynecomastia are present in this man from Venezuela. **B,** A close-up view shows linear elevations suggesting the shapes of the underlying worms. **C,** A longitudinal section through the worm *in situ* shows little inflammatory reaction adjacent to the worm. (*From* Moulinier R, Martinez E, Torres J, *et al.*: Human proliferative sparganosis in Venezuela: A report of a case. *Am J Trop Med Hyg* 1982, 31:358–363; with permission.)

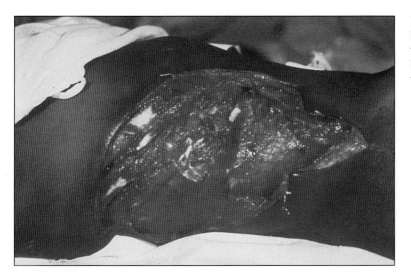

FIGURE 10-45 Amebiasis. Cutaneous ulceration of the right lateral body wall due to *Entamoeba histolytica*. Such lesions may result from extension of a liver abscess or a colonic ulcer. It is also possible for abraded skin to become infected through contact with fecally contaminated substances.

PARASITIC DISEASES ACQUIRED BY DIRECT INOCULATION THROUGH THE SKIN AND MUCOUS MEMBRANES

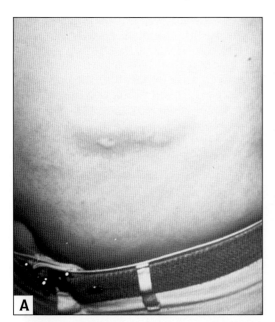

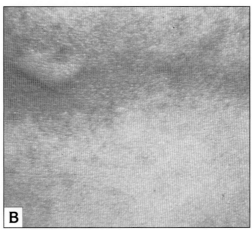

FIGURE 10-46 Cutaneous larva currens. **A**, A linear, migrating, urticarial pruritic rash is present on the abdomen of a patient with a chronic infection with *Stronglyoides stercoralis*. **B**, A close-up view shows details of the lesion. (*From* Pelletier LL Jr: Chronic strongyloidiasis in World War II Far East ex-prisoners of war. *Am J Trop Med Hyg* 1984, 33:55–61; with permission.)

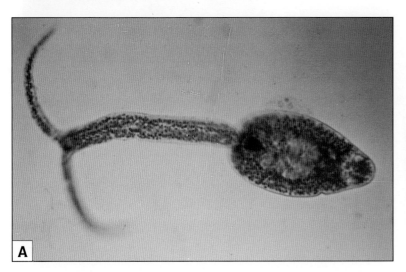

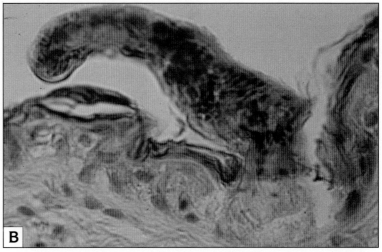

FIGURE 10-47 *Schistosoma* cercaria. **A**, The fork-tailed larval stage of *Schistosoma mansoni*, known as a cercaria, emerges from an infected aquatic snail and swims about seeking contact with the skin of a potential host. **B**, When contact is made, the cercaria initiates infection by penetrating the epidermis, at which time it sheds its tail, and heading deeper into the dermis. (Panel 47B *courtesy of* M.A. Stirewalt, PhD, and R.E. Kuntz, PhD.)

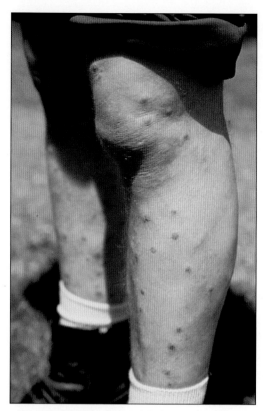

FIGURE 10-48 Cercarial dermatitis of schistosomiasis. Each lesion represents a cercarial invasion site. (*Courtesy of* T. Fritsche, MD, PhD.)

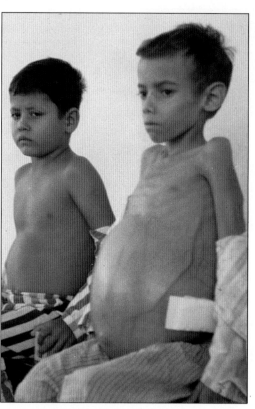

FIGURE 10-49 Hepatosplenic schistosomiasis. These two boys have end-stage hepatosplenic schistosomiasis. The child on the right shows massive ascites, with tremendous engorgement of the enlarged collateral venous structures. He died soon after the photograph was taken. (*Courtesy of* F. Etges, PhD.)

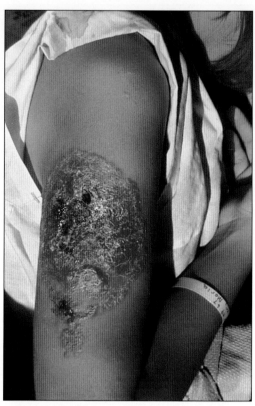

FIGURE 10-50 Acanthamebiasis. A 28-year-old Mexican woman with a 6-month-old skin lesion. A large ulcer shows raised edges with areas of keratosis, hemorrhage, and eschar formation. She also presented with central nervous system signs and symptoms. Autopsy revealed multiple hemorrhagic lesions in the cerebral cortex. (*Courtesy of* G.R. Healy, PhD.)

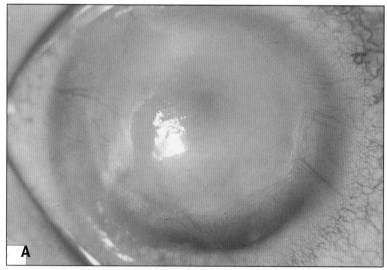

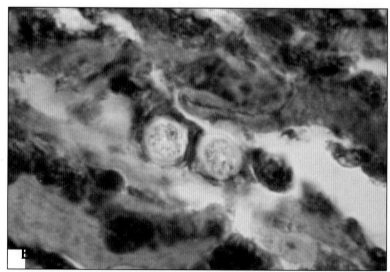

FIGURE 10-51 *Acanthamoeba* keratitis. **A**, Severe keratitis is presented in the eye of a patient. Recently, several miniepidemics of this condition have developed in individuals who used contaminated contact lens fluid or poor cleaning technique. **B**, Corneal scrapings show multiple amebas on microscopic examination. (*Courtesy of* D.B. Jones, MD.)

ACKNOWLEDGMENTS

Many of the slides appearing in this chapter were previously published in *A Pictorial Presentation of Parasites*, edited and published by Herman Zaiman, MD. The authors apologize to those whose contributions may not have been acknowledged due to faulty memory and records (and floods).

SELECTED BIBLIOGRAPHY

Gardner P (ed.): Infectious diseases in international travelers. *Infect Dis Clin North Am* 1992, 6(2).

Markell EK, Voge M, John DT: *Medical Parasitology*, 7th ed. Philadelphia: W.B. Saunders; 1992.

Muller RLJ, Baker J: *Medical Parasitology*. London: Gower Medical Publishing; 1990.

Wilson ME: *A World Guide to Infections*. New York, Oxford University Press; 1991.

Strickland GT (ed.): *Hunter's Tropical Medicine*, 7th ed. Philadelphia: W.B. Saunders; 1991.

CHAPTER 11

Leprosy (Hansen's Disease)

Robert Gelber, Rodolfo M. Abalos,
Roland V. Cellona,
Tranquilino T. Fajardo,
Gerald P. Walsh, Ricardo S. Guinto

CLASSIFICATION

Ridley-Jopling classification of leprosy

Clinical and histologic features	Tuberculoid (TT)	Borderline tuberculoid (BT)	Borderline (BB)	Borderline lepromatous (BL)	Lepromatous (LL)
Skin lesions	Up to 3 in number. Sharply defined asymmetric plaques with tendency for central clearing, elevated borders.	Smaller or larger than in TT. Potentially more numerous than in TT. Usually annular lesions with sharp margination on exterior and interior borders. Borders not as elevated as in TT.	Dimorphic lesions intermediate between BT and BL.	LL type lesions. Ill-defined plaques with an occasional sharp margin. Few or many in number, shiny appearance.	Symmetric. Poorly marginated, multiple infiltrated nodules and plaques or diffuse infiltration. Xanthoma-like or dermatofibroma papules. Leonine facies and eyebrow alopecia.
Nerve lesions	Skin lesions anesthetic early. Nerve near lesion may be enlarged.	Skin lesions anesthetic early. Nerve trunk palsies asymmetric. Nerve abscesses most common in BT.	Anesthetic skin lesions. Nerve trunk palsies.	Skin lesions usually hypoesthetic, may be anesthetic. Nerve trunk palsies common and frequently symmetric.	Hyperesthesia a late sign. Nerve palsies variable. Acral, distal, symmetric anesthesia common.
Lepromin skin test	Positive	Usually positive (80% to 90%).	Negative	Negative	Negative
Lymphocytes	Dense peripheral infiltration about epithelioid tubercle. Infiltration into epidermis well developed.	Less numerous than in TT. Peripheral infiltration about granuloma. Variable epidermal infiltration usually focal.	Lymphopenic	Moderately dense and in the same distribution as macrophages.	Scant, diffuse, or focal in distribution.
Macrophage differentiation	Epithelioid	Epithelioid	Epithelioid	Usually undifferentiated. Epithelioid foci may be present. May show foamy change.	Foamy change the rule. May be undifferentiated in early lesions.
Langhans' giant cells	Present, well developed.	May be present. Usually few in number.	Absent	Absent	Absent
Acid-fast bacilli (AFB)	Rare, < 1/100 OIF or BI=0 (paucibacillary)	Rare, usually BI=0 (paucibacillary). If AFB present, consider a reversal reaction.	1–10/OIF or BI=3–4.	10–100/OIF or BI=4–5.	10–1000/OIF or BI=4–6. Globi present.

FIGURE 11-1 The Ridley-Jopling classification of leprosy. This classification scheme provides a very useful clinical/pathologic framework for understanding the broad spectrum of immune-mediated reactions in leprosy. Possible reactional states, complications, and prognosis are indicated for each form of leprosy. Leprosy has a broad range of clinical manifestations marked by a variable immune response and inflammatory reaction within infected tissues. At one end of the spectrum is tuberculoid (TT) leprosy, in which only a single area of skin and possibly its associated nerve supply are affected. At the opposite end of the spectrum is lepromatous (LL) leprosy, with massive skin infection plus involvement of nerves, nasopharynx, testes, and lymphoreticular system. The intermediate forms are less stable clinically and often progress to the lepromatous form, although regression toward the tuberculoid forms occurs with therapy or sometimes spontaneously. These "upward" and "downward" shifts depend on gains or losses in host resistance. (OIF—oil immersion field; BI—bacteriologic index.) (*From* Kawamura LM, Gelber RH: Leprosy. *In* Arnedt K, LeBoit P, Robinson J, Wintroub BU (eds.): *Cutaneous Medicine and Surgery.* Philadelphia: W.B. Saunders; 1994; with permission.)

Indeterminate Leprosy

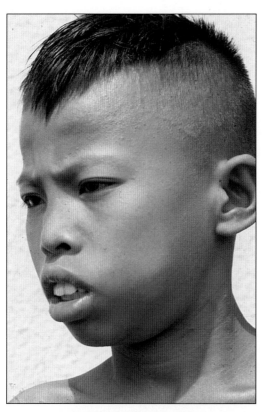

FIGURE 11-2 Indeterminate leprosy is an early stage of leprosy generally found in children. As in this patient, the skin manifestations are solitary (*left cheek*), ill-defined, hypopigmented macules, which are only partially anesthetic. Indeterminate leprosy may progress to either tuberculoid or lepromatous forms of the disease.

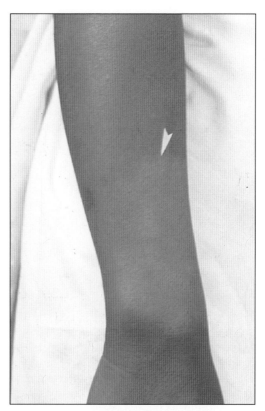

FIGURE 11-3 Indeterminate leprosy is found most commonly on the extensor surface of extremities. The lesion in this patient is a single, faintly hypochromic macule with ill-defined borders. At times, these lesions may be slightly erythematous. Only parts of the lesion may be hypoesthetic, and at times sensation is intact.

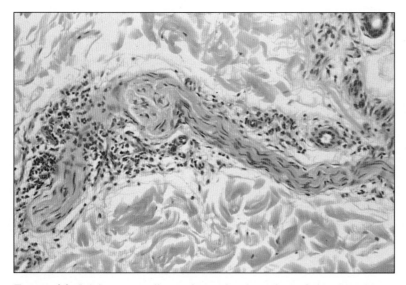

FIGURE 11-4 A hematoxylin-eosin–stained section of the dermis of a patient with indeterminate leprosy, demonstrating a mild perineural infiltrate of mononuclear cells. In indeterminate leprosy, the histopathologic appearance is characterized by the presence of a mild mononuclear cell infiltrate consisting of lymphocytes and epithelioid macrophages around blood vessels, nerves, and dermal appendages.

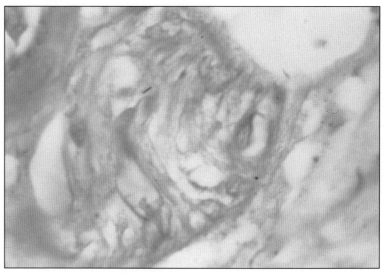

FIGURE 11-5 A Fite-Faraco stain showing a single acid-fast bacillus in a nerve of a patient with indeterminate leprosy. In indeterminate leprosy, acid-fast bacilli may be present and few in number or entirely absent.

Tuberculoid Leprosy

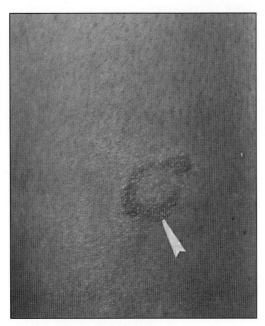

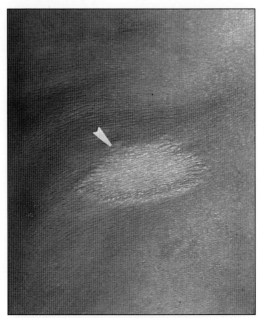

FIGURE 11-6 The typical lesion in tuberculoid (TT) leprosy is a small, single, circinate lesion with a pink, elevated, finely granular, well-defined border. The central hypopigmented macule was insensitive to touch and pain in this patient, which is usually the case. In TT leprosy, lesions may be single or few in number and may be associated with enlarged peripheral nerves, particularly in proximity to skin lesions.

FIGURE 11-7 A well-defined, hypopigmented macule of tuberculoid leprosy with a typical dry surface and a moderately raised, granular, well-defined margin. This lesion is entirely anesthetic. Tuberculoid leprosy is a stable form of disease, which does not evolve to other forms of leprosy nor result in reactional states.

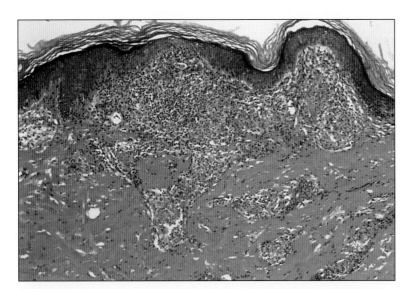

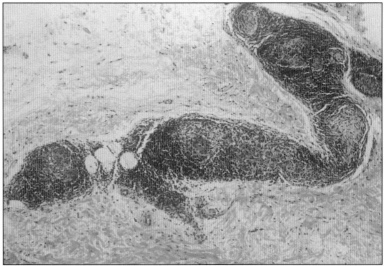

FIGURE 11-8 An epithelioid cell granuloma with large numbers of lymphocytes eroding into the basal layer of the covering epidermis (hematoxylin-eosin stain). The histologic appearance of tuberculoid (TT) leprosy is characterized by focalized epithelioid cell granuloma, particularly of dermal adnexa, which are surrounded by thick zones of lymphocytes and may have Langhans' giant cells. In TT leprosy, as opposed to borderline tuberculoid disease, pathology may extend into the basal layer of the epidermis. In TT leprosy, acid-fast bacilli are invariably absent.

FIGURE 11-9 Tuberculoid leprosy may be associated with invasion and destruction of dermal nerves, which is pathognomonic for leprosy. Pictured is an epithelioid granuloma surrounded by a thick zone of lymphocytes destroying a nerve, which is almost unrecognizable (hematoxylin-eosin stain).

Borderline Tuberculoid Leprosy

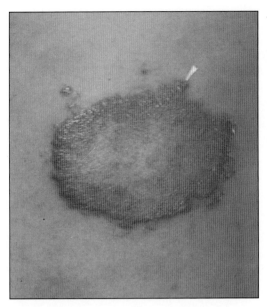

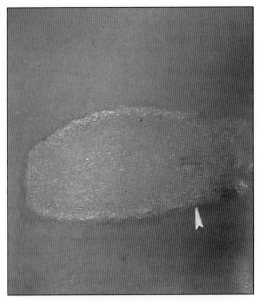

FIGURE 11-10 A single borderline tuberculoid (BT) leprosy lesion in a patient with several BT lesions. The lesion is anesthetic, has a sharp edge, and is largely erythematous with a fairly thick granular margin, which is associated with small satellite lesions. In BT leprosy, lesions may be few or numerous. Although they may be red or brown, most commonly they are hypopigmented macules with raised, well-defined borders or elevated plaques. Lesions are generally hypoesthetic or anesthetic. Patients with BT leprosy may develop lepra type-1 reactions associated with signs of inflammation in preexisting lesions and peripheral nerves, with "satellite" inflamed new lesions at times developing.

FIGURE 11-11 A borderline tuberculoid (BT) skin lesion presenting as a distinct, erythematous-hypochromic macule with a dry surface, which is anesthetic and has a raised, well-defined margin showing satellite lesions. BT leprosy may be unstable and evolve to near-polar lepromatous leprosy.

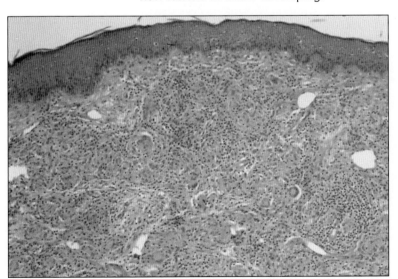

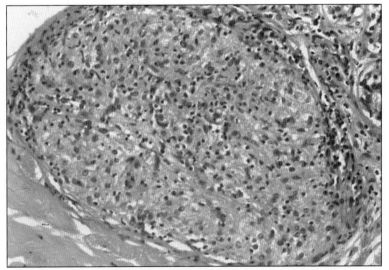

FIGURE 11-12 A hematoxylin-eosin–stained section of the skin from a patient with borderline tuberculoid (BT) leprosy, showing an epithelioid cell granuloma, occasional Langhans' giant cells, and a moderate number of lymphocytes occupying the superficial dermis. As is characteristic in BT leprosy, there is a clear subepidermal zone without pathology. In BT leprosy, there may be a few acid-fast bacilli which, when present, can be demonstrated mostly within nerves.

FIGURE 11-13 A swollen nerve heavily infiltrated by an epithelioid cell granuloma in a patient with borderline tuberculoid leprosy (hematoxylin-eosin stain). There is earlier dermal nerve histopathology near the tuberculoid pole of leprosy than at the lepromatous pole.

Borderline Leprosy

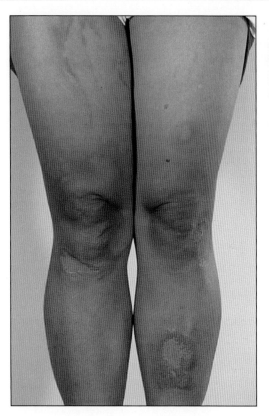

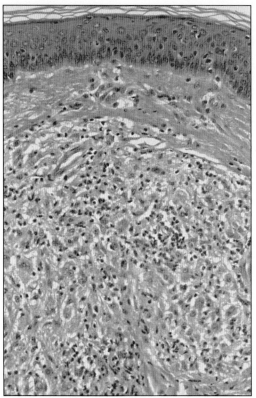

FIGURE 11-14 Borderline (BB) (or mid-borderline) leprosy is an unusual form of the disease. In BB leprosy, lesions may be few or numerous. Lesions are often inflamed and succulent with central clearing, producing a "punched-out" appearance, or they may appear as plaques or bands with peripheral edges fading into normal surrounding skin. When present, sensory deficits are largely confined to central areas. BB patients may develop lepra type-1 reactions.

FIGURE 11-15 An epithelioid granuloma with a few diffusely scattered lymphocytes and a clear subepidermal zone (hematoxylin-eosin stain) from a patient with borderline (BB) leprosy. The histopathologic appearance of BB leprosy is characterized by epithelioid cell granulomata that are diffuse and focalized by a zone of lymphocytes, which, if present, are scattered. In BB leprosy, Langhans' giant cells are conspicuously absent. Dermal nerves may be particularly involved, and lamination of the perineurium may be noted.

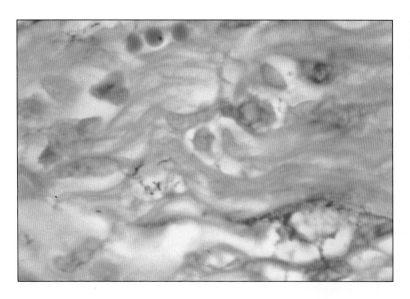

FIGURE 11-16 In borderline (BB) leprosy, acid-fast bacilli may be present in moderate numbers. In this Fite-Faraco–stained section of the skin from a BB patient, moderate numbers of acid-fast bacilli can be seen within a nerve.

Borderline Lepromatous Leprosy

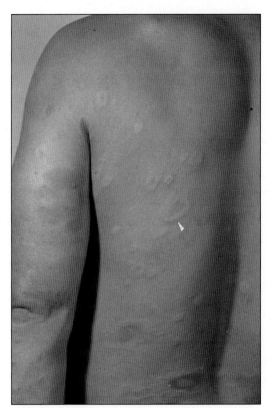

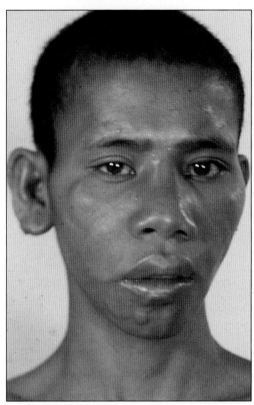

FIGURE 11-17 In borderline lepromatous (BL) leprosy, skin lesions are generally numerous (though rarely they may be singular). Lesions are generally multiform, including ones nearly borderline tuberculoid in appearance to more infiltrated nodules and plaques approximating those in polar lepromatous leprosy. Patients with BL leprosy may develop both lepra type-1 and type-2 reactions. Pictured is a patient with numerous and widespread borderline-type plaques, annular lesions, papules, and macules; the centers of large BT-type lesions have some loss of sensation.

FIGURE 11-18 The face of a patient with borderline lepromatous (BL) leprosy. Thick erythematous plaques can be seen in the nose, right cheek, and chin, with some smaller lesions appearing rather nodular. As is common in BL leprosy, the lesions are not so sharply delineated and show no sensory impairment.

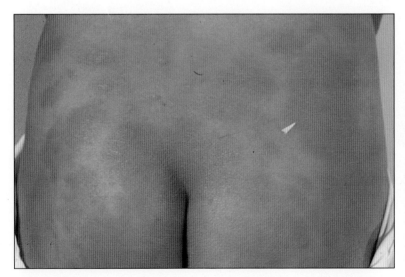

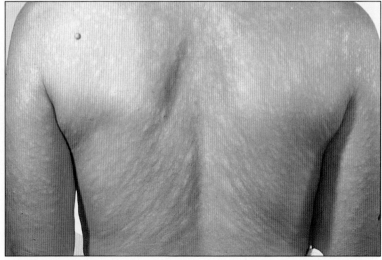

FIGURE 11-19 A somewhat different appearance of borderline lepromatous leprosy. Skin lesions are bilaterally distributed, irregularly shaped, slightly erythematous, and mildly infiltrated. No hypoesthesia was present.

FIGURE 11-20 Another appearance of borderline lepromatous leprosy. The patient's back shows fairly uniformly and symmetrically distributed, infiltrated maculopapular lesions. None of the lesions was sensory-impaired.

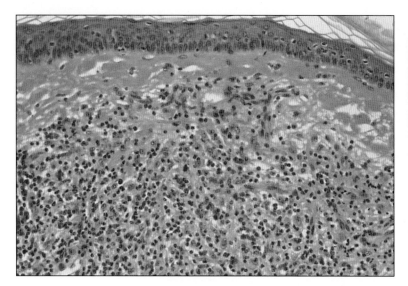

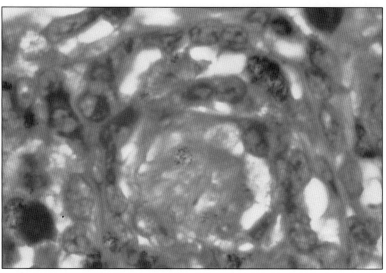

FIGURE 11-21 Borderline lepromatous leprosy is characterized by the presence of histiocytic cell granulomata, some having an epithelioid-like pattern and others with foamy cytoplasm ("foam cells"), admixed in areas with large numbers of lymphocytes (hematoxylin-eosin stain). Foam cells are the result of the presence of large amounts of *Mycobacterium leprae*–derived, largely fatty material, particularly the *M. leprae*–specific glycolipid 1.

FIGURE 11-22 In borderline lepromatous (BL) leprosy, there are numerous acid-fast bacilli. A Fite-Faraco–stained section of the dermis of a BL patient shows numerous acid-fast bacilli within a nerve.

Lepromatous Leprosy

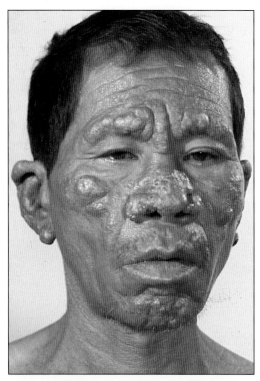

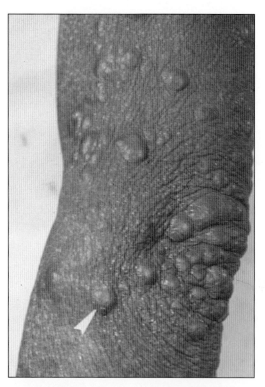

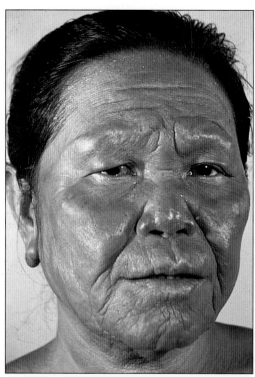

FIGURE 11-23 A man with far-advanced, nodular lepromatous (LL) leprosy. Diffuse infiltration coupled with nodules over the eyebrows, cheeks, ear lobes, nose, and chin are observed. Patients demonstrate *M. leprae*–specific anergy (cell-mediated responses) but have high levels of circulating antibody to *M. leprae* and a diffuse polyclonal hyperglobulinemia, which may lead to a variety of false-positive serologic tests, including VDRL, antinuclear antibodies, and rheumatoid factor.

FIGURE 11-24 The arm of a patient with lepromatous leprosy demonstrates multiple, typical nodules of far-advanced disease.

FIGURE 11-25 A woman with advanced lepromatous (LL) leprosy with marked, diffuse infiltration, madarosis, and loss of eyelashes. There is a similar expression of LL leprosy seen almost exclusively in Mexico, where no visible skin lesions are observed but only diffuse, dermal infiltration and loss of body hair, termed *diffuse lepromatosis*.

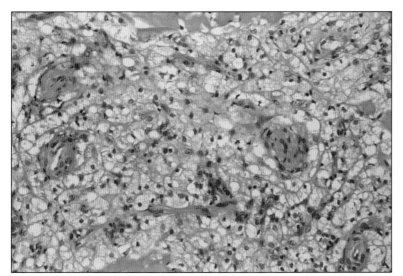

FIGURE 11-26 A hematoxylin-eosin–stained section of skin is typical of a patient with active lepromatous leprosy and demonstrates highly vacuolated foam cells, normal-appearing nerves, and a histiocytic granuloma. In the dermis, nerves may appear normal, hyalinized, with pathology of the perineurium, or fibrosed. Lymphocytes, if present, are usually scanty.

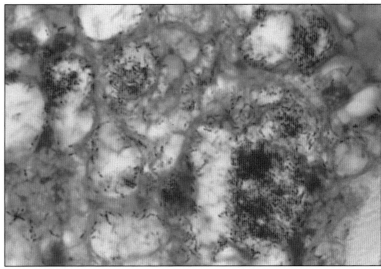

FIGURE 11-27 As in the Fite-Faraco stain shown in Fig. 11-22, lepromatous leprosy patients have enormous numbers of acid-fast bacilli, often in huge clumps, termed *globi*. It has been estimated that at times 10% of the dry weight of the skin in these patients may be bacilli. In lepromatous patients, acid-fast bacilli are most plentiful in the skin, peripheral nerves, upper airways, and anterior chamber of the eye, but they are also present in every organ system except the central nervous system and lungs.

REACTIONAL STATES, RELAPSE, AND COMPLICATIONS

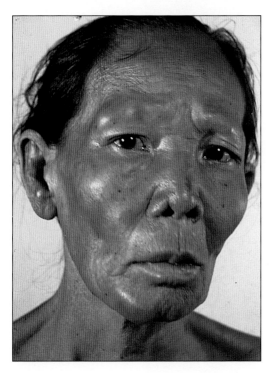

FIGURE 11-28 Erythema nodosum leprosum (ENL) (lepra type-2 reaction). This woman has manifestations of lepromatous leprosy and deep-seated ENL lesions over her chin, eyebrows, and ears. ENL skin lesions may be single or multiple and may occur in recurrent crops, with individual lesions lasting only a few days to 1 week. ENL occurs generally on therapy and may also be associated with neuritis, fever, lymphadenitis, orchitis, uveitis, arthritis, and/or frank glomerulonephritis.

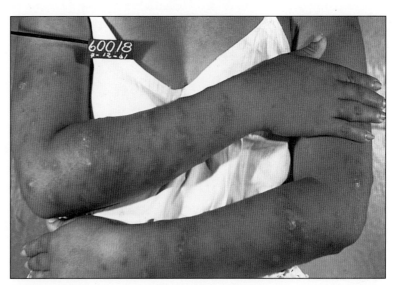

FIGURE 11-29 A patient with several cutaneous and subcutaneous inflammatory erythema nodosum leprosum (ENL) lesions. As in this patient, at times these lesions may pustulate and ulcerate. ENL appears to be caused by circulating immune complexes. It is associated with elevated levels of tumor necrosis factor (TNF) and a local increase in cell-mediated immunity, as manifested by increased numbers of T-helper cells, interleukin-2, interferon-γ, and a loss of suppressor T-cell activity. Corticosteroids or thalidomide is effective therapeutically, with thalidomide acting by inhibiting TNF synthesis. (Sampaio EP, Sarno EN, Galilly R, *et al.*: Thalidomide selectively inhibits tumor necrosis factor alpha production by stimulated human monocytes. *J Exp Med* 1991, 173:669–703.)

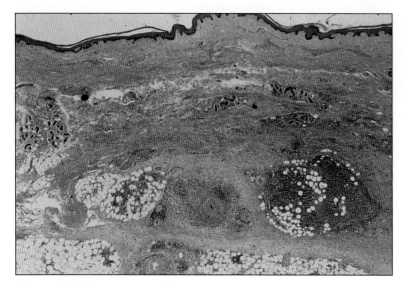

FIGURE 11-30 A hematoxylin-eosin–stained section of the dermis from a patient with erythema nodosum leprosum demonstrates a severe inflammatory process involving the lower dermis and subcutaneous tissue. Obliterative arteriolitis, microabscesses, and edema are evident.

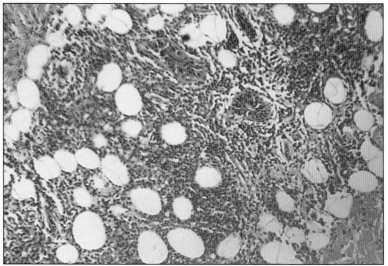

FIGURE 11-31 An acute inflammatory process, rich in polymorphonuclear leukocytes, involving the sweat glands in a patient with erythema nodosum leprosum (ENL) (hematoxylin-eosin-stain). Although lymphocytes and macrophages may be present histologically in ENL skin lesions, their hallmark is neutrophils and a leukocytoclastic vasculitis involving the dermis and subcutis. The histologic appearance of ENL is remarkably similar to that of an Arthus reaction. Bacilli in ENL are usually few and degenerate. This reactional state generally occurs after the initiation of effective antimicrobial therapy and therefore is thought to be associated with the release of antigen from dead and dying bacilli.

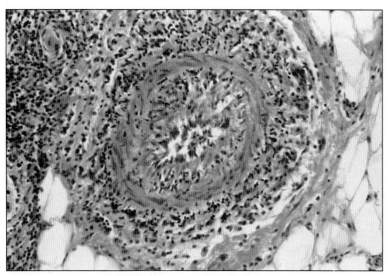

FIGURE 11-32 A blood vessel in erythema nodosum leprosum (ENL) exhibits edema and infiltration of the vascular wall with acute inflammatory cells as well as endothelial cell hyperplasia and narrowing of the lumen. In ENL, complement and immunoglobulin G can be demonstrated in the walls of small blood vessels.

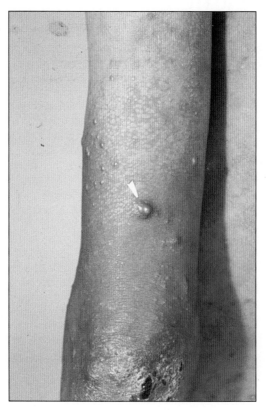

FIGURE 11-33
Histoid nodules of lepromatous leprosy. Histoid nodules and papules are seen on the arm of a patient previously treated with dapsone. These characteristic, shiny, asymmetric lesions are generally seen in relapsed lepromatous leprosy and not in *de novo* disease.

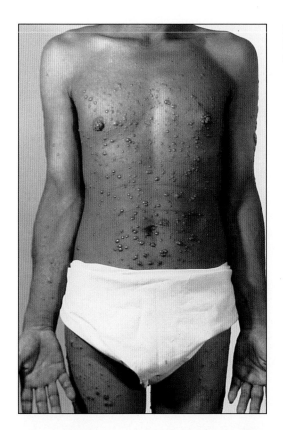

FIGURE 11-34 Florid and atypically widespread and symmetric distribution of discrete, "shiny" histoid lesions is seen in a relapsed lepromatous patient, who had previously been treated with dapsone.

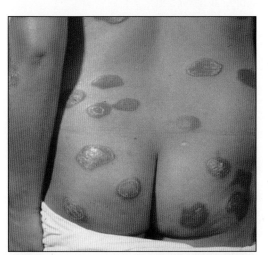

FIGURE 11-35 Lepra type-1 reaction (reversal reaction): multiple, moderately inflamed, sharply demarcated, subsiding reactional lesions are seen in a patient with borderline tuberculoid leprosy. Lepra type-1 reactions may occur prior to therapy as patients are becoming more lepromatous (downgrading reactions), or during therapy as the histopathologic picture is shifting toward the tuberculoid end of the spectrum (reversal reaction). Symptoms of lepra type-1 reactions are confined to skin inflammation (generally in old borderline lesions, but new "satellite" lesions may also appear), neuritis, and occasionally low-grade fever. If neuritis is untreated for as little as 24 hours, irreversible sensory or motor defects may occur.

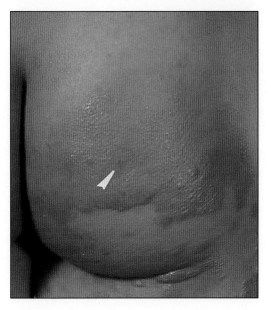

FIGURE 11-36 In a lepra type-1 reaction, an extensive and succulent inflamed plaque with a sharply demarcated, clear central area is seen in a patient with borderline (BB) leprosy. The peripheral edges of this lesion are sloping into surrounding normal skin with a central uninvolved, anesthetic area. Lepra type-1 reactions affect only borderline patients (borderline tuberculoid, BB, and borderline lepromatous) and not tuberculoid or lepromatous patients. Reversal reactions are associated with locally increased numbers of CD-4+ γ-T-helper cells and γ/δ cells, as well as increased levels of interferon-γ and interleukin-2. (Modlin RL, Pirmez C, Hofman FM, *et al.*: Lymphocytes bearing antigen-specific γ/δ T-cell receptors in human infectious disease lesions. *Nature* 1989, 339:544–548.) Corticosteroids are the only effective therapy for lepra type-1 reactions, and therapy must be maintained for a minimum of 2 months lest relapse commonly occur. The strict indications for therapy of lepra type-1 reactions are inflammation on cosmetically important places, such as the face, severe inflammation threatening to ulcerate, or neuritis.

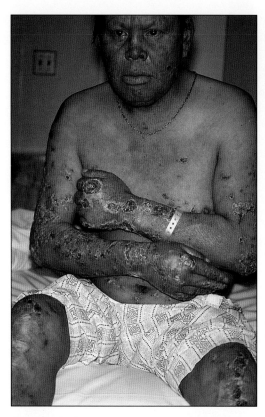

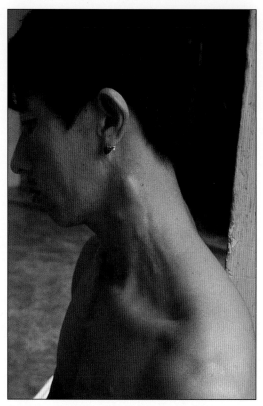

FIGURE 11-37 Lucio's reaction. A patient from Mexico has this almost exclusively Mexican reaction. The shallow ulcerations generated by this reaction may be confined to the legs or generalized as in this patient; often they occur prior to therapy in lepromatous patients with diffuse lepromatosis and may become secondarily infected, resulting in bacteremia and commonly death. This dermal ischemic infarction may result from a leukocytoclastic vasculitis or, alternatively, thrombosis of superficial vessels. The Lucio's phenomenon has been associated with extraordinarily high levels of circulating cryoglobulins. Neither thalidomide nor corticosteroids are effective therapy, but plasmapheresis has occasionally been successful.

FIGURE 11-38 Large peripheral nerves in leprosy. The swelling in the neck is a huge posterior auricular nerve, this nerve generally being neither visible nor palpable. Leprosy is the only disease (except for a few rare hereditary neuropathies) that results in enlarged peripheral nerves. Almost all the morbidity of leprosy is due to *M. leprae's* unique tropism, among bacteria, for peripheral nerves and its resultant peripheral neuropathy. In leprosy, large nerve trunks, small superficial nerve twigs, and microscopic dermal nerves may be pathologically enlarged. The most commonly involved and enlarged peripheral nerve trunks include the ulnar nerve at the elbow, superficial radial nerve at the wrist, peroneal nerve just below the knee, sural nerve in the posterior calf, and posterior tibial nerve just behind the medial malleolus at the ankle.

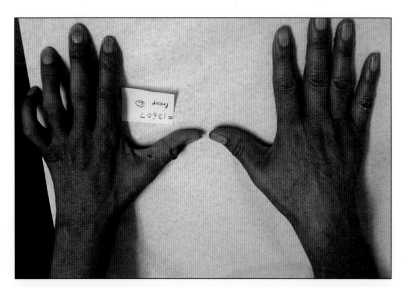

FIGURE 11-39 Clawed hand deformity in leprosy. This patient shows clawing of the left fourth and (particularly) fifth fingers, loss of left dorsal interosseous musculature (especially first dorsal interosseous muscle), and anesthesia of the fourth and fifth fingers. This deformity and malfunction are a consequence of leprous involvement of the ulnar nerve, the most common trunk involved pathologically in leprosy. If the joints of the hand are flexible, tendon transfers can straighten the fingers and improve function.

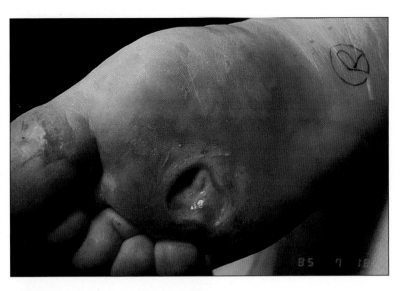

FIGURE 11-40 Plantar ulceration in leprosy. Plantar ulcerations, generally seen over the metatarsal heads, are one of the major causes of morbidity in leprosy and occur in patients with insensitive feet. As in this patient, they may become secondarily infected, result in osteomyelitis, and at times even require amputation. Therapy for plantar ulceration requires nonweight-bearing, ideally in a total-contact walking cast, and appropriate antibiotics. When plantar ulcers are healed, shaving recurrent callus formation and providing patients with specially molded shoes assist in preventing recurrences.

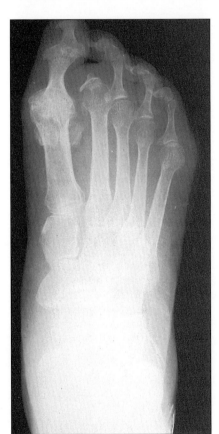

FIGURE 11-41 Bone abnormalities in leprosy. A radiograph of the right foot of a woman with lepromatous leprosy demonstrates loss of bony architecture of distal digits, including amputation of the second digit distal to the base of the proximal phalanx and tapering of the distal phalanges of digits 3–5. These processes are believed to be a consequence of insensitivity and trauma. An additional process seen in leprosy is subarticular collapse, which results in a moderate hallux valgus deformity and lateral plantar subluxation. Patients with leprosy may also develop osteomyelitis and Charcot joints. Patients with lepromatous leprosy have destructive lesions of bones, most commonly of the small bones of the hands and feet.

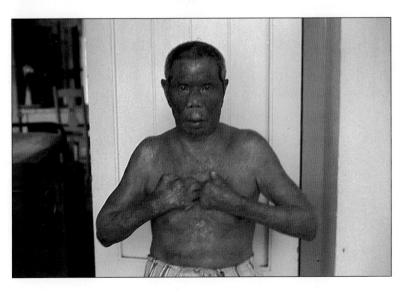

FIGURE 11-42 Among other complications of lepromatous leprosy are loss of digits and a saddle-nose deformity, seen in a patient whose disease went long untreated. Clofazimine pigmentation of the skin is evident, wherein it may accumulate in a patchy distribution, particularly evident in lesional areas. This discoloration is often unacceptable to certain lighter-skinned patients.

TREATMENT

Treatment of adult leprosy

Source	Paucibacillary, no AFB present (generally TT and BT)	Multibacillary, AFB present (generally BL and LL)
WHO	Dapsone, 100 mg/d, and supervised rifampin, 600 mg/mo for 6 mo	Dapsone 100 mg/d, with clofazimine, 50 mg/d, and supervised rifampin, 600 mg, plus clofazimine, 300 mg/mo; therapy to be continued at least 2 yr or until smears negative (generally 5 yr)
Gelber	Dapsone, 100 mg/d for 5 yr	Dapsone, 100 mg/d for life, and rifampin, 600 mg/d for 3 yr or until AFB skin smears negative

FIGURE 11-43 Two commonly advocated antimicrobial regimens to treat leprosy. The intensity of therapy proposed depends on the levels of bacteria present and the presence or absence of effective cell-mediated immunity. Multibacillary leprosy requires multidrug therapy for a prolonged time. The course of therapy for paucibacillary disease can be significantly shorter, and one effective antimicrobial is generally considered sufficient. (AFB—acid-fast bacilli; BL—borderline lepromatous; BT—borderline tuberculoid; LL—lepromatous; TT—tuberculoid.) (World Health Organization Expert Committee on Leprosy: *Sixth Report* [Technical Report Series no. 768]. Geneva: WHO; 1988. Gelber RH: The chemotherapy of lepromatous leprosy: Recent developments and prospects for the future. *Eur J Clin Microbiol Infect Dis* 1994, in press.)

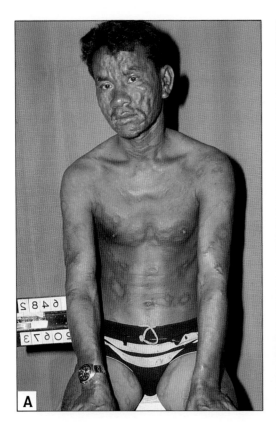
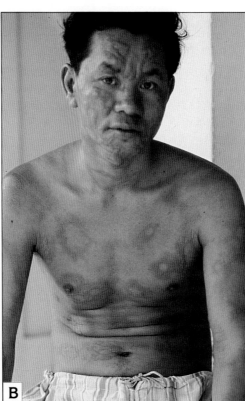

FIGURE 11-44 Response to therapy. **A,** A patient with borderline lepromatous leprosy; his face is infiltrated and, indeed, as in lepromatous leprosy, "leonine," whereas the trunk has a more borderline appearance. **B,** The same patient is shown after several months of effective antimicrobial therapy. There is a dramatic reduction of the dermal infiltration of the face. Indeed, lepromatous nodules and plaques regularly resolve with effective treatment, whereas tuberculoid lesions may resolve entirely, partially, or change little on therapy.

EPIDEMIOLOGY AND PATHOGENESIS

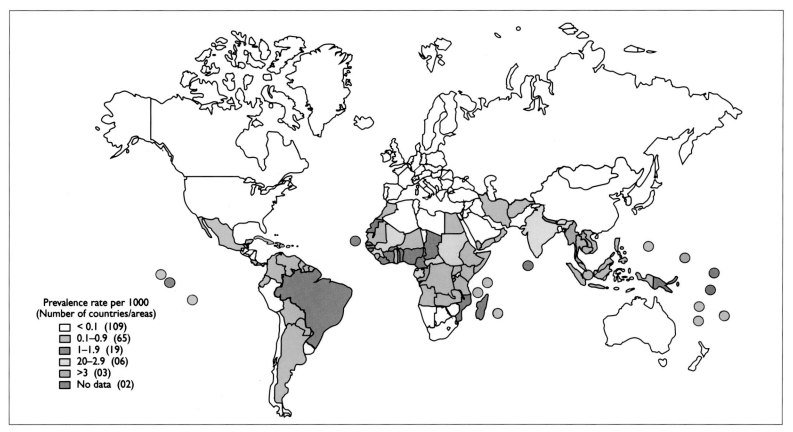

Prevalence rate per 1000
(Number of countries/areas)
- ☐ < 0.1 (109)
- ☐ 0.1–0.9 (65)
- ☐ 1–1.9 (19)
- ☐ 20–2.9 (06)
- ☐ >3 (03)
- ☐ No data (02)

FIGURE 11-45 The worldwide distribution of leprosy. Five to 6 million patients worldwide require therapy. Leprosy is a disease of the developing world, where 80% of patients live in five countries: India (60%), Myanmar, Indonesia, Brazil, and Nigeria. The tuberculoid form of leprosy is equally divided among the sexes, whereas the lepromatous form is twice as common in men.

In India and Africa, roughly 90% of the patients have tuberculoid leprosy; in China and Southeast Asia, the ratio of tuberculoid to lepromatous patients is approximately 1:1; whereas in Mexico, almost 90% of patients have lepromatous disease. (Noordeen SK: A look at world leprosy. *Lepr Rev* 1991, 62:72–86.)

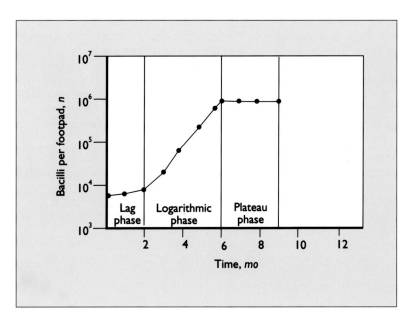

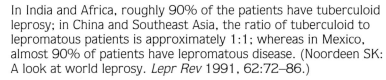
FIGURE 11-46 *Mycobacterium leprae* multiples in mouse footpads. Unfortunately, the organism cannot be grown on artificial media or in tissue culture. When 5000 *M. leprae* are inoculated into the hind footpads of mice, they multiply to 10^6 bacilli in 6 months. (Shepard CC: The experimental disease that follows the injection of human leprosy bacilli into foot-pads of mice. *J Exp Med* 1960, 112:445–454.) This model has proved useful in evaluating antimicrobials for potential activity against *M. leprae*, providing "drug sensitivities" for clinical isolates, monitoring viability of *M. leprae* in clinical trials, and evaluating potential vaccine candidates. In the nude mouse and neonatally thymectomized Lewis rat (NTLR), *M. leprae* grows to much greater levels and disseminates, providing a model more akin to the lepromatous patient; the NTLR provides the most sensitive means to monitor *M. leprae* viability in clinical trials.

Phenolic glycolipid I

$$O - \langle\bigcirc\rangle - (CH_2)_{18} - CH - CH_2 - CH - (CH_2)_4 - CH - CH - CH_2 - CH$$

with OCH_3, Trisaccharide, Acyl, Acyl, CH_3 labels

Trisaccharide

Trisaccharide
3,6 di O Me Glu (1-4) 2,3 di Me Rha (1-2) 3 O Me Rha

FIGURE 11-47 *M. leprae*–specific glycolipid. Almost 2% of *M. leprae* is composed of this unique phenolic glycolipid (PG), which is largely contained in *M. leprae's* outer capsule and is also excreted extracellularly. (Hunter SW, Fujiwara T, Brennan PJ: Structure and antigenicity of the major specific glycolipid antigen of *Mycobacterium leprae. J Biol Chem* 1982, 257:15072–15078.) The unique nature of the terminal trisaccharide, and particularly the terminal sugar, has provided the means to develop a serologic test for leprosy. (Cho SN, Fujiwara T, Gelbert RH, *et al.*: Use of an artificial antigen containing the 3,6-di-O-methyl-beta-D-glycopyranosyl epitope for the serodiagnosis of leprosy. *J Infect Dis* 1984, 150:311–322.) Almost all untreated lepromatous patients have serum antibody to PG-1, which is mostly immunoglobulin M and antibody to PG-1. However, 60% of tuberculoid and borderline tuberculoid patients have antibody, and patients without disease in endemic countries may have circulating antibody. Skin testing with killed *M. leprae* (lepromin) also has little utility, because lepromatous patients have negative skin tests, tuberculoid patients are positive, and unaffected individuals in endemic countries may be either positive or negative.

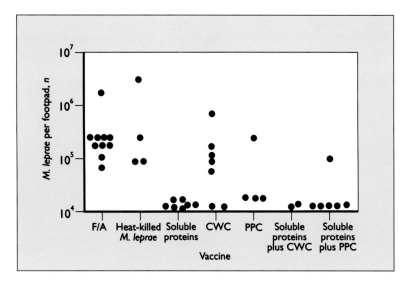

FIGURE 11-48 Leprosy vaccines effective in mice. The long-term protection of mice from the local footpad multiplication of *M. leprae* was achieved by vaccination with certain *M. leprae* subunits, largely proteins (soluble proteins) emulsified in Freund's incomplete adjuvant. Bacille Calmette-Guérin (BCG) has been at best moderately effective as a leprosy vaccine. (Noordeen SK: Vaccination against leprosy: Recent advances and practical applications. *Lepr Rev* 1985, 56:703–710.) As a leprosy vaccine, heat-killed *M. leprae* together with BCG has proved no more effective than vaccination with BCG alone. (Convit J, Sampson C, Zuniga M, *et al.*: Immunoprophylactic trial with combined *Mycobacterium leprae*/BCG vaccine against leprosy: Preliminary results. *Lancet* 1992, 339:446–450.) Vaccination with soluble proteins of *M. leprae* has proved to provide more solid and long-lasting protection than *M. leprae* itself, various single *M. leprae* proteins, cell wall core (CWC), or protein peptidoglycan complex (PPC) in the murine model. (Gelber RH, Murray L, Siu P, *et al.*: Vaccination of mice with a soluble protein fraction of *Mycobacterium leprae* provides consistent and long-term protection against *M. leprae* infection. *Infect Immun* 1992, 60:1840–1844. Gelber RH, Mehra V, Bloom B, *et al.*: Vaccination with pure *M. leprae* proteins inhibits *M. leprae* multiplication in mouse footpads. *Infect Immun* 1994, in press.) Perhaps these findings are due to the presence in mycobacteria of certain fats and carbohydrates known to be immunosuppressant *in vitro* to both lymphocytes and macrophages. A newer generation mycobacterial vaccine devoid of these products and containing important protein epitopes may yet prove effective against leprosy and perhaps even tuberculosis.

T-cell cytokine patterns

T_H1	**Augments CMI**
IFN-γ	Macrophage activation
IL-2	T-cell growth
LT	Cytotoxicity
T_H2	Augments humoral immunity
IL-4	B-cell activation, IgE production
	Macrophage suppression
IL-5	Eosinophil differentiation
IL-10	Inhibits IFN-γ production
	Macrophage suppression
	B-cell activation
	Inhibits CMI

FIGURE 11-49 Functional types of T cells determine their cytokine production and immune activity. The T_H1 pattern, as exemplified by interferon-γ, interleukin-2 (IL-2), and lymphotoxin (LT), augments delayed-type hypersensitivity. In contrast, the T_H2 pattern augments humoral immunity and inhibits delayed-type hypersensitivity. (CMI—cell-mediated immunity.)

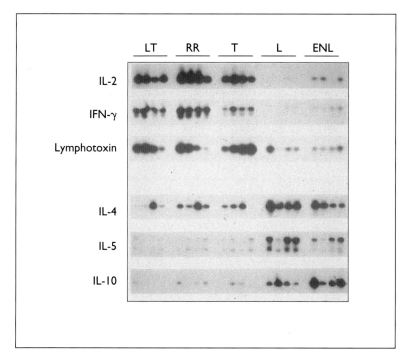

Figure 11-50 Gels of "cytokine-coding mRNA." A cDNA product is obtained by applying reverse transcriptase to dermal tissue slices, then amplifying the cDNA by polymerase chain reaction using probes coding for the cytokine of interest. Visualization and quantification are by hybridization with radioactive cDNA probes. Normalization for cell number is by measuring mRNA for β-actin. Normalization for T-cell numbers is by measuring mRNA coding for the CD3 delta peptide. By inspection, the T_H1 pattern is dominant in lepromin skin tests (LT), reversal reactions (RR), and tuberculoid (T) lesions, and the T_H2 pattern is dominant in lepromatous (L) lesions and erythema nodosum leprosum (ENL). (Yamamura M, Wang X-H, Ohmen J, *et al.*: Cytokine patterns of immunologically mediated tissue damage. *J Immunol* 1992, 149:1470–1475.)

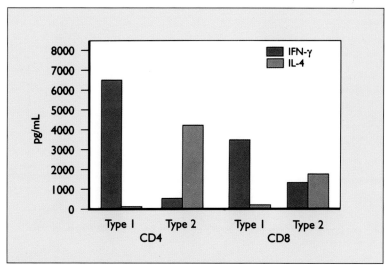

Figure 11-51 Interferon-γ (IFN-γ) and interleukin-4 (IL-4) produced by anti-CD3-stimulated CD4[+] clones from tuberculoid skin lesions and CD8[+] clones from lepromatous lesions. When IFN-γ is used as a marker for T_H1 and IL-4 as a marker for T_H2, it is evident that both CD4[+] and CD8[+] clones may be either T_H1 or T_H2 in cytokine pattern. (Yamamura M, Uyemura K, Deans RJ, *et al.*: Defining protective responses to pathogens: Cytokine profiles in leprosy lesions. *Science* 1991, 254:277–279.)

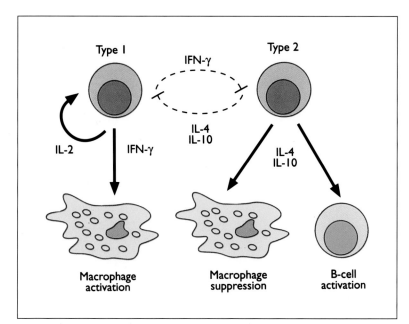

Figure 11-52 Patterns of T-cell cytokine activity. The T_H1 cytokines stimulate CD4 cells, activate macrophages, and inhibit T_H2 pattern expression. Reciprocally, T_H2 cytokines stimulate antibody production, suppress macrophages, and inhibit T_H1 pattern expression.

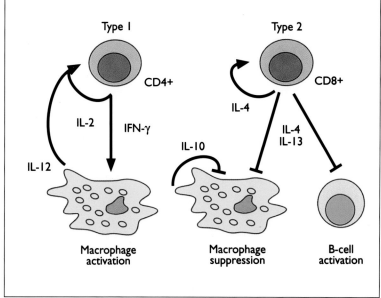

Figure 11-53 A more detailed accounting of T-cell cytokine patterns shows (1) autocrine stimulation of T_H1 and T_H2 patterns by IL-2 and IL-4, respectively; (2) stimulation of T_H1 response by IL-12; and (3) inhibition of macrophages by IL-4, IL-10, and IL-13.

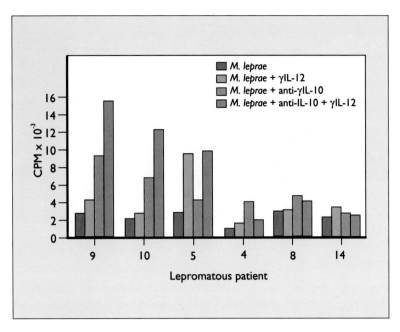

FIGURE 11-54 In peripheral blood mononuclear cells (PBMCs) from three lepromatous patients (patients 9, 10, and 5), the addition γIL-12, anti-IL-10, or the combination of γIL-12 and anti-IL-10 augments the proliferative response to *M. leprae*. In three lepromatous patients (patients 4, 8, and 14) whose PBMCs respond to purified protein derivative (PPD), no such augmentation is seen, suggesting that *M. leprae's* unresponsiveness may involve other cytokines as well. (Modlin RL, Personal communication.)

ACKNOWLEDGMENTS

Slides 1–36 are reproduced with courtesy of the Leonard Wood Memorial/Eversley Child's Sanatorium Laboratory for Leprosy Research, and the Sasakawa Memorial Health Foundation, Cebu, the Philippines. These illustrations originally appeared in *An Atlas of Leprosy*, published in 1983 by these organizations.

SELECT BIBLIOGRAPHY

Hastings RC (ed.): *Leprosy.* New York: Churchill-Livingstone; 1985.

Gelber RH: Leprosy (Hansen's disease). *In* Mandell GL, Douglas RG Jr., Bennett JE (eds.): *Principles and Practice of Infectious Disease*, 4th ed. New York: Churchill-Livingstone; 1994.

Ridley DS, Jopling WH: Classification of leprosy according to immunity. *Int J Lepr Other Mycobact Dis* 1966, 31:255–273.

Waters MFR, Rees RJW, McDougall AC, *et al.*: Ten years of dapsone in lepromatous leprosy: Clinical, bacteriological and histological assessment and the findings of viable leprosy bacilli. *Lepr Rev* 1974, 45:288–298.

Pattyn SF: Search for effective short-course regimens for the treatment of leprosy. *Int J Lepr Other Mycobact Dis* 1993, 61:76–81.

CHAPTER 12

Spirochetal Infections of the Skin

Michael J. Chiu
Clay J. Cockerell
Karen R. Houpt
Justin D. Radolf

SYPHILIS (*TREPONEMA PALLIDUM* SSP. *PALLIDUM*)

Primary Syphilis

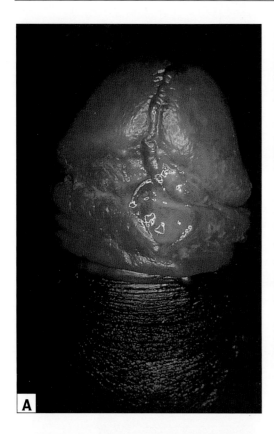

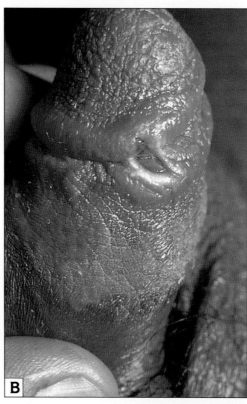

FIGURE 12-1 Classical chancre. **A** and **B**, The chancre represents the first clinical manifestation of syphilis. It begins as a papule that appears after an incubation period averaging 21 days (range, 30–90 days). The typical lesion is a solitary painless ulcer with a clean base and discrete borders that have a rubbery or cartilaginous consistency. In men, penile chancres are found typically on the coronal sulcus, penile shaft, frenulum, or urinary meatus. Chancres may also occur in the anal canal, mouth, and extragenital sites.

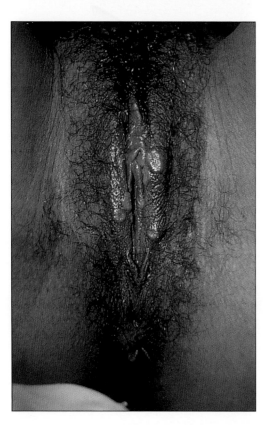

FIGURE 12-2 Multiple chancres in a woman. In women, chancres typically occur on the vulva, labia, or cervix. Painless, nonsuppurative regional adenopathy may develop in half the patients with primary syphilis. Diagnosis of primary syphilis is best confirmed by darkfield examination of lesion exudate. Serologic tests may be negative in as many as 20% to 40% of patients with primary lesions. Multiple lesions occur in up to 30% of patients.

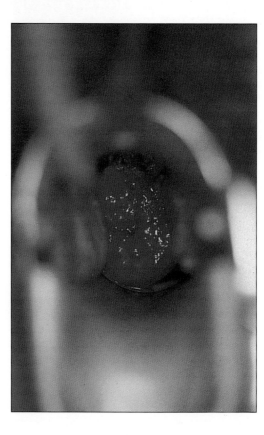

FIGURE 12-3 Cervical chancre. Vaginal or cervical chancres in women are often asymptomatic. Primary syphilis is often not diagnosed in women or homosexual men because lesions are asymptomatic or unrecognized by the patient.

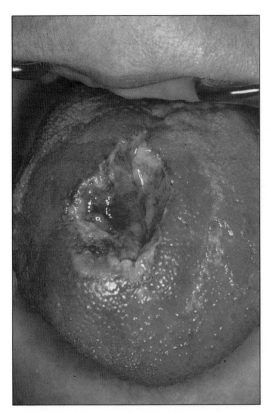

FIGURE 12-4
Tongue chancre. Chancres may appear extragenitally in a small proportion of patients. They occur most commonly in the mouth area, followed in frequency by the chin, cheek, fingers, and nipples. This patient initially presented with a tongue ulcer that was thought to be a malignancy. Biopsy showed histopathologic changes consistent with primary syphilis, and serologic syphilis tests were positive. The patient subsequently admitted to having oral sex with a man with primary syphilis.

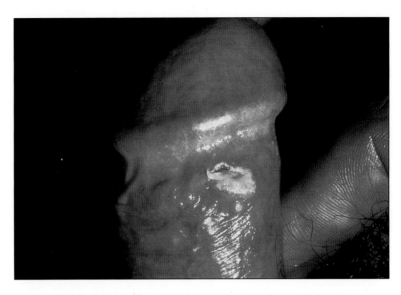

FIGURE 12-5 Superinfected chancre. Although most chancres are painless, superinfected lesions may be painful and have irregular borders. Atypical chancres are quite common, and it is important to have a high index of suspicion that any genital lesion may be syphilitic. Any indolent indurated lesion on the body, especially if accompanied by unilateral adenopathy, should arouse suspicion of syphilis.

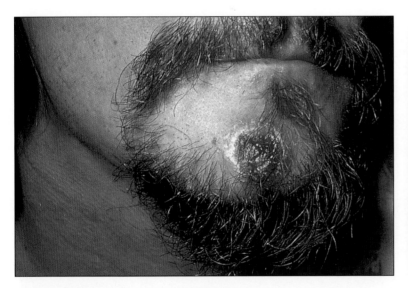

FIGURE 12-6 Healing chancre of the chin. Even without treatment, chancres heal in approximately 4–6 weeks. Lymphadenopathy may persist for months after the chancre disappears.

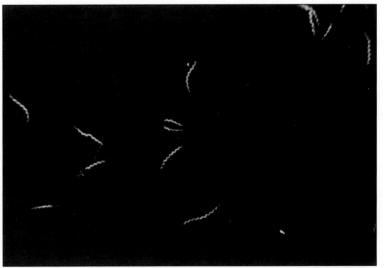

FIGURE 12-7 Darkfield examination. Darkfield microscopy should be performed on specimens taken from lesions on nonmucosal sites, because lesions on mucosal surfaces can yield commensal treponemes that may be mistaken for *Treponema pallidum.* Material for darkfield examination should be obtained from the suspected lesion by cleansing gently with saline and gauze. Exudate from the lesion is then placed on a glass slide and covered with a cover slip. If the specimen is thick, a drop of saline may be added to prevent drying during transit to a microscope fitted with darkfield condenser. The slide should be examined immediately for motile spirochetes. Identification of as few as one motile spirochete is enough to make the diagnosis of syphilis. A negative examination does not eliminate syphilis as a diagnostic possibility, because a minimum of 10,000 organisms/mL of exudate is required for them to be visible with darkfield microscopy.

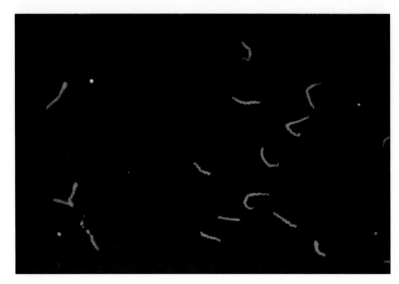

FIGURE 12-8 Direct fluorescent antibody test for *Treponema pallidum*. In this test, spirochetes are detected in clinical material using a *T. pallidum*–specific monoclonal antibody conjugated to fluorescein. Smears from lesions are air-dried and fixed with heat or acetone. After application of the antibody, the slide is examined with fluorescence microscopy. This technique is both more sensitive and specific than darkfield microscopy. Other major advantages of this technique are its ability to detect spirochetes even after they are dead and to differentiate pathogenic from commensal spirochetes. (*Courtesy of* S.A. Lukehart, PhD.)

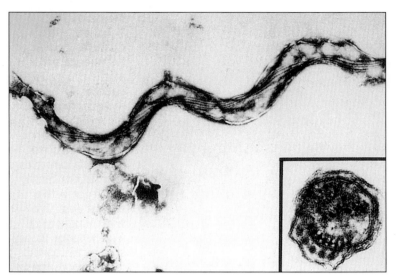

FIGURE 12-9 Electron micrography of virulent *T. pallidum*. Negative-stained whole mount and ultrathin section (*inset*) of a virulent *T. pallidum* from rabbit testes. *T. pallidum* is one of the few human pathogens that cannot be cultivated on artificial media. The organism can be isolated from clinical specimens (blood and cerebrospinal fluid) by intratesticular inoculation of rabbits.

Secondary Syphilis

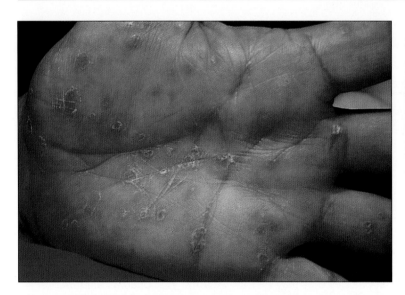

FIGURE 12-10 Palmar lesions of secondary syphilis. Approximately 6–24 weeks after initial infection, usually when chancres are healing or disappeared, clinical manifestations of disseminated disease may appear. Disseminated syphilis can affect virtually any organ but is most commonly recognized by its dermatologic manifestations. One half to two thirds of patients have lesions on the palms and soles, including characteristic erythematous scaly papules.

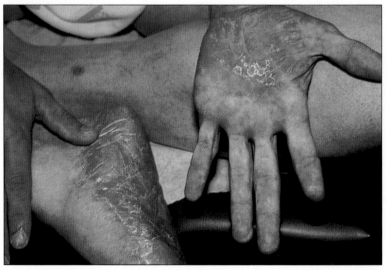

FIGURE 12-11 Secondary syphilis with involvement of the palms and soles. Syphilitic skin involvement is usually described as macular, maculopapular, papular, or papulosquamous. Lesions may be confused with psoriasis, lichen planus, or pityriasis rosea. Even if no treatment is given, signs and symptoms of secondary syphilis will disappear after a period of a few weeks to 12 months. Twenty-five percent of untreated patients will have a clinical relapse within the next few years that is usually less severe than the initial manifestation of secondary syphilis.

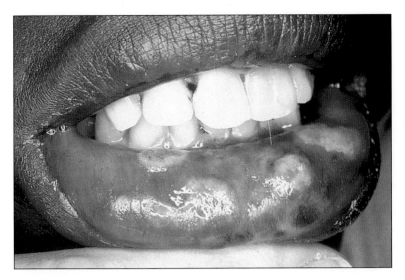

FIGURE 12-12 Mucous patches. Mucous patches are superficial erosions of the oral or genital mucosa. These are the most infectious lesions of secondary syphilis and may be seen in up to 35% of patients with secondary syphilis. Lesions are typically painless. Darkfield examination of these lesions is complicated by the fact that normal commensal spirochete species may be confused with *T. pallidum*.

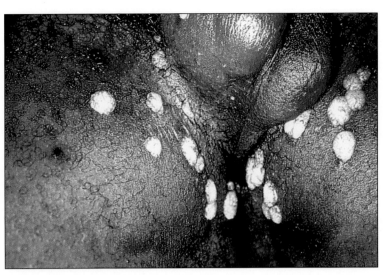

FIGURE 12-13 Condyloma lata. In a small percentage of patients, moist, papular, erythematous plaques known as condyloma lata develop. Typically, these lesions developed in intertriginous areas and are highly infectious. Invariably spirochetes are identified with darkfield microscopy.

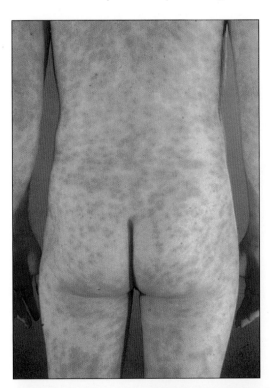

FIGURE 12-14 Diffuse maculopapular eruption of secondary syphilis. Approximately 60% to 70% of secondary syphilis rashes are either macular or maculopapular. Vesicular or bullous lesions do not occur in the adult forms of secondary syphilis.

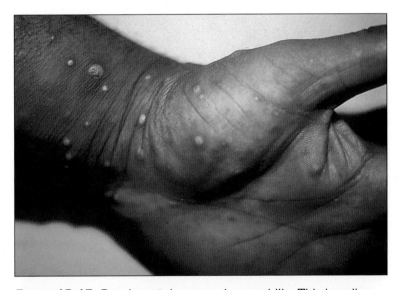

FIGURE 12-15 Papulopustular secondary syphilis. This is a distinctly uncommon appearance for secondary syphilis. This type of eruption is seen in < 1% of secondary syphilis patients with cutaneous involvement. This appearance tends to appear in more debilitated patients. (Chapel T: The signs and symptoms of secondary syphilis. *Sex Trans Dis* 1980, 7:161–164.)

FIGURE 12-16 Nodular secondary syphilis. Nodular skin lesions are a very uncommon manifestation of secondary syphilis. This patient was misdiagnosed by a number of physicians until tests for serologic syphilis were finally done. The patient's facial appearance had improved markedly 2 weeks after beginning treatment with 2.4 MU of benzathine penicillin G. (*Courtesy of* M. Eason, RN.)

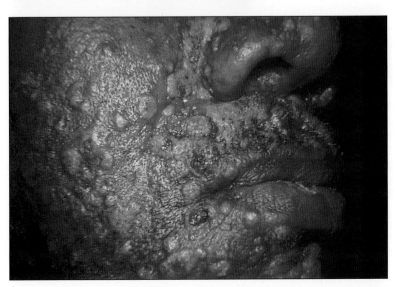

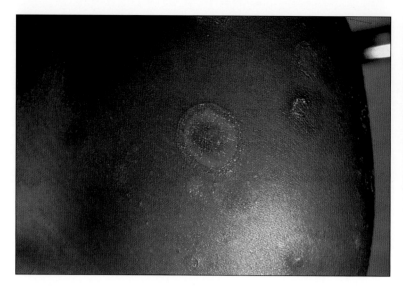

FIGURE 12-17 Annular secondary syphilis. Annular lesions occasionally may occur in secondary syphilis, being present in < 6% of patients with skin involvement. This appearance is more commonly seen in patients of African descent. Lesions are usually seen on the anogenital areas, palms and soles, axilla, and particularly the face. Lesions may be misdiagnosed as sarcoidosis, granuloma annulare, or tinea corporis. (Crissey JT, Denenholz DA: Clinical picture of infectious syphilis. *Clin Dermatol* 1984, 2(1):56.)

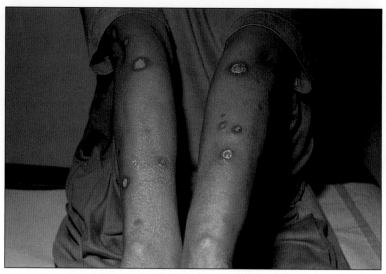

FIGURE 12-18 Lues maligna in an HIV-seropositive patient. Lues maligna (malignant syphilis or syphilis maligna praecox) is a rare, severe form of secondary syphilis. In the prepenicillin era, this severe form of syphilis could progress to death from multiple organ involvement. Histopathologically, a necrotizing vasculitis is seen, which often leads to necrotizing skin lesions and ulcers. This condition is usually seen in debilitated or immunocompromised individuals. (Crissey JT, Denenholz DA: Clinical picture of infectious syphilis. *Clin Dermatol* 1984, 2(1):58–59.)

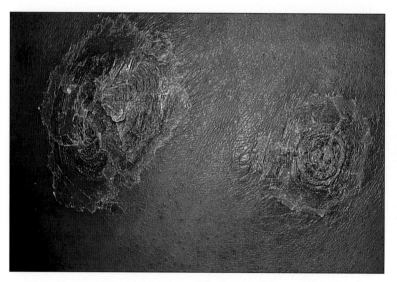

FIGURE 12-19 Rupial secondary syphilis. A very uncommon (< 1%) manifestation of secondary syphilis, rupia describes the thick, dark, raised, amellated, adherent crusts on the skin, which resemble oyster shells.

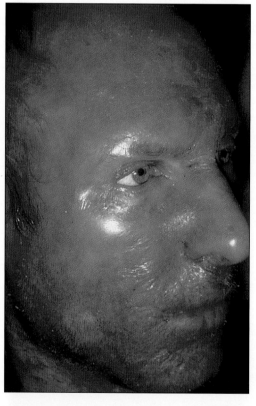

FIGURE 12-20 Eruption of secondary syphilis in a patient with AIDS. Due to the weakened immune system in HIV infection, patients with HIV and syphilis may have more atypical or florid skin rashes. This patient presented with shiny indurated plaques and patchy alopecia. His CD4 count was 92 cells/mm³; VDRL was positive at 1:32. Biopsy revealed a mixed inflammatory cell infiltrate, and Warthin-Starry stain revealed numerous spirochetes in the superficial dermis and epidermis. A number of other case reports exist of very unusual appearances of syphilitic lesions in HIV-seropositive patients. (*From* Glover R, Piaquadio D, Kern S, Cockerell C: An unusual presentation of secondary syphilis in a patient with human immunodeficiency virus infection. *Arch Dermatol* 1992, 128:550–534; with permission.)

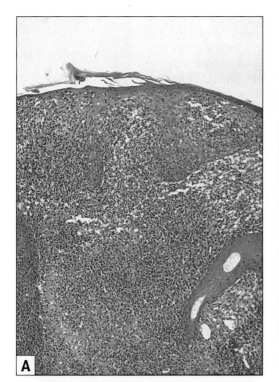

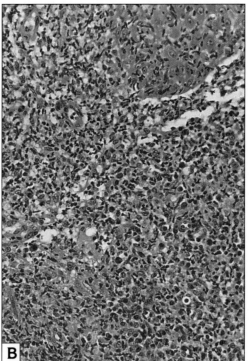

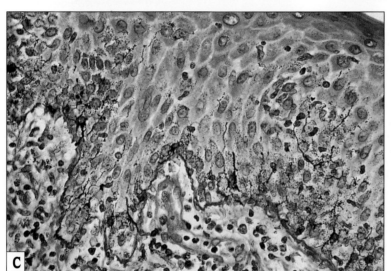

FIGURE 12-21 Histologic appearance of secondary syphilis. **A**, Hematoxylin-eosin staining reveals a superficial and deep, psoriasiform, lichenoid infiltrate comprised of lymphocytes, histiocytes, and numerous plasma cells. (Original magnification, × 20.) **B**, On higher magnification, numerous plasma cells are evident. (Hematoxylin-eosin stain; original magnification, × 400.) **C**, Warthin-Starry staining demonstrates numerous coiled argyrophilic structures in the epidermis and dermis that represent spirochetes. (Original magnification, × 400.)

Tertiary Syphilis

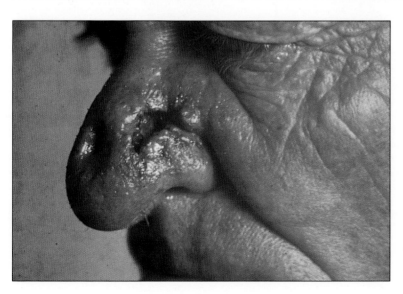

FIGURE 12-22 Gumma of the nose. Gummas, a manifestation of tertiary syphilis, may affect virtually any part of the body. They are typically indolent and painless and develop from 2 to as late as 35 years after initial infection. Manifestations may range from small nodules to deep necrotizing ulcerative lesions. Spirochetes are very difficult to detect in gummas, and it is thought that gummas represent a hypersensitivity reaction to *T. pallidum* antigens in foci of persistent infection. Diagnosis may be confirmed by serologic testing and therapeutic trials. Biopsy specimens can show histopathologic changes suggestive of syphilis (coagulative necrosis with surrounding monocytes and lymphocytes), but findings are not specific for gummatous syphilis. (*Courtesy* of the Centers for Disease Control and Prevention.)

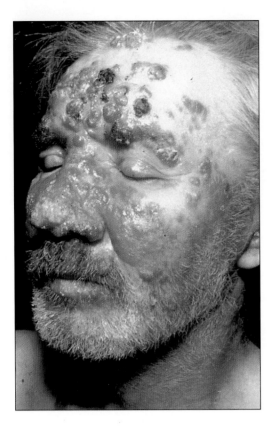

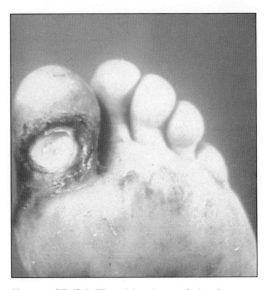

FIGURE 12-23 Nodular gummatous syphilis. Nodules in this form of syphilis may range in size from microscopic to large nodules measuring many centimeters. The nodules are pink or purplish red and tend to appear on the face, upper body, and extremities. The nodules may break down into an ulcerative form. If untreated, the lesion may heal over many weeks or months with significant scarring.

FIGURE 12-24 Trophic ulcer of the foot due to tabes dorsalis. Tabes dorsalis refers to demyelinization of the posterior columns of the spinal cord, dorsal roots, and dorsal root ganglia usually seen 20–25 years after initial syphilitic infection. In advanced stages, loss of vibratory, position, and temperature sensation may develop. Traumatic ulceration of the lower extremities may subsequently develop. (*Courtesy of* the Centers for Disease Control and Prevention.)

Congenital Syphilis

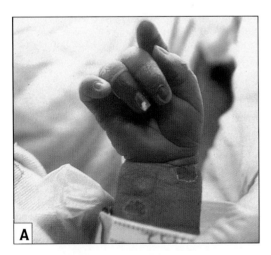
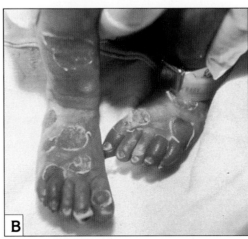
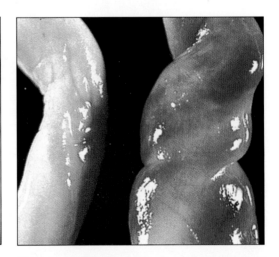

FIGURE 12-25 Vesiculobullous eruption of congenital syphilis. Congenital syphilis is divided into early and late stages. In the early stages, infants may have skin and other systemic manifestations that are similar to those of adult secondary syphilis. The vesiculobullous eruption is virtually pathognomonic for congenital syphilis and is the only bullous skin lesion seen in syphilitic infections. Lesions have a predilection for the palms and soles and may appear very soon after or even at birth. Lesions begin as bullae that may rupture, leaving a macerated, dusky red surface that may dry and form crusts. Fluid in the bullae often yields easily identified spirochetes on darkfield examination. (*Courtesy* of P. Sanchez, MD.)

FIGURE 12-26 Funisitis. A normal umbilical cord (*left*) is compared with a segment of umbilical cord with necrotizing funisitis (*right*). An inflammatory process within the umbilical cord, necrotizing funisitis may produce phlebitis and thrombosis. The gross "barber pole" appearance of the umbilical cord as seen here is highly suggestive of congenital syphilis. (*From* Fojaco RM, Hensley GT, Moskowitz L: Congenital syphilis and necrotizing funisitis. *JAMA* 1989, 261:1788–790; with permission.)

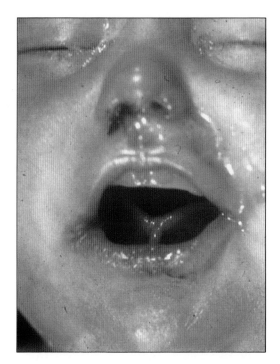

FIGURE 12-27 Snuffles. A syphilitic rhinitis termed "snuffles" may occur in 50% to 60% of infants with early congenital syphilis and is often the first manifestation of early congenital syphilis. Initially, the rhinitis produces a thin, mucoid nasal discharge that is usually attributed to a "cold." The rhinitis responds poorly to symptomatic treatment and progressively becomes more purulent and even blood-tinged. The diagnosis may be made by darkfield examination of the nasal discharge, as the discharge is teeming with virulent organisms.

ENDEMIC TREPONEMATOSES

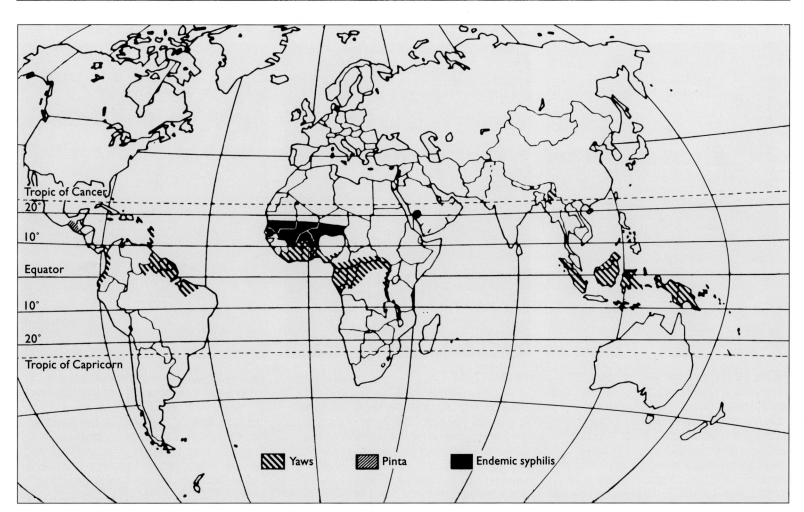

FIGURE 12-28 Geographic distribution of the endemic treponematoses (early 1980s). Endemic treponematoses are infections due to members of the genus *Treponema*. Yaws is caused by *T. pallidum* ssp. *pertenue*, pinta by *T. carateum*, and endemic syphilis by *T. pallidum* ssp. *endemicum*. Aggressive control campaigns since the 1950s have resulted in a decline in the prevalence of the endemic treponematoses. The only known reservoir of these infections is humans. (*From* Perine PL: *Handbook of Endemic Treponematoses: Yaws, Endemic Syphilis, and Pinta*. Geneva: World Health organization; 1984; with permission.)

Yaws (*Treponema pallidum* ssp. *pertenue*)

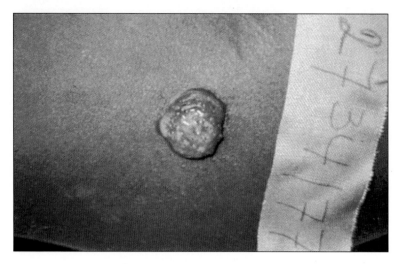

FIGURE 12-29 Initial papillomatous yaws of the upper thigh. This lesion is also called primary frambesioma (raspberry), mother yaw, and chancre pianique. Children are the main reservoir of yaws, and transmission is via direct nonsexual contact. The primary infection begins as a papule that enlarges to become a papillomatous lesion containing many treponemes. The lesion may last for 3–6 months and may heal spontaneously before the appearance of further lesions. (*From* Perine PL: *Handbook of Endemic Teponematoses: Yaws, Endemic Syphilis, and Pinta.* Geneva: World Health Organization; 1984; with permission.)

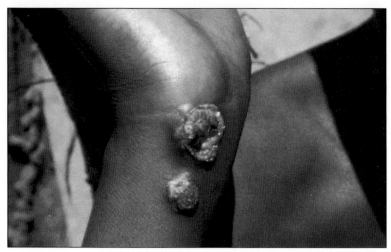

FIGURE 12-30 Early yaws papilloma on the wrist. The site of the initial infection is often a preexisting disruption of the skin, such as lacerations, abrasions, or insect bites. Early lesions are often pruritic, and scratching facilitates spread of the infection to other areas of the body by autoinoculation. Lesions may heal spontaneously, only to recur again at other sites. (*From* Perine PL: *Handbook of Endemic Teponematoses: Yaws, Endemic Syphilis, and Pinta.* Geneva: World Health Organization; 1984; with permission.)

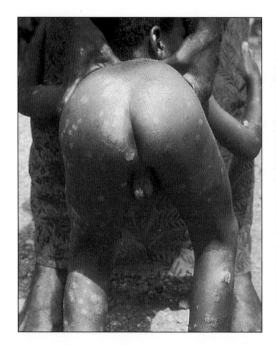

FIGURE 12-31 Polymorphous yaws. Early yaws lesions may have papillomatous, macular, papular, squamous, or nodular appearance. Multiple relapses may occur during the 5 years after initial infection. Osteitis and periostitis may also be seen. Histologic examination characteristically shows an infiltrate of mononuclear and plasma cells with many treponemes visualized using special stains. (*From* Perine PL: *Handbook of Endemic Teponematoses: Yaws, Endemic Syphilis, and Pinta.* Geneva: World Health Organization; 1984; with permission.)

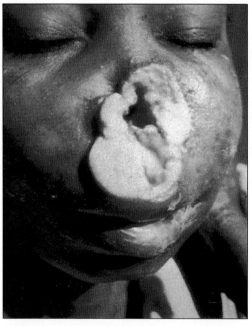

FIGURE 12-32 Gangosa (rhinopharyngitis mutilans). Gangosa in a late complication of yaws, leprosy, leishmaniaisis, or endemic syphilis. The term describes grossly mutilating, ulcerative destruction of the nose, soft and hard palates, and pharynx. Although gangosa is classified as a late yaws lesion, this patient's lesion actually occurred by direct extension of early mucocutaneous yaws lesions into the borders of the nose and mouth, followed by bacterial superinfection and ulceration. (*From* Perine PL: *Handbook of Endemic Teponematoses: Yaws, Endemic Syphilis, and Pinta.* Geneva: World Health Organization; 1984; with permission.)

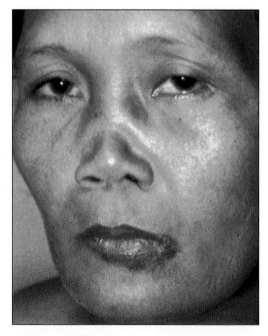

FIGURE 12-33 Goundou. Goundou is a hypertrophic osteitis of the nasal process of the maxilla, which produces bony, hornlike exostoses at the sides of the nose and results in a distinctive facial appearance. Goundou may be seen in yaws or endemic syphilis. The treatment of yaws is a single 2.4-MU dose of intramuscular benzathine penicillin G. (*From* Perine PL: *Handbook of Endemic Teponematoses: Yaws, Endemic Syphilis, and Pinta.* Geneva: World Health Organization; 1984; with permission.)

Pinta (*Treponema carateum*)

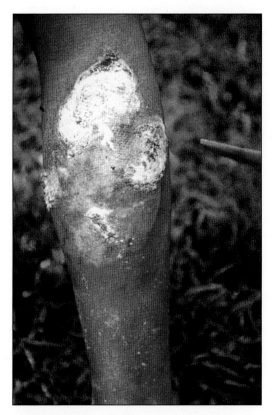

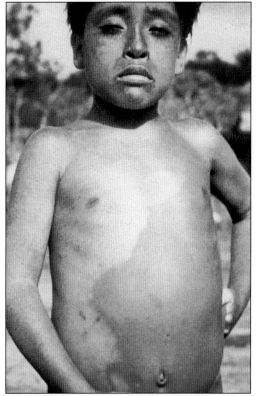

FIGURE 12-34 Violaceous psoriasiform plaque of early pinta on the forearm. Also known as *mal del pinto*, *carate*, or *azul*, pinta is caused by *T. carateum*. Unlike the other treponemal infections, pinta's manifestations are confined only to the skin. The initial lesion is a small papule that increases in size slowly and evolves into a psoriasiform plaque. The main reservoir for pinta is young adults aged 15–30 yrs. Disease transmission is believed to be by contact of broken skin with infectious lesions. (*From* Perine PL: *Handbook of Endemic Treponematoses: Yaws, Endemic Syphilis, and Pinta.* Geneva: World Health Organization; 1984; with permission.)

FIGURE 12-35 Late pigmented pinta-blue variety. Late pinta is characterized by pigmentary changes, with lesion colors changing slowly from a copper color to lead gray or slate blue. The pigmentation changes may progress at different rates in the same lesion, resulting in differing degrees of dyschromia. Pinta produces no disability other than skin disfigurement. Treatment is 2.4 MU of intramuscular benzathine penicillin G, but pinta lesions respond more slowly than other treponematoses. (*From* Perine PL: *Handbook of Endemic Treponematoses: Yaws, Endemic Syphilis, and Pinta.* Geneva: World Health Organization; 1984; with permission.)

LYME DISEASE (*BORRELIA BURGDORFERI*)

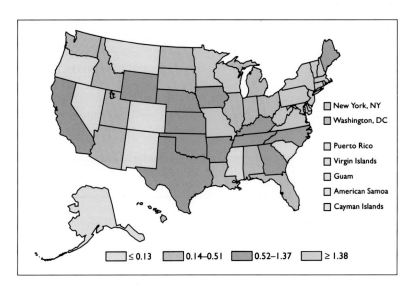

New York, NY
Washington, DC

Puerto Rico
Virgin Islands
Guam
American Samoa
Cayman Islands

≤ 0.13   0.14–0.51   0.52–1.37   ≥ 1.38

FIGURE 12-36 Geographic distribution of Lyme disease, United States, 1992. Lyme disease (or lyme borreliosis) is a multisystem illness due to *Borrelia burgdorferi*. This spirochetal illness is transmitted via ticks of the genus *Ixodes*. Currently, Lyme disease is the most prevalent arthropod-borne infection in the United States with 14,000 cases reported to the Centers for Disease Control and Prevention between 1980 and 1990. (*From* the Centers for Disease Control and Prevention: Summary of notifiable disease, United States, 1992. *MMWR* 1992, 41(55):37; with permission.)

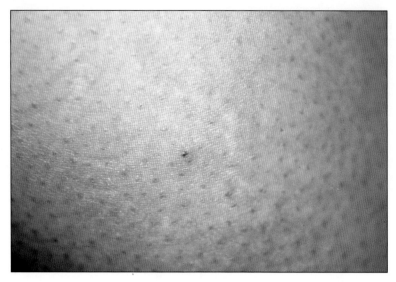

FIGURE 12-37 Tick *in situ* with surrounding erythema migrans. The major reservoirs of *B. burgdorferi* are the white-footed mouse and white-tailed deer. Humans are infected via *ixodid* ticks incidentally. The ixodid ticks are very small, and the preceding tick bite is often unnoticed by the patient. Three to 30 days after the tick bite, *B. burgdorferi* migrates outward, producing a characteristic, centrifugally expanding annular lesion know as erythema migrans. Lesions may become quite large (occasionally 60 cm in diameter), and central clearing occurs in may cases.

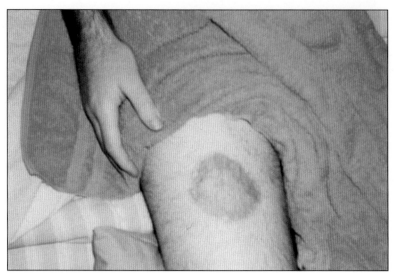

FIGURE 12-38 Erythema migrans. A burning sensation, itching, or pain may be noted over the lesion. Approximately 75% of patients with Lyme disease manifest this pathognomonic skin finding. Constitutional symptoms, such as fever, chills, headache, myalgias, arthralgias, fatigue, and lymphadenopathy, are often seen in association with erythema migrans and probably represent hematogenous dissemination of *B. burgdorferi* and systemic release of cytokines. A small percentage of untreated patients experience recurrences of erythema migrans from 1–14 months after the original lesion.

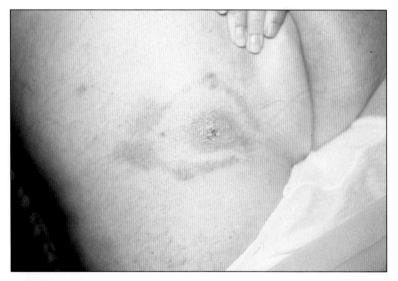

FIGURE 12-39 Erythema migrans with central and vesicle formation. The thigh, groin, and axilla (where ticks characteristically feed) are the most common sites of erythema migrans. Central portions of erythema migrans may have scaling, vesicles, induration, ulceration, or purpura. Erythema migrans may be confused with cellulitis, contact dermatitis, brown recluse spider bite, fixed drug eruptions, or granuloma annulare. Histologic findings in erythema migrans show a superficial and deep perivascular lymphocytic infiltrate that may contain plasma cells, histiocytes, and infrequently mast cells and neutrophils.

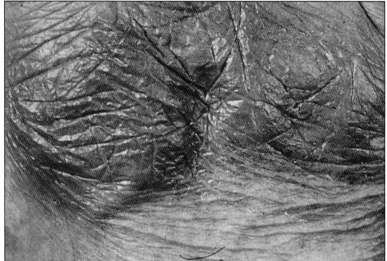

FIGURE 12-40 Acrodermatitis chronica atrophicans (ACA). ACA is a patchy, erythematous, doughy swelling usually seen on the extremities. It is associated with late Lyme disease and has been seen primarily in European patients. Lesions appear 6 months to 8 years after initial infection. Over time, the skin becomes atrophic with a glistening appearance ("cigarette paper skin"). Histologic findings are dermal perivascular lymphocytic infiltrate with plasma cells, telangiectatic endothelial-lined spaces, and mild epidermal thinning. (*From* Malane MS, Grant-Kels JM, Feder HM, Luger SW: Diagnosis of Lyme disease based on dermatologic manifestations. *Ann Intern Med* 1991, 114:490–498; with permission.)

SELECTED BIBLIOGRAPHY

Perine PL: *Handbook of Endemic Treponematoses: Yaws, Endemic Syphilis, and Pinta.* Geneva: World Health Organization; 1984.

Lukehart SA, Holmes KK: Syphilis. *In* Isselbacher KJ, Braunwald E, Wilson JD, *et al.* (eds.): *Harrison's Principles of Internal Medicine,* 13th ed. New York: McGraw-Hill; 1944:726–737.

Holmes KK, Mardh P, Sparling PF, Wiesner PJ: *Sexually Transmitted Diseases,* 2nd ed. New York: McGraw-Hill; 1984.

Steere AC: *Lyme disease.* N Engl J Med 1989, 321:586–596.

CHAPTER 13

Clostridial Infections

Dennis L. Stevens

MICROBIOLOGY

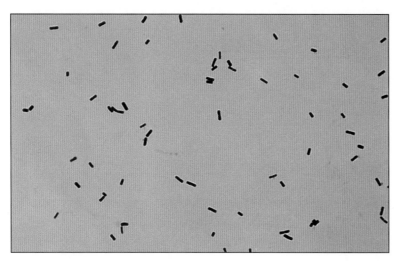

FIGURE 13-1 Gram stain shows large, slender, gram-positive rods characteristic of *Clostridium perfringens*.

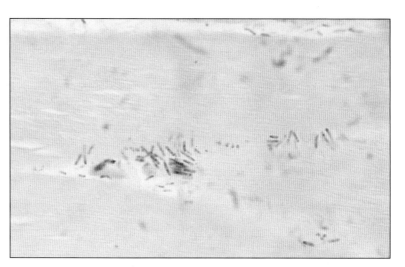

FIGURE 13-2 Tissue Gram stain showing slender rods with subterminal spores. Note that *in vivo C. perfringens* are gram-variable and may be confused with gram-negative rods.

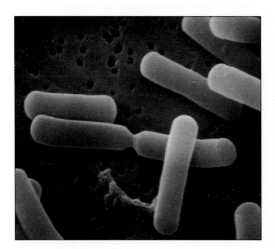

FIGURE 13-3 Scanning electron micrograph of *C. perfringens*.

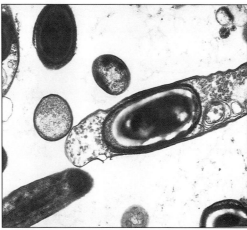

FIGURE 13-4 Transmission electron micrograph showing internal structure of *C. perfringens*. Note the prominent subterminal endospore. Although the bacteria is readily killed by modest heat, endospores are resistant to boiling for several hours and succumb only to a combination of heat and high pressure (autoclaving).

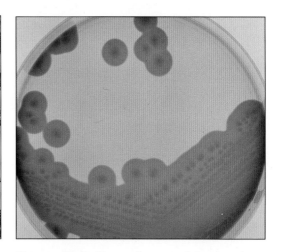

FIGURE 13-5 Egg yolk agar plate showing a positive lecithinase reaction. Lecithin (phosphatidylcholine) is hydrolyzed to phosphorylcholine and diacylglycerol. Diacylglycerol is insoluble and forms the white precipitate in the egg yolk emulsion. The test is positive in strains producing α-toxin (phospholipase C).

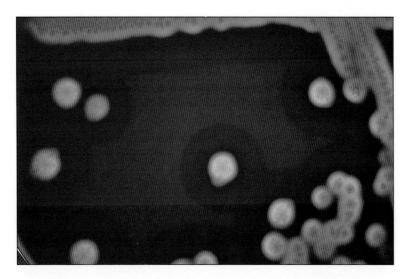

FIGURE 13-6 Blood agar plate incubated with *C. perfringens*. Note the double zone of hemolysis. The outer zone of incomplete hemolysis is due to α-toxin, and the inner zone of clear hemolysis is due to θ-toxin.

GAS GANGRENE (MYONECROSIS)

Types of *Clostridium*-associated gas gangrene

Traumatic
> Caused by *C. perfringens*, *C. septicum*, and *C. histolyticum*
> Trauma is usually crush injury or associated with compromise of blood supply

Spontaneous
> More commonly due to *C. septicum*
> Often associated with metastatic seeding from bowel portal
> Predisposing factors are intra-abdominal tumor, acute leukemia, neutropenia, cancer chemotherapy, or radiation therapy

Recurrent
> More than one episode of gas gangrene

FIGURE 13-7 Gas gangrene caused by *Clostridium* species can occur in three different settings. Traumatic is clearly the most common type of gas gangrene.

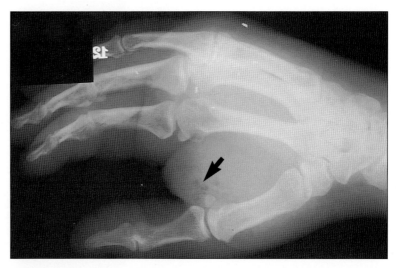

FIGURE 13-8 Recurrent gas gangrene. This patient developed gas gangrene twice. He lost both legs and part of his hand following gas gangrene related to shrapnel wounds in Vietnam. Fourteen years later, he sustained blunt trauma to the palm of his hand. Gas gangrene recurred at the site of retained shrapnel. Note the gas in the tissues (*arrow*).

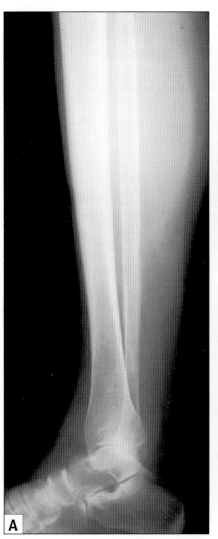

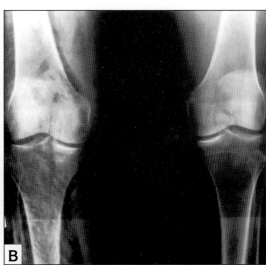

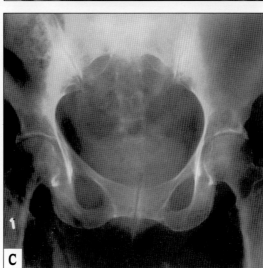

FIGURE 13-9 Traumatic gas gangrene. **A**, A radiograph demonstrates no gas in the tissue of a patient who suffered minor, nonpenetrating trauma to the foot 2 days previously. The patient complained of increasing pain and fever but had no evidence of local infection on physical examination. **B**, Same patient 6 hours later shows that gas (which is now also present in the calf) has extended to the knee. **C**, Four hours later, there is rapid progression with evidence of gas in the soft tissue of the pelvis. The patient died of fulminant shock and renal failure. (*continued*)

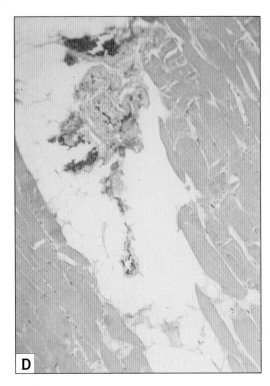

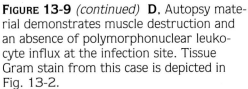

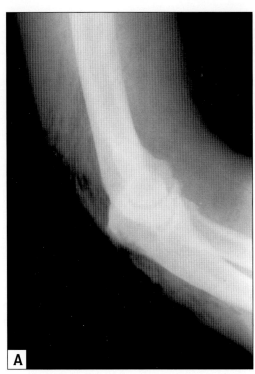

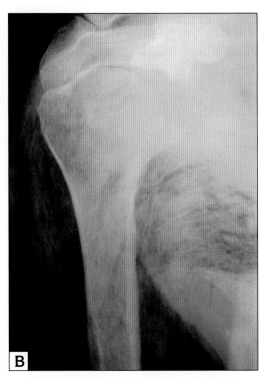

FIGURE 13-9 *(continued)* **D.** Autopsy material demonstrates muscle destruction and an absence of polymorphonuclear leukocyte influx at the infection site. Tissue Gram stain from this case is depicted in Fig. 13-2.

FIGURE 13-10 Spontaneous gas gangrene. **A** and **B,** Radiographs of the elbow (*panel 10A*) and shoulder (*panel 10B*) show gas in tissue. The patient developed spontaneous gas gangrene of the hand, which spread rapidly up the arm and onto the thorax. *C. septicum* was grown from blood and necrotic tissue of the arm.

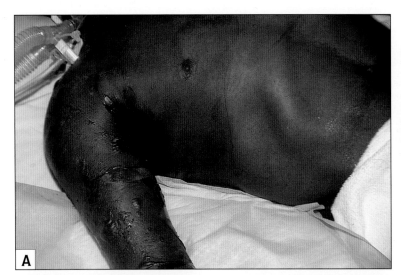

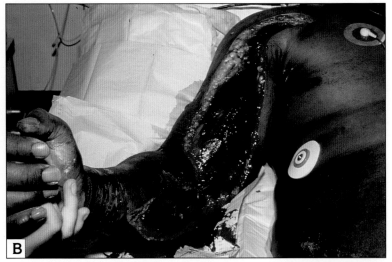

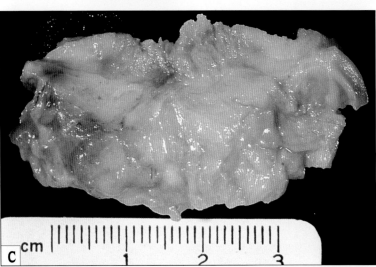

FIGURE 13-11 A, The line of demarcation in the patient shown in Fig. 13-10. The causative organism was *C. septicum*. **B,** The patient received hyperbaric oxygen therapy, antibiotics, and aggressive surgical debridement with disarticulation of the arm at the shoulder. **C,** Two months after recovery, a barium enema demonstrated carcinoma of the colon. (*Courtesy of J. Mader, MD.*)

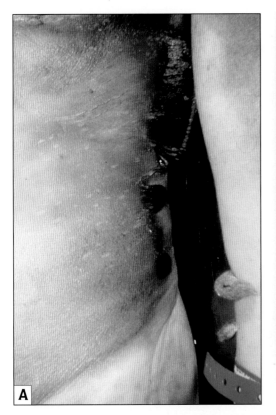
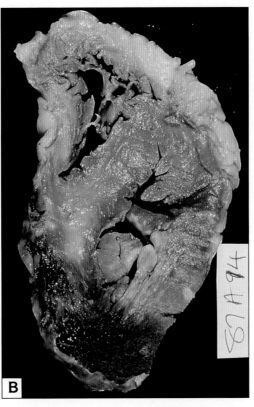

FIGURE 13-12 A, Hemorrhagic bullae formation at the leading edge of progressive gas gangrene in an elderly woman with *C. septicum* bacteremia who died suddenly. **B,** Autopsy revealed gas gangrene of the heart. (*Courtesy* of H. Rosen, MD.)

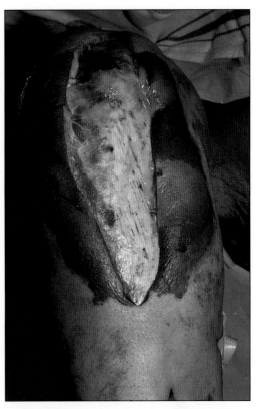

FIGURE 13-13 Spontaneous necrotizing fasciitis due to *C. septicum* in a patient with known carcinoma of the colon. Note the maroon/violaceous color of the skin. This photograph was taken immediately after fasciotomy.

CLOSTRIDIUM SORDELLI–ASSOCIATED TOXIC SHOCK SYNDROME

Clinical features of *Clostridium sordellii*–associated toxic shock syndrome

Massive edema
Hemoconcentration (hematocrit = 60% to 80%)
Leukemoid reaction (leukocytes = 50–90,000/mm³)
Absence of fever
Absence of pain
Late hypotension

FIGURE 13-14 Clinical features of *Clostridium sordellii*–associated toxic shock syndrome.

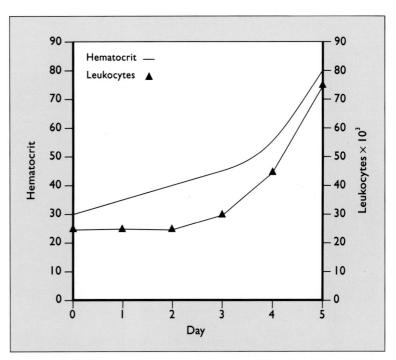

FIGURE 13-15 The dramatic hemoconcentration (*solid line,* HCT—hematocrit) and leukemoid reaction (*triangles*) seen in patients with *C. sordellii* infection. Hemoconcentration is secondary to diffuse capillary leak with loss of albumin and water into the interstitial space. The mechanism of profound leukocytosis is unknown.

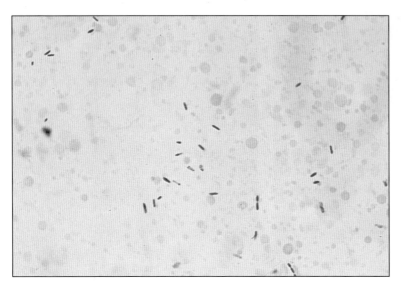

FIGURE 13-16 Tissue Gram stain of edematous tissue from a patient with *C. sordellii* infection. There is an absence of inflammation at the site of infection despite the presence of gram-positive rods.

NONCLOSTRIDIAL NECROTIZING SOFT TISSUE INFECTIONS

Nonclostridial necrotizing soft tissue infections

Gram-negative aerobic infections
    Pasteurella multocida (*see* Chapter 5)
    Pseudomonas
Streptococcal gangrene (*see* Chapter 3)
Mixed staphylococcal/streptococcal infection
Halophilic *Vibrio* infection
Mixed aerobic/anaerobic infections
    Diabetic gangrene
    Postsurgical gangrene
    Fournier's gangrene

FIGURE 13-17 Possible causes of necrotizing soft tissue infections other than *Clostridium* species.

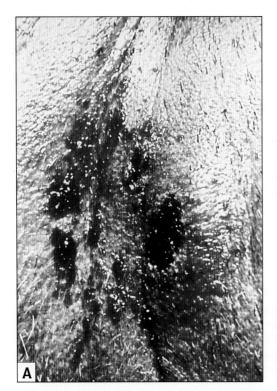

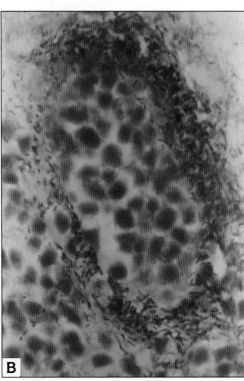

FIGURE 13-18 Cellulitis caused by *Pseudomonas aeruginosa*. **A,** A cutaneous lesion on a patient. Frequently, there is no evidence of necrotizing fasciitis. Often, *Pseudomonas* cellulitis is associated with bacteremia in compromised hosts or with skin lesions in regions such as the axilla and groin or at the site of intravenous drug abuse. **B,** A tissue biopsy specimen demonstrating that ecthyma gangrenosum in *panel 18A* is a venous vasculitis.

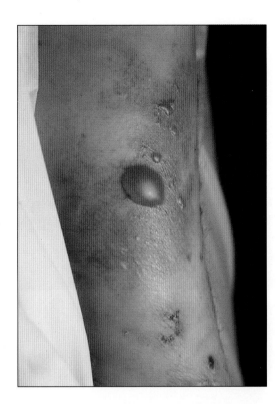

FIGURE 13-19
Bullous lesion from a patient with halophilic vibrio infection (*Vibrio vulnifica*) acquired in the Gulf of Mexico.

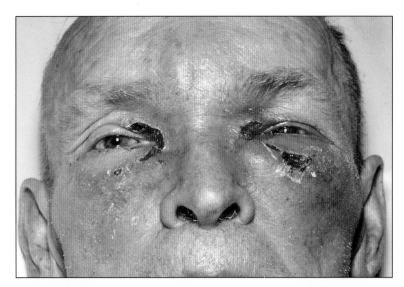

FIGURE 13-20 Mixed staphylococcus/streptococcus soft tissue infection (*see also* Fig. 3-35 in Chapter 3).

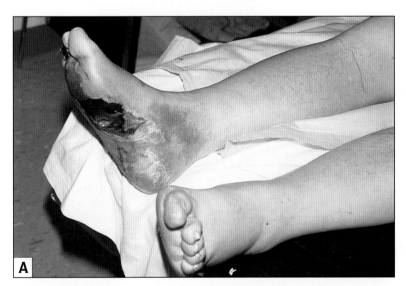

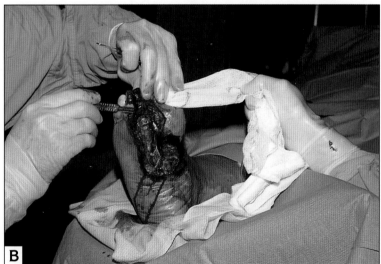

FIGURE 13-21 A, Mixed aerobic/anaerobic infection occurred in this diabetic patient with peripheral neuropathy and peripheral vascular disease. **B**, Emergent surgical debridement was necessary. *Escherichia coli*, group B streptococcus, *Enterococcus faecalis*, *Bacteroides fragilis*, and *Proteus mirabilis* were grown from the biopsy specimen.

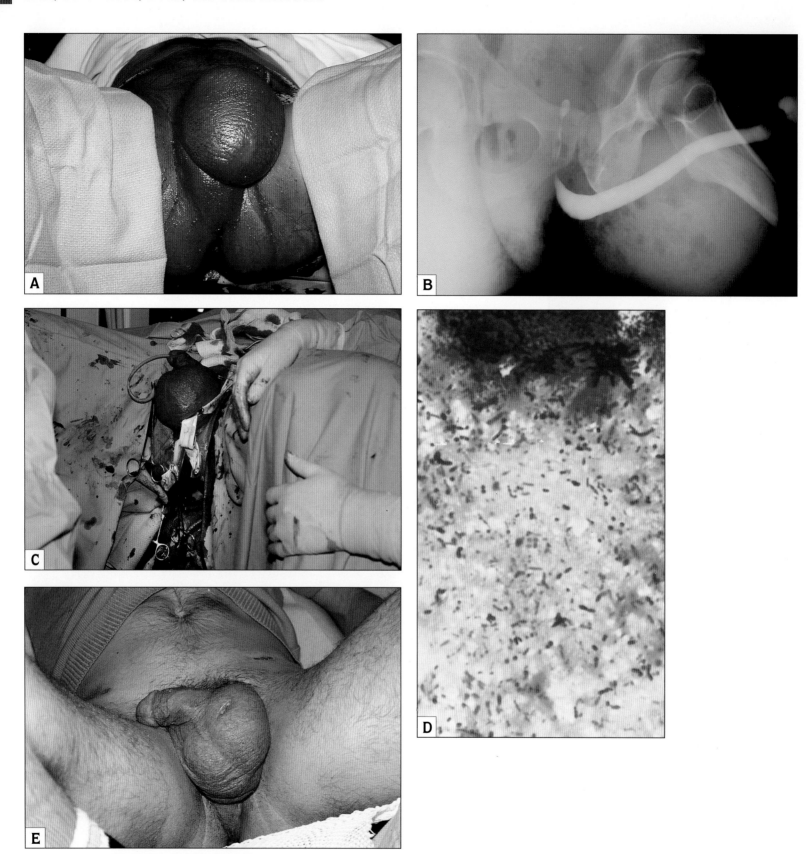

FIGURE 13-22 Fournier's gangrene. **A**, Scrotal swelling in a young man with Fournier's gangrene. The brown color is due to povidone-iodine surgical preparation. **B**, A urethrogram in the same patient demonstrates normal urethral mucosa but gas in the tissues of the thigh, buttocks, and anterior abdominal wall. Infection began in the rectal mucosa at the site of an inflamed hemorrhoid and extended along fascial planes. **C**, Surgical drainage of the scrotal contents revealed blackish material. Penrose drains were placed in the incisions in the anterior abdominal wall, buttocks, and scrotum. The underlying musculature was normal and was not debrided. **D**, Gram stain of the scrotal fluid demonstrates many types of gram-positive and gram-negative bacteria. Cultures grew *Enterococcus faecalis*, *Bacteroides* sp., *Escherichia coli*, and anaerobic streptococci. **E**, After 3 weeks of antibiotic therapy (gentamicin, ampicillin, and clindamycin), the infection has resolved. However, in many cases of Fournier's gangrene, aggressive radical surgery may be indicated.

ACKNOWLEDGMENTS

The author is grateful for the assistance of John Mangan and Michael Wyett for the photography and medical illustrations.

SELECTED BIBLIOGRAPHY

Dellinger EP: Necrotizing soft tissue infections. *In* Davis JM, Shires T (eds.): *Principles and Management of Surgical Infections.* Philadelphia: J.B. Lippincott; 1991:23–31.

Kasper DL, Zaleznik DF: Gas gangrene and other clostridial infections. *In* Braunwald E, *et al.* (eds.): *Harrison's Principles of Internal Medicine,* 13th ed. New York: McGraw-Hill; 1994:636–640.

McGregor JA, Soper DE, Lovell G, Todd JK: Maternal deaths associated with *Clostridium sordellii* infection. *Am J Obstet Gynecol* 1989, 161:987.

Stevens DL: Soft tissue infections. *In* Braunwald E, *et al.* (eds.): *Harrison's Principles of Internal Medicine,* 13th ed. New York: McGraw-Hill; 1994:561–563.

Stevens DL, Musher DM, Watson DA, *et al.*: Spontaneous, nontraumatic gangrene due to *Clostridium septicum. Rev Infect Dis* 1990, 12:286–296.

CHAPTER 14

Osteomyelitis

Jon T. Mader
Rajendra Kumar
David Simmons
Jason Calhoun

Osteomyelitis: Clinical types

Hematogenous osteomyelitis
Osteomyelitis 2° to continuous focus of infection
No generalized vascular disease
Generalized vascular disease
Chronic osteomyelitis (necrotic bone)

FIGURE 14-1 Clinical types of osteomyelitis. Bone infections are currently classified by the Waldvogel system as either hematogenous osteomyelitis or osteomyelitis secondary to a contiguous focus of infection. Contiguous-focus osteomyelitis is subdivided into osteomyelitis with or without vascular insufficiency. Hematogenous and contiguous-focus osteomyelitis are further divided into acute or chronic disease. (Waldvogel FA, Medoff G, Swartz MN: Osteomyelitis: A review of clinical features, therapeutic considerations, and unusual aspects [pts 1–3]. *N Engl J Med* 1970, 282:198–206, 260–266, 316–322.)

BONE INFECTIONS

Hematogenous Osteomyelitis

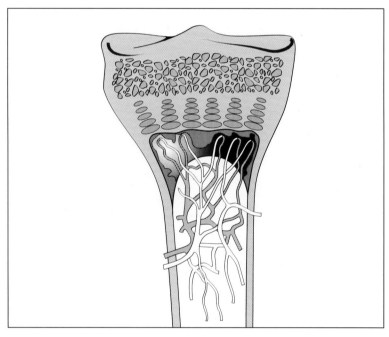

FIGURE 14-2 Pathogenesis of hematogenous osteomyelitis. The location of hematogenous osteomyelitis is explained by the bone anatomy in the metaphysis of the long bone. Nonanastomosing capillary ends of the nutrient artery make sharp loops under the growth plate and enter a system of large venous sinusoid, where the blood flow becomes slow and turbulent. These capillary loops are essentially "end-artery" branches of the nutrient artery. Any end-capillary obstruction can lead to an area of avascular necrosis. The patient is predisposed to infection by minor trauma that produces a small hematoma, vascular obstruction, and subsequent bone necrosis. The area is then susceptible to inoculation from a transient bacteremia. (Trueta J, Morgan JD: The vascular contribution to osteogenesis: I. Studies by the injection method. *J Bone Joint Surg* 1960, 42B:97–109. Hobo T: Zur pathogenese de akuten haematogenen Osteomyelitis, mit Berucksichtigung der Vitalfarbungslehre. *Acta Sch Med Univ Kioto* 1922, 4:1–29.)

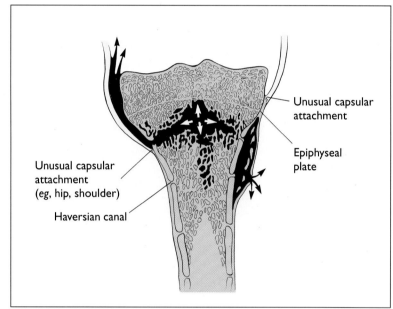

Unusual capsular attachment

Unusual capsular attachment (eg, hip, shoulder)

Epiphyseal plate

Haversian canal

FIGURE 14-3 Routes of spread. The infection may proceed from the metaphysis laterally through the haversian and Volkmann canal systems, perforate the bony cortex, and separate the periosteum from the surface of the bone. When this occurs in the presence of medullary extension, both the periosteal and endosteal circulations are lost and large segments of dead cortical and cancellous bone, termed sequestrum, are formed. The infection may also spread down the intramedullary canal. Because of the anatomy, the joint is usually spared unless the metaphysis is intracapsular. Cortical perforation at the proximal radius, humerus, or femur infects the elbow, shoulder, or hip joint, respectively, regardless of the age of the patient.

Hematogenous osteomyelitis long bone

Age	Localization	Growth plate	Factors spread
Infant (< 1 yr)	Metaphysis	± Capillary perforation	Epiphysis Joint space Diaphysis Subperiosteal space
Child (1–16 yrs)	Metaphysis	No capillary perforation	Diaphysis Subperiosteal space
Adult (> 16 yrs)	Diaphysis	Reabsorption	Diaphysis Periosteal perforation ± Joint space

FIGURE 14-4 Location of hematogenous osteomyelitis by age. In infants, medullary infection may spread to the epiphysis and joint surfaces through capillaries that cross the growth plate. In children over 1 year of age, the growth plate is avascular, and the infection is confined to the metaphysis and diaphysis. In adults, the infection usually begins in the diaphysis but may spread to involve the entire medullary canal. Extension into the adjacent joint may occur because the growth plate has matured and once again shares vessels with the metaphysis. The infection may also spread to the subperiosteum. Infants and children may form large subperiosteal abscess(es) because the periosteum is not firmly attached to the bone. Because the periosteum is firmly adherent to the bone in adults, the infection may erode through the periosteum and lead to a soft-tissue abscess or a draining sinus.

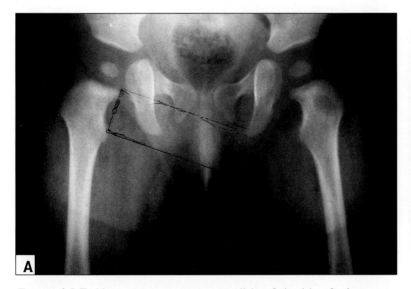
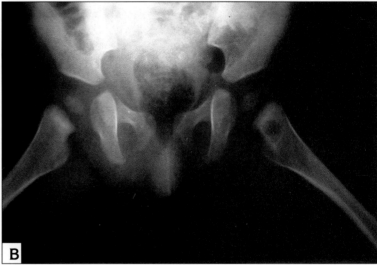

FIGURE 14-5 Hematogenous osteomyelitis of the hip. **A**, Antero-posterior radiograph of the pelvis in a 4-year-old child shows a lytic lesion with minimal sclerosis in the metaphysis of the left proximal femur. **B**, A frog-leg radiograph better demonstrates the lytic lesion in the proximal femur.

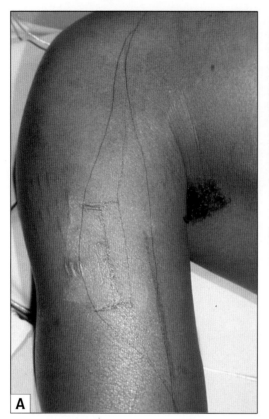

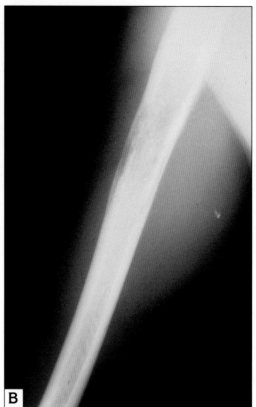

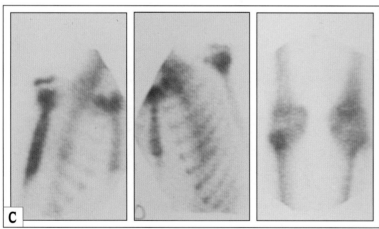

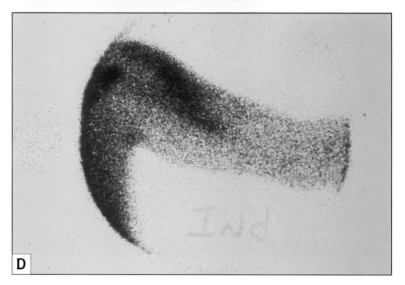

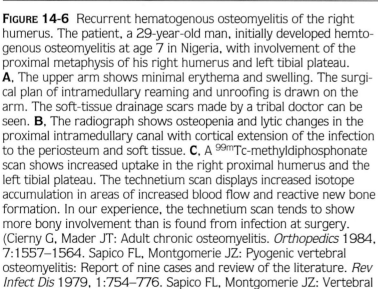

FIGURE 14-6 Recurrent hematogenous osteomyelitis of the right humerus. The patient, a 29-year-old man, initially developed hemtogenous osteomyelitis at age 7 in Nigeria, with involvement of the proximal metaphysis of his right humerus and left tibial plateau. **A,** The upper arm shows minimal erythema and swelling. The surgical plan of intramedullary reaming and unroofing is drawn on the arm. The soft-tissue drainage scars made by a tribal doctor can be seen. **B,** The radiograph shows osteopenia and lytic changes in the proximal intramedullary canal with cortical extension of the infection to the periosteum and soft tissue. **C,** A ^{99m}Tc-methyldiphosphonate scan shows increased uptake in the right proximal humerus and the left tibial plateau. The technetium scan displays increased isotope accumulation in areas of increased blood flow and reactive new bone formation. In our experience, the technetium scan tends to show more bony involvement than is found from infection at surgery. (Cierny G, Mader JT: Adult chronic osteomyelitis. *Orthopedics* 1984, 7:1557–1564. Sapico FL, Montgomerie JZ: Pyogenic vertebral osteomyelitis: Report of nine cases and review of the literature. *Rev Infect Dis* 1979, 1:754–776. Sapico FL, Montgomerie JZ: Vertebral osteomyelitis in intravenous drug abusers: Report of three cases and review of the literature. *Rev Infect Dis* 1980, 2:196–206.) **D,** An indium-111 chloride scan shows increased uptake in the intramedullary canal of the right proximal humerus with extension to the adjacent soft tissues. Indium and gallium attach to transferrin, which leaks from the blood stream into areas of inflammation. Indium and gallium scans also show increased isotope uptake in areas concentrating polymorphonuclear leukocytes, macrophages, and malignant tumors. Because these scans do not show bone detail well, it is often difficult to distinguish between bone and soft-tissue inflammation; a comparison with a ^{99m}Tc scan helps resolve this problem. In contrast to gallium-67 citrate, indium-111 chloride is more heavily concentrated by hematopoietic tissue and is not found to accumulate in areas of reactive bone, including old fractures. (Lisbang R, Rosenthall L: Observations of the sequential use of ^{99m}Tc phosphate complex and ^{67}Ga imaging in osteomyelitis, cellulitis, and septic arthritis. *Radiology* 1977, 123:123–129. Sayle BA, Fawcett HD, Wilkey DJ, *et al.*: Indium-111 chloride imaging in chronic osteomyelitis. *J Nucl Med* 1985, 26:225–229.) *(continued)*

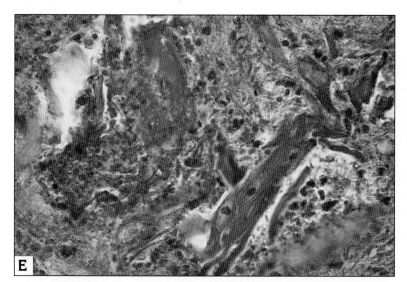

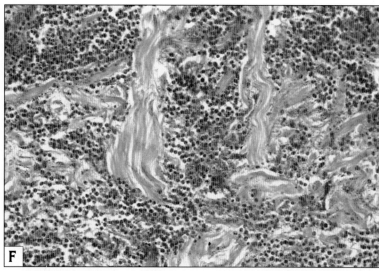

FIGURE 14-6 *(continued)* **E,** A surgical bone specimen (× 400) shows an abscess containing necrotic bone trabeculum infiltrated by viable polymorphonuclear leukocytes and surrounded by an accumulation of nonviable leukocytes (suppuration). Note the development of intramedullary sinuses. (Hematoxylin-eosin stain.)

F, Another surgical bone specimen (× 160) shows an abscess containing foci of degraded bone collagen. Most of the inflammatory cells can be identified as polymorphonuclear leukocytes. (Hematoxylin-eosin stain.)

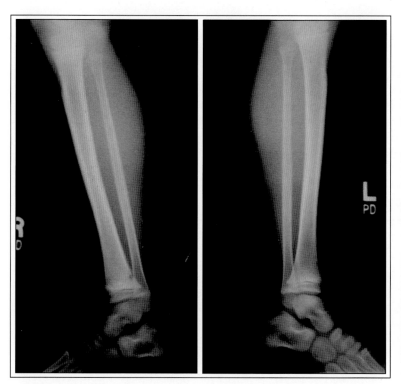

FIGURE 14-7 Hematogenous osteomyelitis of the right tibia. A radiograph of both legs of a 6-year-old child shows a small lytic lesion in the distal metaphysis of the right tibia with periosteal reaction.

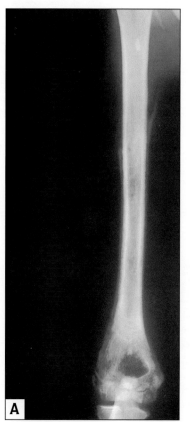

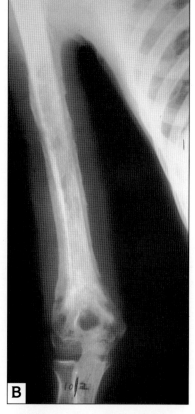

FIGURE 14-8 Hematogenous osteomyelitis of the right humerus. **A,** A radiograph of a 16-year-old girl shows lytic changes and periosteal elevation in the middle and distal humeral shaft. **B,** At 1.5 months later, the osteomyelitis has progressed with the development of involucrum. More bony destruction is noted in the distal humerus. Extensive involucrum lends stability to osteomyelitic bone in the pediatric age group.

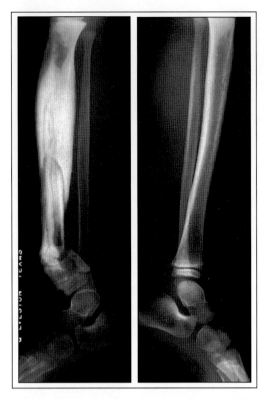

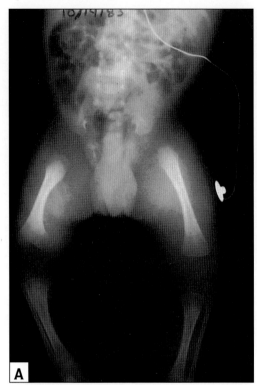

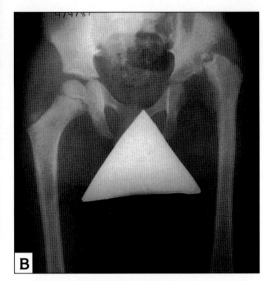

FIGURE 14-9 Hematogenous osteomyelitis of the right tibia in a 7-year-old child. There is a large involucrum in the right tibial shaft. An old fracture of the distal tibia with a fibrous union is also present.

FIGURE 14-10 Septic arthritis of the left hip and early osteomyelitis of the left femoral head. **A**, The radiograph shows joint space widening of the hip, osteopenia of the femoral head, and diffuse soft-tissue swelling in a neonate. The infant developed a cellulitis around an intravenous line with a subsequent methicillin-resistant *Staphylococcus aureus* line infection and bacteremia. One week later, the neonate refused to move his left hip. The clinical picture, hip tap, and radiographs were consistent with a diagnosis of a left hip joint infection with early osteomyelitis of the femoral head. **B**, A radiograph 4 years later shows destruction of the left femoral head and shortening of the proximal femur. There is superior displacement of the left femoral head, resulting in pseudoarthrosis.

Vertebral Osteomyelitis

Vertebral osteomyelitis	
Hematogenous	**Spinal arteries**
Age of onset	< 20 and > 50 yrs
Bone	Lumbar > thoracic > cervical
Bacteriology	*Staphylococcus aureus*
	Gram-negative bacilli
	Streptococcus spp.
Clinical findings	Nonspecific back pain
	Spasm of the paraspinal muscles
	± Fever
Hallmark finding	Exquisite tenderness on pressure or percussion of the spinal process of the involved vertebra

FIGURE 14-11 Characteristics of vertebral osteomyelitis. The infection is usually hematogenous in origin but may be secondary to trauma. There is often a preceding history of urinary tract infection or intravenous drug abuse. The lumbar vertebral bodies are most often involved, followed in frequency by the thoracic and cervical vertebrae. Spreading of infection to adjacent vertebral bodies may occur rapidly through the rich venous network in the spine. (Sapico FL, Montgomerie JZ: Pyogenic vertebral osteomyelitis: Report of nine cases and review of the literature. *Rev Infect Dis* 1979, 1:754–776. Sapico FL, Montgomerie JZ: Vertebral osteomyelitis in intravenous drug abusers: Report of three cases and review of the literature. *Rev Infect Dis* 1980, 2:196–206.)

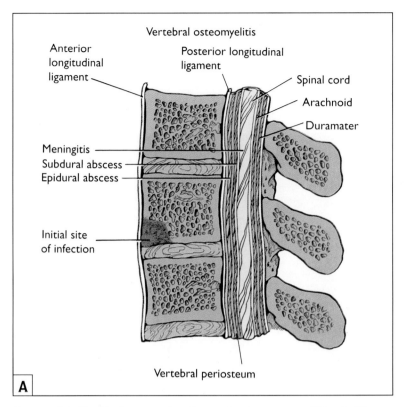

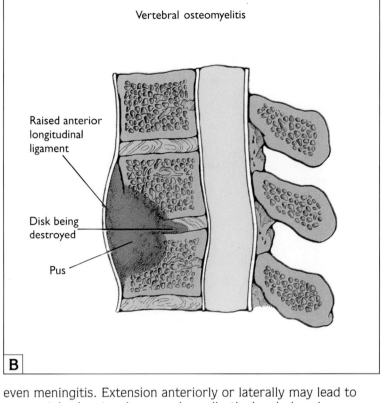

FIGURE 14-12 Pathogenesis of vertebral osteomyelitis. **A**, The initial infection involves the anterior-inferior portion of a vertebral body, suggesting spread from the bony entrance of the anterior spinal artery. However, retrograde infection through Batson's plexus of veins is also postulated. Posterior extension of the infection may lead to epidural and subdural abscesses or even meningitis. Extension anteriorly or laterally may lead to paravertebral, retropharyngeal, mediastinal, subphrenic, psoas, or retroperitoneal abscesses. **B**, Established vertebral osteomyelitis may result in collapse of the vertebral body. Successful treatment usually results in fusion of the involved vertebral bodies.

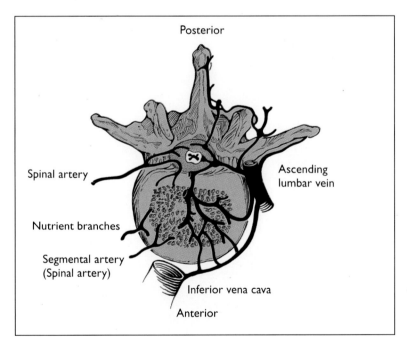

FIGURE 14-13 Routes of spread. The segmental arteries supplying the vertebrae usually bifurcate to supply two adjacent bony segments. Therefore, the infection usually involves two adjacent vertebrae and the intervening intervertebral disk. Vascular drainage is through a venous plexus that interconnects the vertebral bodies. Spreading of the infection to adjacent vertebral bodies can occur through these anastomosing venous channels.

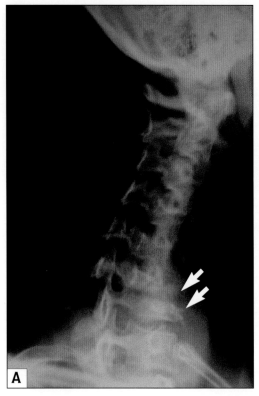
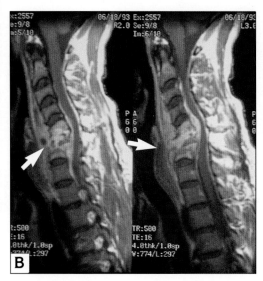
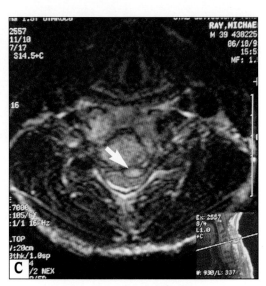

FIGURE 14-14 Septic spondylitis of C5–6 and C6–7. **A**, Cervical spine films of a 39-year-old man show septic spondylitis of C5–6 and C6–7 disk spaces (*arrows*). Narrowing of affected intervertebral disk space and destruction of the adjoining endplates are present. **B**, T1-weighted (TR/TE 500/15 ms) magnetic resonance (MR) image of the cervical and thoracic vertebrae shows involvement of C5–6 and C6–7 disk spaces (*arrows*). There are destructive changes in the bodies of C6 and C7 and extension of the infection into the prevertebral and epidural areas. **C**, T1-weighted (TR/TE 7000/105 ms) MR image cross-section at C6 shows destruction of the C6 vertebral body due to osteomyelitis and epidural extension of the infection (*arrow*).

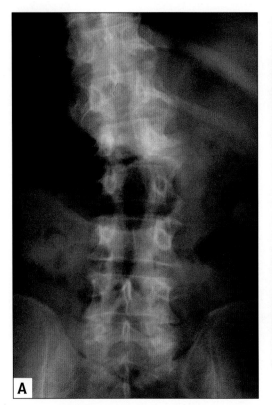
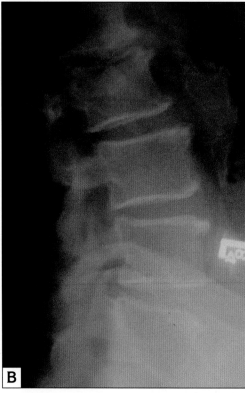
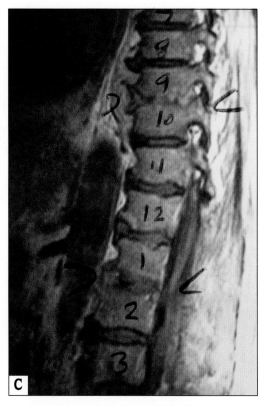

FIGURE 14-15 Vertebral osteomyelitis in a 70-year-old man. **A**, An anteroposterior radiograph of the thoracolumbar spine shows compression of the body of L1, disk-space narrowing, and angulation deformity at L1–2. *Staphylococcus aureus* was isolated from a fine needle biopsy specimen of the L1–2 disk space. The patient has scoliosis of the thoracic spine. **B**, A lateral view of the lumbar spine shows joint-space narrowing at L1–2 with destructive changes at the apposing endplates of these vertebrae. **C**, T1-weighted (TR/TE 600/20 ms) MR image shows destructive changes at L1 and L2. Degenerative changes are also present at T9–10.

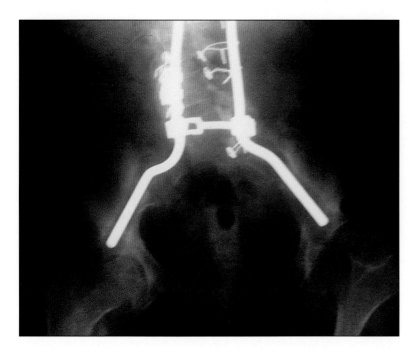

FIGURE 14-16 Vertebral osteomyelitis in a 12-year-girl. Hardware has been placed to stabilize a progressive scoliosis. The radiograph shows hardware loosening, as demonstrated by loss of bone around the distal parts of the hardware.

Contiguous-Focus Osteomyelitis Without Generalized Vascular Insufficiency

Contiguous-focus osteomyelitis with no generalized vascular disease	
Interval	**< 1 mo after injury**
Bones	Tibia, femur
Age	15–35, > 50 yrs
Bacteriology	Multiple organisms isolated
	Staphylococcus aureus
	Staphylococcus epidermidis
	Streptococcus pyogenes
	Gram-negative rods
	Anaerobes

FIGURE 14-17 Characteristics. Organisms are directly inoculated into the bone at the time of trauma and spread by nosocomial contamination during perioperative or intraoperative procedures or by extension from an adjacent soft-tissue infection. Common predisposing factors include open fractures, surgical reduction and internal fixation of fractures, prosthetic devices, and chronic soft-tissue infections. In contrast to hematogenous osteomyelitis, multiple organisms are usually isolated from the infected bone, with *Staphylococcus aureus* being the most commonly isolated pathogen. (Mader JT: Osteomyelitis. *In* Stein JH (ed.): *Internal Medicine*, 4th ed. St. Louis: Mosby-Year Book; 1994:1925–1931.)

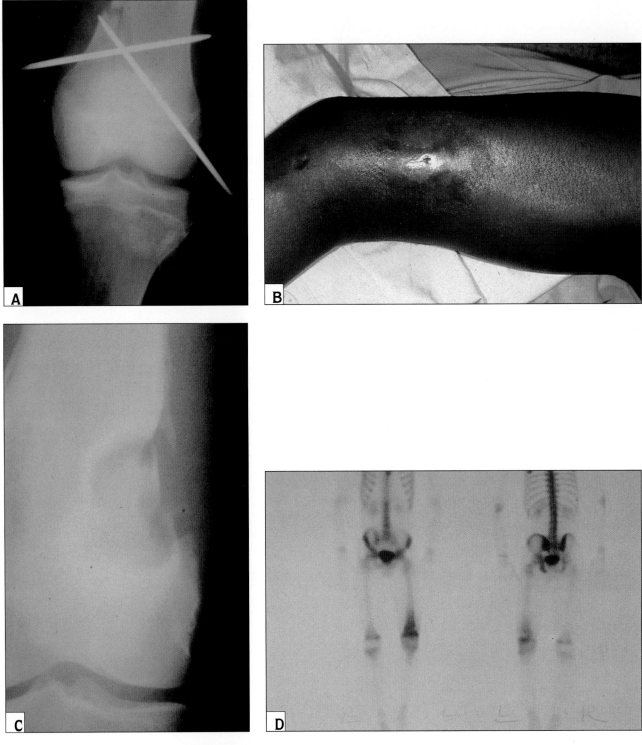

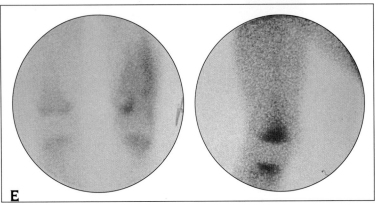

FIGURE 14-18 Contiguous-focus osteomyelitis in a 16-year-old boy. **A**, A football player from eastern Texas suffered a fracture of his left distal femur while playing football. Surgery was performed with a closed reduction and percutaneous pinning of the fracture. The leg was in a cast for 2 months. The anteroposterior knee radiograph shows percutaneous pinning of the distal femur fracture with two Steinmann pins. **B**, One month after removal of the cast, a draining sinus developed with soft-tissue discoloration in the distal thigh. **C**, A radiograph of the distal femur shows bony destructive changes with a large sequestrum in the distal left femur. There is bony sclerosis around the sequestrum. **D**, A 99mTc-methyldiphosphonate scan shows increased uptake in the left distal femur. **E**, Indium-111 chloride scan shows increased uptake in the left distal femur. *(continued)*

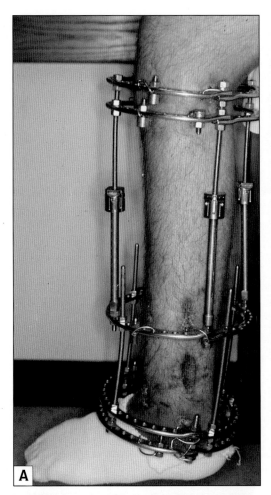

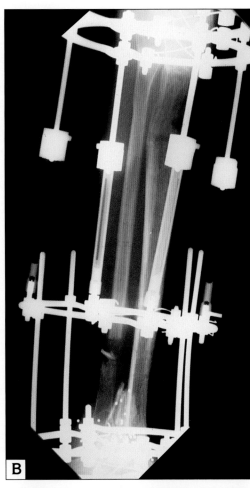

FIGURE 14-29 Ilizarov fixation for osteomyelitis. **A**, A 32-year-old man with osteomyelitis of his distal left tibia shows a Ilizarov device in place. The proximal tibial corticotomy is being expanded at a rate of 1 mm a day. **B**, An oblique radiograph shows that the distal tibial defect is being brought together by new bone formation in the proximal tibia. The new bone formation is noted radiographically in the proximal tibia at the site of the corticotomy.

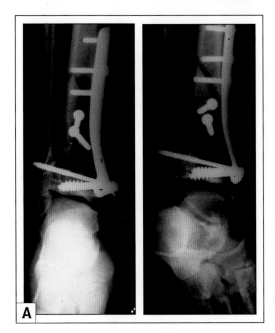

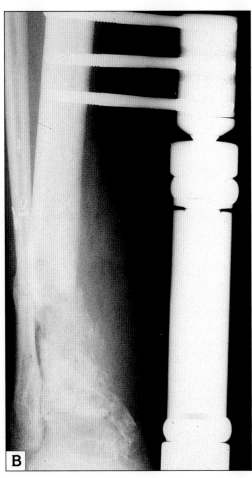

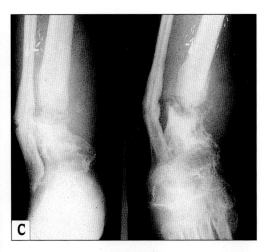

FIGURE 14-30 Complicated plate and screw fixation for osteomyelitis. **A**, Anteroposterior and oblique radiographs of the ankle in a 35-year-old man show a nonunited fracture of the distal tibia held together by orthopedic hardware (side plate and screws). The patient developed osteomyelitis in the distal tibia following an open fracture. Cultures were positive for methicillin-sensitive *Staphylococcus aureus*. **B**, The hardware from the distal tibia was removed, and the infected bone resected and debrided and an external fixator placed across the ankle. A cancellous bone graft was placed into the distal tibia following debridement surgery. **C**, The bone graft failed, resulting in nonunion of an infected fracture in the distal tibia. Debridement bone cultures were positive for methicillin-sensitive *Staphylococcus aureus*, *Streptococcus pyogenes*, and *Pseudomonas aeruginosa*. *(continued)*

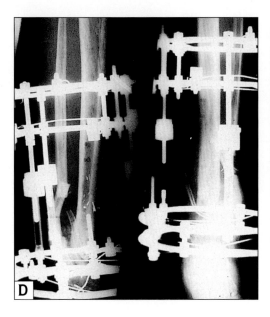

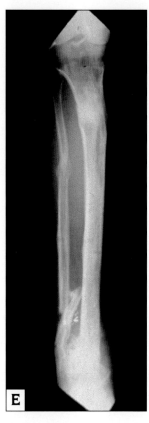

FIGURE 14-30 *(continued)* **D,** The infected bone graft was resected, leaving a segmental defect in the distal tibia. The leg was placed into an Ilizarov external fixator for 8 months and the defect closed with new bone growth from a corticotomy (fracture) in the middle tibia. **E,** After 1.5 years, the distal tibia has been reconstructed with the Ilizarov device, and the ankle has been fused. The osteomyelitis of the distal tibia is arrested. An osteotomy is present in the distal fibula.

CIERNY-MADER STAGING SYSTEM

Cierry-Mader staging system

Disease
  I. Medullary
  II. Superficial
  III. Localized
  IV. Diffuse
Host
  A. Good immune system and delivery
  B. Compromised locally or systemically
  C. Requires no or merely suppressive treatment

FIGURE 14-31 Cierny-Mader classification. Four major factors influence treatment and prognosis of osteomyelitis: Disease factors include (1) the degree of necrosis and (2) the site and extent of involvement; host factors include (3) the condition of the host and (4) the disabling effects on the host of the disease itself. These factors must be considered when assessing treatment results and efficacy of treatment alternatives. The Cierny-Mader classification includes these factors and stages the infection and host using four anatomic types (I–IV) and three physiologic classes (A–C). (Cierny G, Mader JT, Pennick H: A clinical staging system of adult osteomyelitis. *Contemp Orthop* 1985, 10:17–37.)

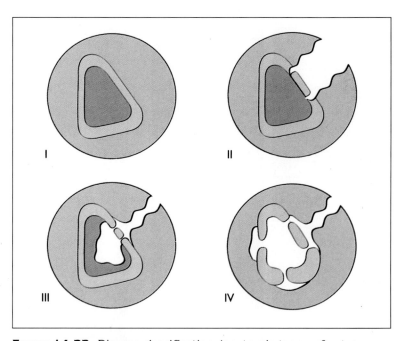

FIGURE 14-32 Disease classification (anatomic types of osteomyelitis). Medullary osteomyelitis (I) denotes infection confined to the intramedullary surfaces of the bone. Superficial osteomyelitis (II), a true contiguous-focus infection of bone, occurs when an exposed infected necrotic surface of bone lies at the base of a soft-tissue wound. Localized osteomyelitis (III) is usually characterized by a full-thickness cortical sequestration, which can be removed surgically without compromising bony stability. Diffuse osteomyelitis (IV) is a through-and-through process that usually requires an intercalary resection of the bone for cure. Diffuse osteomyelitis includes those infections associated with a loss of bony stability either before or after debridement surgery. (Cierny G, Mader JT, Pennick H: A clinical staging system of adult osteomyelitis. *Contemp Orthop* 1985, 10:17–37.)

Host factors that affect treatment	
Local compromise	Systemic compromise
Chronic lymphoedema	Malnutrition
Venous stasis	Immune deficiency
Major vessel disease	Immunosuppressive therapy
Arteritis	Malignancy
Extensive scarring	Diabetes mellitus
Radiation fibrosis	Extremes of age
Extensive small vessel	Renal failure
Compromise	Hepatic failure
Insensate region	Active cigarette abuse

FIGURE 14-33 Host classification. The patient is classified as an A, B, or C host according to the status of his or her physiologic, metabolic, and immunologic capabilities. The A host represents a patient with normal capabilities. The B host is either systemically or locally compromised, or both; coexistent diseases and factors compromising the host's status are listed. When the morbidity of treatment is worse than that imposed by the disease itself, the patient is given the C host classification. The terms acute and chronic osteomyelitis are not used in this staging system because areas of macronecrosis must be removed regardless of the acuity or chronicity of an uncontrolled infection. The stages are dynamic and interact according to the pathophysiology of the disease; they may be altered by successful therapy, host alteration, or treatment. (Cierny G, Mader JT, Pennick H: A clinical staging system of adult osteomyelitis. *Contemp Orthop* 1985, 10:17–37.)

Stage I Osteomyelitis

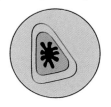

Stage I
(Medullary osteomyelitis)

Necrosis limited to medullary contents and endosteal surfaces
Etiology: Hematogenous
Treatment:
  Early: Antibiotics / host alteration
  Late: Unroofing, intramedullary reaming

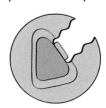

Stage II
(Superficial osteomyelitis)

Necrosis limited to exposed surfaces
Etiology:
  Early: Antibiotics / host alteration
  Late: Superficial debridement / coverage, possible ablation

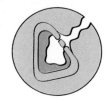

Stage III
(Localized osteomyelitis)

Well marginated and stable before and after debridement
Etiology: Trauma, evolving stages I and II, Iatrogenic
Treatment:
  Antibiotics / host alteration
  Debridement, dead space management
  Temporary stabilization, bone graft optional

Stage IV
(Diffuse osteomyelitis)

Circumferential and/or permeative
Unstable prior to or after debridement
Etiology: Trama, evolving stages I and II and III, Iatrogenic
Treatment:
  Antibiotics / host alteration
  Stabilization-ORIF, external fixation (Ilsizarov)
  Deabridement, dead space management
  Possible ablation

FIGURE 14-34 Treatment summary of the Cierny-Mader staging system.

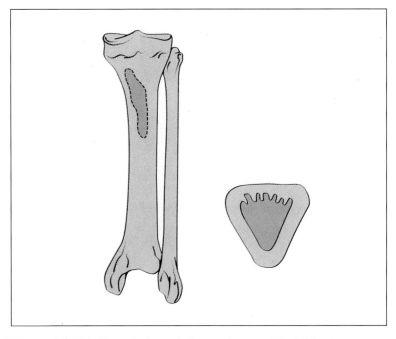

FIGURE 14-35 Stage I or medullary osteomyelitis. This stage equates with early hematogenous osteomyelitis. The primary lesion is endosteal.

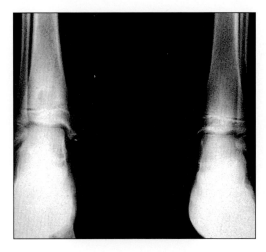

FIGURE 14-36 Stage I or hematogenous osteomyelitis of the distal tibia. Antero-posterior radiograph of the ankles of an 8-year-old boy shows a lytic lesion in the distal tibia just above the growth plate. Note the well-defined intramedullary tract extending superior to the lytic defect.

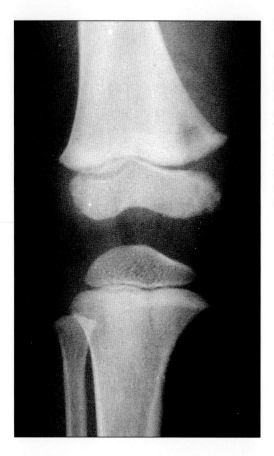

FIGURE 14-37 Stage I or hematogenous osteomyelitis of the distal femur. Antero-posterior radiograph of the right knee of a 4-year-old girl. There is a small lytic lesion of the distal femur just above the growth plate with diffuse soft-tissue swelling.

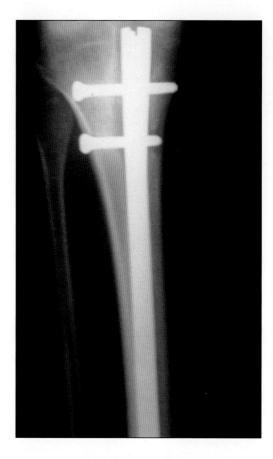

FIGURE 14-38 Stage I osteomyelitis of the proximal tibia. Anteroposterior radiograph of a 24-year-old man shows an infected intra-medullary rod in place in the tibia. Note the lucencies surrounding the proximal rod and around the distal ends of the two screws.

Medullary osteomyelitis stage I

Simple dead space
Simple closure

FIGURE 14-39 Treatment summary for Cierny-Mader Stage I osteomyelitis. Pediatric Stage I usually can be treated with antibiotics alone. Adult Stage 1 osteomyelitis is usually treated with cortical unroofing and intramedullary reaming.

Stage II Osteomyelitis

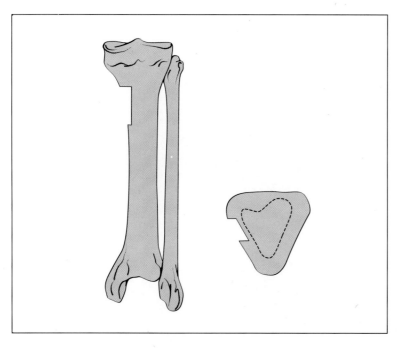

FIGURE 14-40 Stage II or superficial osteomyelitis. The bone infection results from an adjacent soft-tissue infection and represents a true contiguous-focus lesion. An exposed, infected necrotic outer surface of the bone lies at the base of a soft-tissue wound.

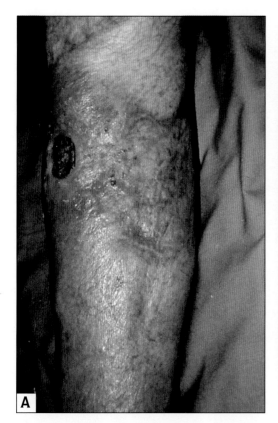

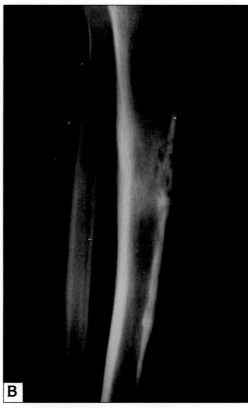

FIGURE 14-41 Stage II or superficial osteomyelitis of the proximal tibia. **A**, A 66-year-old man had developed a medial draining lesion following a tick bite 30 years prior to admission. Because of the persistent, purulent foul-smelling discharge, he or his wife had to change the dressing several times a day. His wife became tired of the dressing changes and requested that he be treated. **B**, Lateral radiograph shows superficial involvement of the tibia. The patient was taken to surgery for superficial debridement and a local muscle flap. Following surgery and antibiotic therapy, the osteomyelitis was arrested.

Superficial osteomyelitis stage II
No dead space Complex closure

FIGURE 14-42 Treatment summary for Cierny-Mader Stage II osteomyelitis. Stage II osteomyelitis requires superficial debridement and coverage with a local or microvascular flap.

Stage III Osteomyelitis

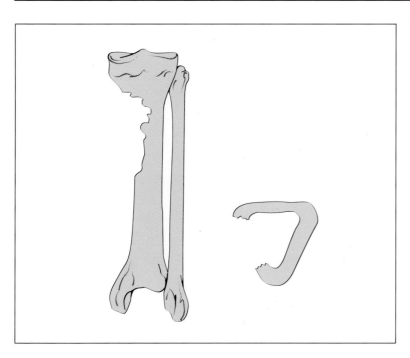

FIGURE 14-43 Stage III or localized osteomyelitis. Stage III osteomyelitis is characterized by full-thickness cortical sequestration, which can be removed surgically without compromising the stability of the infected bone.

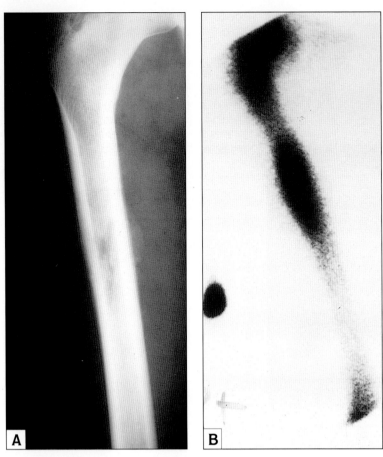

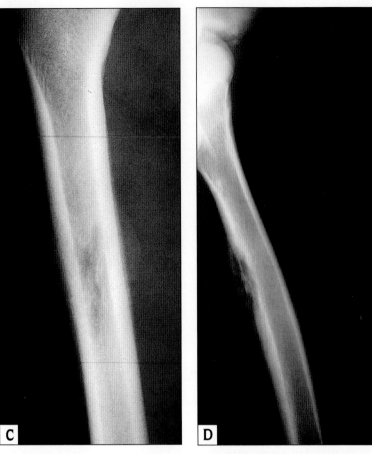

FIGURE 14-44 Stage III or localized osteomyelitis of the femur. **A,** An anteroposterior radiograph of a 48-year-old man shows a lytic lesion in the proximal femur. **B,** A 3-hour ^{99m}Tc-methyl-diphosphonate scan shows increased uptake in the proximal femur. **C,** Lateral radiograph of the femur reveals lytic changes in the femur and a small subperiosteal abscess posteriorly. **D,** The side view of the femur lesion reveals the localized intracortical nature of the osteomyelitis. The patient was treated with surgical saucerization of the osteomyelitis and 4 weeks of parenteral antibiotic therapy. The osteomyelitis was arrested.

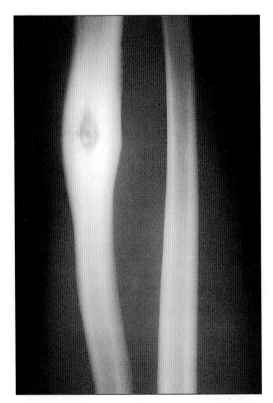

FIGURE 14-45 Stage III or localized osteomyelitis of the right forearm. Anteroposterior radiograph of a 14-year-old boy shows a lytic lesion surrounding a sequestrum in the distal radius. Reactive sclerosis about the lesion indicates chronicity of the infection.

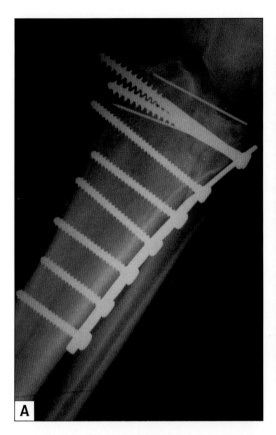

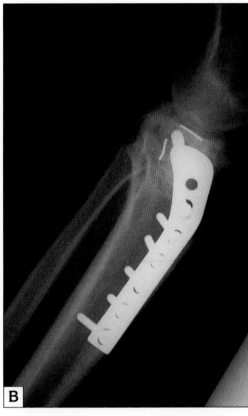

A **B**

FIGURE 14-46 Stage III or localized osteomyelitis of the tibial plateau. **A,** Anteroposterior radiograph of the left upper leg of a 35-year-old man. The fracture of the left upper leg is well healed, but there is a lucency under the tibial plate and around the proximal pin. The hardware was removed, and the cultures were positive for methicillin-sensitive *Staphylococcus aureus.* The osteomyelitis was arrested. **B,** Lateral radiograph of the left upper leg again shows radiolucency about the proximal pin, and there are also lytic changes in the proximal tibia. Hardware infection in a healed and stable bone is an example of Stage III osteomyelitis.

Localized osteomyelitis stage III

Complex dead space
Complex closure
Simple stabilization

FIGURE 14-47 Treatment summary for Cierny-Mader Stage III osteomyelitis. Stage III osteomyelitis requires surgical debridement, saucerization or hardware removal, and possibly a bone graft to augment stability.

Stage IV Osteomyelitis

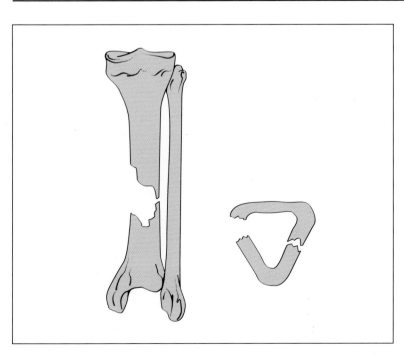

FIGURE 14-48 Stage IV or diffuse osteomyelitis. Stage IV osteomyelitis represents a through-and-through infection of the bone and usually requires segmental resection of the bone. A Stage IV patient may also have bone infection on both sides of a nonunion or major joint. Diffuse osteomyelitis includes those infections associated with a loss of bony stability either before or after debridement surgery.

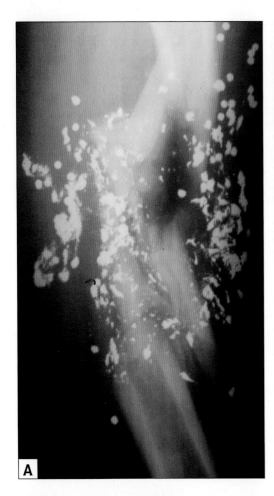

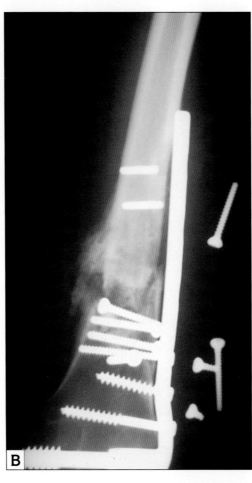

FIGURE 14-49 Stage IV or diffuse osteomyelitis of the femur. **A**, An antero-posterior radiograph of a 26-year-old man shows an infected nonunited fracture of the femur with shotgun wadding and pellets. **B**, The plate affixing the nonunited fracture is infected and loose with screws lying freely in the soft tissues.

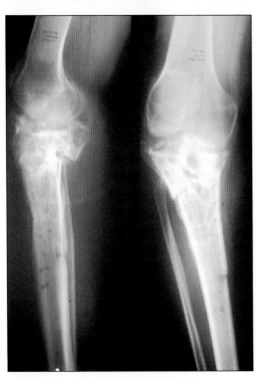

FIGURE 14-50 Stage IV or diffuse osteomyelitis of the proximal tibia and distal femur. Antero-posterior radiograph of the right knee of a 45-year-old man shows bony destructive changes about the joints and a healed proximal tibial fracture. The osteomyelitis developed after an open fracture of the tibia. *Pseudomonas aeruginosa* was isolated on multiple occasions from the bone. The patient had undergone multiple surgical procedures previously.

Diffuse osteomyelitis stage IV
Complex dead space
Complex closure
Complex stabilization

FIGURE 14-51 Treatment summary for Cierny-Mader Stage IV osteomyelitis. Stage IV osteomyelitis requires debridement, dead-space management, and stabilization.

SPECIAL CLINICAL SITUATIONS

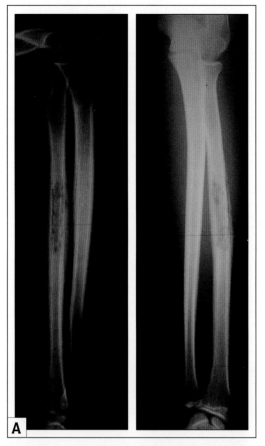

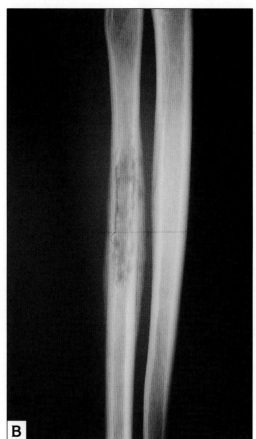

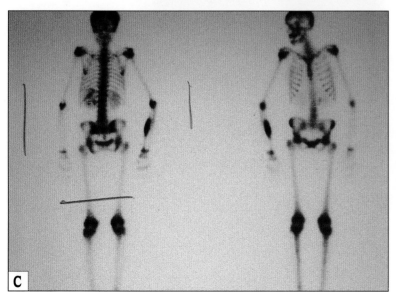

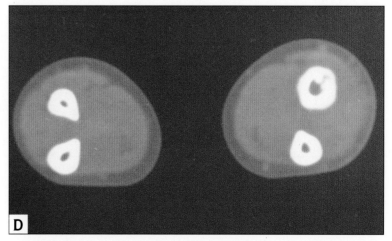

FIGURE 14-52 Osteomyelitis in sickle cell disease. **A,** Anteroposterior and lateral radiographs of the right forearm of a 22-year-old woman with sickle cell disease show a lytic lesion in the midshaft of the radius. It is often difficult to differentiate thrombotic marrow crisis from osteomyelitis in patients with sickle cell disease. (Epps CH Jr, Bryant DD III, Coles MJ, Castro O: Osteomyelitis in patients who have sickle-cell disease: Diagnosis and management. *J Bone Joint Surg* 1991, 73A:1281–1294.) This patient presented with a history of bone pain and low-grade fever, followed 2 weeks later by the onset of spiking fever, chills, and leukocytosis. **B,** The close-up view better delineates the lytic bone changes, new bone formation, and periosteal thickening in the midshaft to the radius. Surgical cultures were positive for *Salmonella* species. **C,** A 3-hour ^{99m}Tc-methyldiphosphonate scan shows increased uptake in the right radius, corresponding to the lesion seen on the plain radiographs. **D,** The CT scan shows cortical thickening with an intracortical sinus tract in the right radius. Note the diffuse soft-tissue swelling of the right forearm. Bone marrow edema is present in most instances.

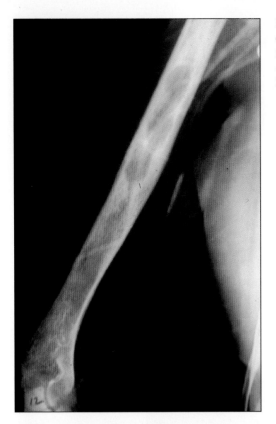

FIGURE 14-53 Osteomyelitis in heroin addiction. Lateral radiograph of the right humerus of a 25-year-old woman with a history of intravenous heroin abuse shows diffuse intra-medullary lytic lesions in the right humeral shaft. Cultures were positive for *Staphylococcus aureus* and *Serratia marcescens*. (Chandrasekar PH, Narula AP: Bone and joint infections in intravenous drug abusers. *Rev Infec Dis* 1986, 8:904–911.)

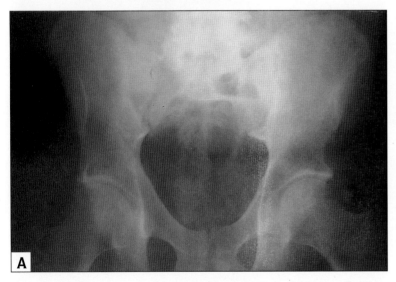

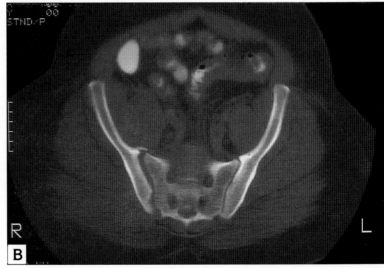

FIGURE 14-54 Osteomyelitis in heroin addiction. **A**, An anteroposterior radiograph of the pelvis of a 27-year-old man with a history of active heroin and cocaine abuse shows widening with adjacent bony destruction at the right sacroiliac joint secondary to septic arthritis and osteomyelitis. **B**, The CT scan shows widening and bony destructive changes at the right sacroiliac joint. Note the soft-tissue swelling in the right iliopsoas region.

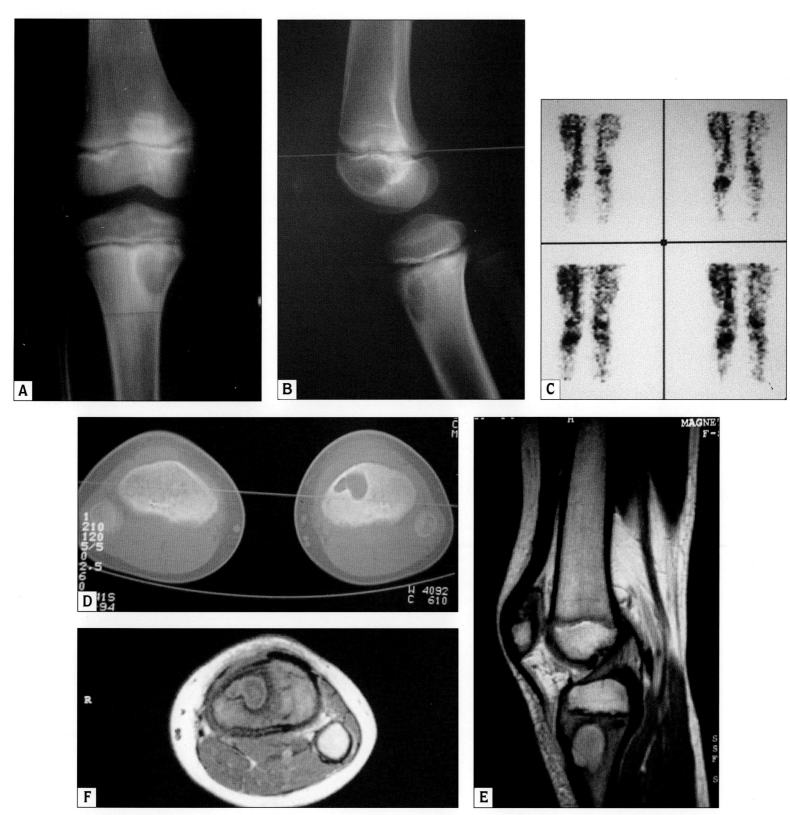

FIGURE 14-55 Brodie's abscess. **A**, An anteroposterior radiograph of the right knee in a six-year-old girl with a subacute Brodie's abscess shows a single lucent lesion located in the tibial metaphysis. Brodie's abscess is the name given to a chronic localized bone abscess. The patient presented with a 6-week history of knee pain and low-grade fever. Subacute cases may present with fever, pain, and periosteal elevation, whereas chronic cases are often afebrile and present with longstanding dull pain. The lesion is typically single and located near the metaphysis when seen in children. Seventy-five percent of these patients are less than 25 years of age. (Dunn EC, Singer L: Operative treatment of Brodie's abscess. *J Foot Surg* 1991, 30:443–445.) **B**, Lateral radiograph shows a lucent area representing an abscess in the anterior tibial metaphysis. The surgical bone culture was positive for methicillin-sensitive *Staphylococcus aureus*. **C**, 99mTc-methyldiphosphonate scan (immediate film) shows increased uptake in the proximal right tibia. **D**, CT scan through both proximal legs shows a lytic lesion in the right proximal tibia with a well-defined, sclerotic border. **E**, T2-weighted (TR/TE 2000/80 ms) sagittal MR image of the right tibia shows a bone abscess in the proximal tibia manifested by increased signal intensity in the area of osteomyelitis. **F**, T1-weighted (TR/TE 600/15 ms) axial MR image shows an area of decreased signal intensity in the proximal tibia. The bone marrow of the fibula gives the normal bright signal of intramedullary fat.

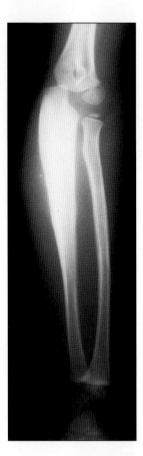

FIGURE 14-56
Garré's osteo-myelitis. An anteroposterior radiograph of the forearm in a 4-year-old girl with Garré's osteomyelitis shows increased bone density and marked thicken-ing in the proxi-mal ulnar shaft.

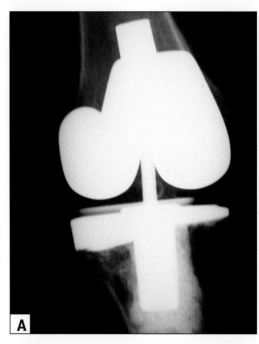

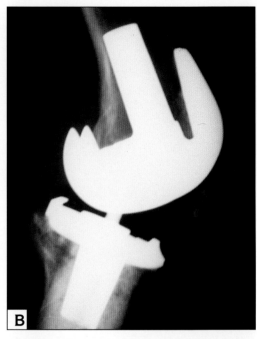

FIGURE 14-57 Prosthetic joint osteomyelitis. **A,** Anteroposterior radiograph of the right knee in a 60-year-old man with a prosthetic knee infection shows bony destruction along the medial aspect of the tibial component of the total knee arthroplasty at the bone-cement interface. **B,** Lateral radiograph of the right knee shows bony destruction along the posterior aspect of the tibial component of the prosthesis. (Ivey FM, Hicks CA, Calhoun JH, Mader JT: Treatment options for infected knee arthroplasties. *Rev Infect Dis* 1990, 12:468–478.)

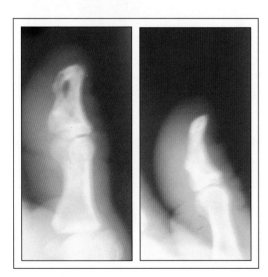

FIGURE 14-58 Hand osteomyelitis. Antero-posterior and lateral radiographs of the right thumb in a 33-year-old man with *Staphylococcus aureus* osteomyelitis. The radiographs show a lytic lesion in the distal phalanx with diffuse soft-tis-sue swelling.

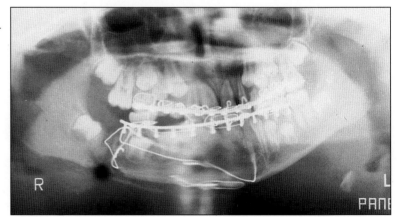

FIGURE 14-59 Mandibular osteomyelitis. Panorex radiograph of the mandible of an 8-year-old girl shows infected hardware. An infected nonunited fracture is present in the body of the right mandible. One year prior, the patient had suffered an open mandibular fracture in a horseback accident. Cultures were posi-tive for *Streptococcus pyogenes* and *Prevotella melaninogenicus*. (Calhoun KH, Shapiro RD, Stiernberg CM, *et al.*: Osteomyelitis of the mandible. *Arch Otolaryngol* 1988, 114:1157–1162.)

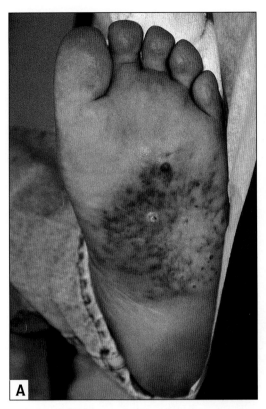

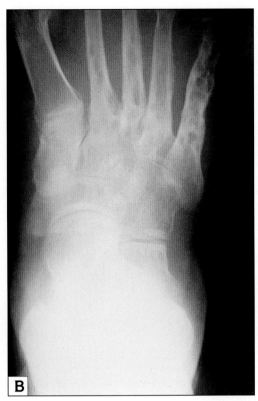

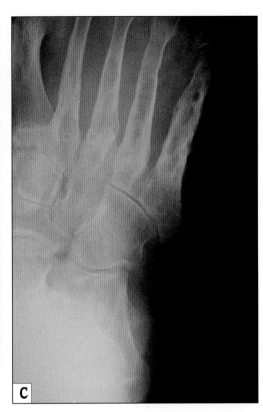

FIGURE 14-60 Anaerobic *Actinobacillus* osteomyelitis. **A,** The Plantar aspect of the left foot of a 26-year-old man from south Texas with Madura foot (mycetoma) shows hyperkeratosis and discoloration. Cultures from surgical debridement grew *Actinobacillus* species. **B,** Anteroposterior radiograph shows bony destruction and sclerosis of the second through fifth metatarsals. The patient was begun on oral clindamycin. **C,** Four months later, the radiograph shows improvement of the osteomyelitis in the second through fourth metatarsals.

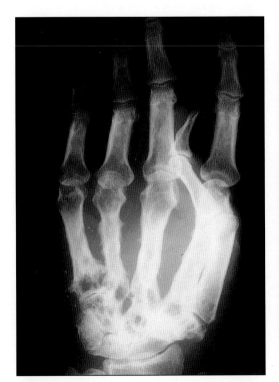

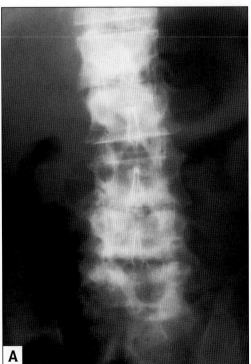

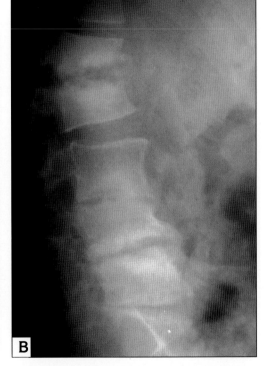

FIGURE 14-61 Anaerobic (*Actinomycetes*) osteomyelitis. Anteroposterior radiograph of the right hand of a 60-year-old man with actinomycosis shows marked bony destruction of the carpal bones and the bases of the second through fifth metacarpals. Lytic and sclerotic changes are noted at these sites. *Actinomycetes israelii* was isolated from bone cultures.

FIGURE 14-62 Fungal (*Candida*) osteomyelitis of the spine. **A,** An anteroposterior radiograph of the lumbar spine in a 27-year-old man with a current history of intravenous drug abuse shows narrowing of the L1–2, L3–4, and L4–5 disk spaces. Changes of spondylosis are also present. **B,** Lateral radiograph of the lumbosacral spine shows narrowing and bony destruction at the L1–2, L3–4, and L4–5 disk spaces. A fine needle biopsy specimen from L2–3 and L4–5 showed pseudohyphae on histologic examination. The culture grew *Candida albicans*. (Gathe J Jr, Harris R, Garland B, *et al.*: *Candida* osteomyelitis: Report of 5 cases and review of the literature. *Am J Med* 1987, 82:927–937.)

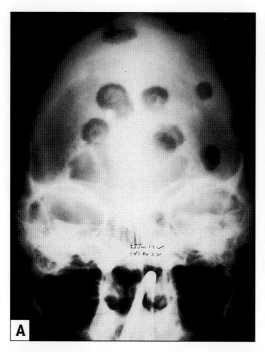
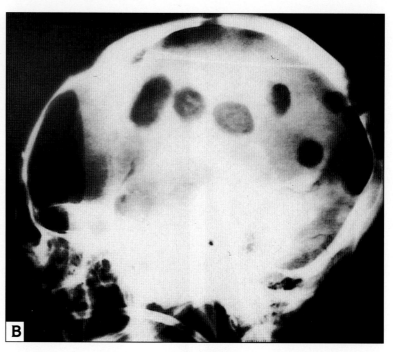

FIGURE 14-63 Fungal (*Coccidioidomycosis*) osteomyelitis of the skull. **A**, An anteroposterior radiograph of the skull of a 30-year-old man from south Texas shows multiple, punched-out, lytic lesions containing sequestra. *Coccidioidomycosis immitis* was isolated from a bone biopsy specimen. **B**, Lateral radiograph also shows multiple punched-out lytic lesions with sequestra. Many of the bone lesions penetrate to the dura. Note the intracranial air from pneumoencephalogram in the frontal region.

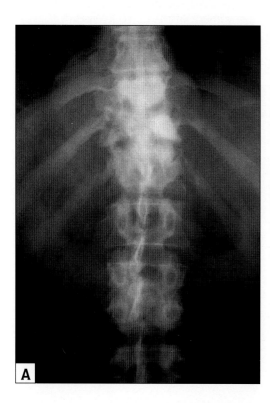
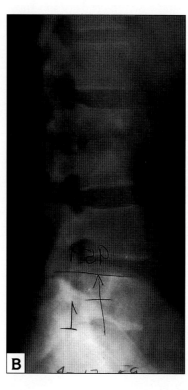

FIGURE 14-64 Fungal (*Coccidioidomycosis*) osteomyelitis of the spine. **A**, Anteroposterior radiograph of the lumbosacral spine in a 33-year-old woman from west Texas shows narrowing of T10–11, T11–12, and L2–3 disk spaces with destructive changes at the endplates. *C. immitis* was isolated from a bone biopsy specimen of the T10–11 disk space. **B**, Lateral radiograph shows narrowing of L2–3 disk space with destructive changes at the apposing endplates.

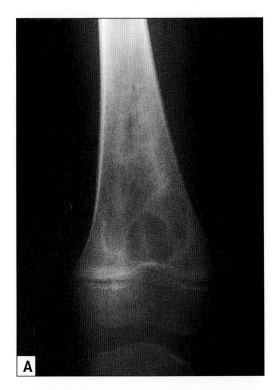

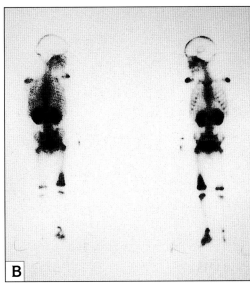

FIGURE 14-65 Fungal (*Coccidioidomycosis*) osteomyelitis of the femur. **A,** Antero-posterior radiograph of the right femur of a 10-year-old boy from west Texas shows a large lytic lesion in the distal right femur. *C. immitis* was isolated from a bone biopsy specimen of the distal femur. **B,** Three-hour ^{99m}Tc-methyldiphosphonate scans show increased uptake in the distal right femur.

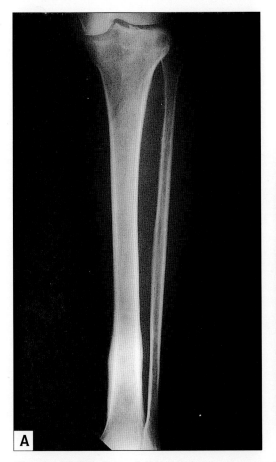

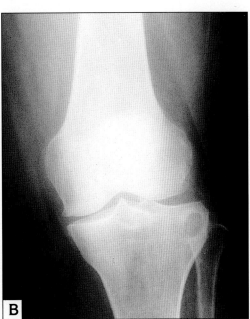

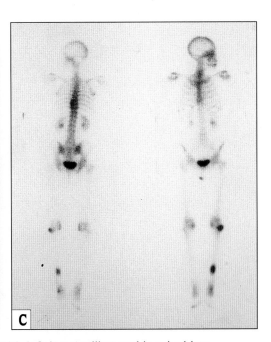

FIGURE 14-66 Fungal (*Sporothrix*) osteomyelitis of the leg. **A,** Anteroposterior radiograph of the left leg in a 32-year-old woman shows a punched-out lesion in the proximal tibia and scle-rotic changes in the distal tibia. *Sporothrix schenckii* was isolated from a bone biopsy specimen of the proximal tibia. The woman grew roses in her garden, where she probably acquired the infec-tion. She presented with left leg swelling and inguinal lym-phadenopathy. **B,** Anteroposterior radiograph of the left knee shows a close-up view of the punched-out lesion in the proximal tibia. **C,** Three-hour total-body ^{99m}Tc-methyldiphosphonate scans show increased uptake in the proximal and distal tibia.

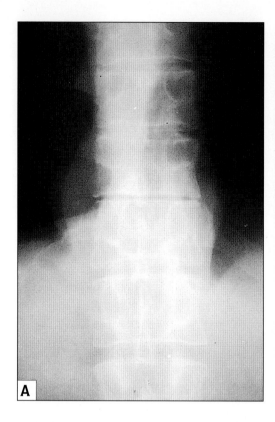
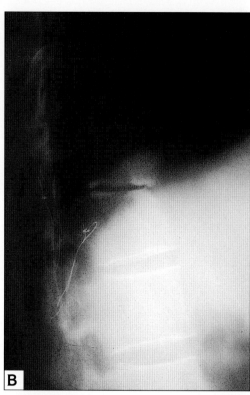

FIGURE 14-67 Skeletal tuberculosis of the spine. **A**, An anteroposterior radiograph of the thoracolumbar spine in a 40-year-old man shows narrowing of T11–12 disk space with preserved bone height. Note the paravertebral abscess along the lower thoracic spine. *Mycobacterium tuberculosis* was isolated by a fine needle aspiration. Vertebral infection from *M. tuberculosis* usually begins in the anterior portion of a vertebral body adjacent to the intervertebral disk. The infection produces destruction of the nearby bone and the intervertebral disk. Adjacent vertebral bodies may become infected, and a paravertebral abscess may develop. **B**, Lateral radiograph of the thoracic spine shows narrowing of T11–12 disk space. Note the bony destruction at the anterior aspect of the body of T12. (Gorse GJ, Pais MJ, Kusske JA, Cesario TC: Tuberculous spondylitis: A report of six cases and a review of the literature. *Medicine* 1983, 62:178–193.)

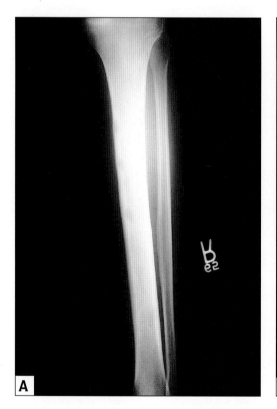
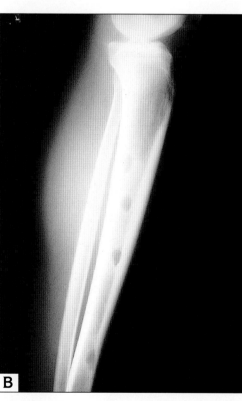

FIGURE 14-68 Skeletal tuberculosis of the leg. **A**, Anteroposterior radiograph of the right tibia in a 43-year-old man shows lytic lesions with minimal new bone formation in the tibia. Bone cultures were positive for *M. tuberculosis*. **B**, A lateral radiograph better delineates the lytic lesions with minimal new bone formation in the proximal and right tibial shaft.

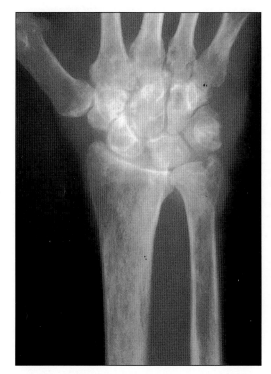

FIGURE 14-69 Nontuberculous mycobacterial infection. Anteroposterior radiograph of the left wrist of a 34-year-man with AIDS shows osteopenia and bony erosions in the wrist, proximal metacarpals, and the adjacent ulna and radius with joint-space narrowing. Cultures were positive for *Mycobacterium avium intracellulare.* The radiographic features may mimic rheumatoid arthritis. (Marchevsky A, Damsker B, Green S, Tepper S: The clinicopathological spectrum of nontuberculous mycobacterial osteoarticular infection. *J Bone Joint Surg* 1985, 67A:925–929.)

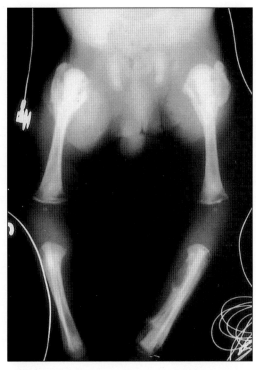

FIGURE 14-70 Viral (rubella) osteomyelitis. Anteroposterior radiograph of the lower extremities of an infant with congenital rubella shows destructive bone changes and new bone formation in the left and right femoral heads and tibias. In rubella, the bone lesions tend to be self-limiting.

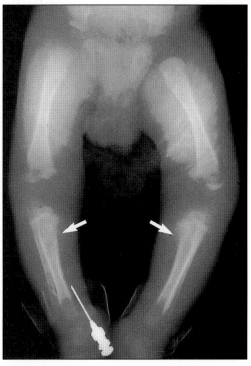

FIGURE 14-71 Syphilitic osteomyelitis (congenital syphilis). Anteroposterior radiograph of the lower extremities of an infant with congenital syphilis shows bony changes in both proximal tibias. Congenital syphilis causes obliterative endarteritis and perivascular mononuclear cuffing. The syphilitic lesions are usually teaming with spirochetes. As a result of the histologic changes, there may be generalized osteochondritis and perichondritis, which may affect the architecture of any of the bones of the skeletal system. Note the lytic lesions in the medial aspect of the proximal tibia bilaterally (*arrows*). This characteristic finding of the disease is known as Wimberger's sign.

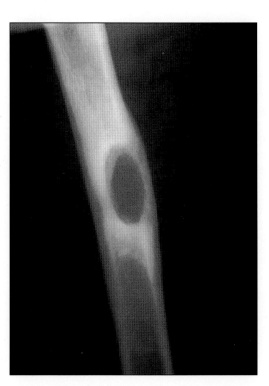

FIGURE 14-72 Syphilitic osteomyelitis (gumma). Anteroposterior radiograph of the femur of a 62-year-old man with late syphilis reveals a punched-out lesion in the midshaft occupied by a gumma. The gumma is a nonspecific granulomatous-like lesion occurring in late syphilis. Deep granulomatous lesions may break down to form punched-out lesions. Gummas of the bone may result in a pathologic fracture or joint destruction.

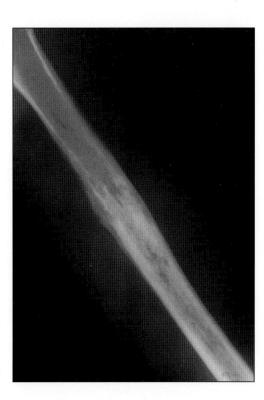

FIGURE 14-73 Syphilitic osteomyelitis (late syphilis). Anteroposterior radiograph of a femur of a 70-year-old man with late syphilis shows diffuse lytic and sclerotic changes in the shaft consistent with chronic osteomyelitis.

ACKNOWLEDGMENTS

The authors thank Diane Staebler and Donna Milner-Mader for manuscript research and preparation.

SELECTED BIBLIOGRAPHY

Calhoun JH, Mader JT: Osteomyelitis of the diabetic foot. *In* Frykberg RG (ed.): *The High Risk Foot in Diabetes Mellitus.* New York: Churchill Livingstone; 1991:213–239.

Cierny G, Mader JT, Pennick H: A clinical staging system of adult osteomyelitis. *Contemp Orthop* 1985, 10:17–37.

Mader JT: Osteomyelitis. *In* Stein JH (ed.): *Internal Medicine*, 4th ed. St. Louis: Mosby-Year Book; 1994:1925–1931.

Mader JT, Cobos JA, Calhoun JH: Osteomyelitis. *In* Rakel RE (ed.): *Conn's Current Therapy.* New York: WB Saunders; 1994:973–978.

CHAPTER 15

Joint Infections and Rheumatic Manifestations of Infectious Diseases

Bruce C. Gilliland
Mark H. Wener

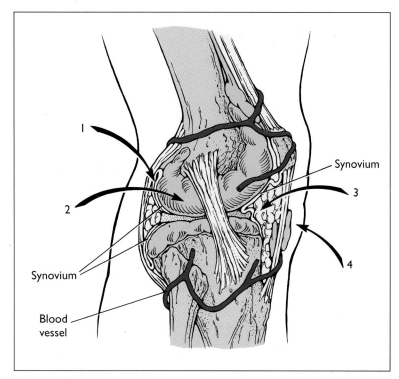

Figure 15-1 Routes of microbial invasion of the joint. Micro-organisms can be carried by the circulation from a distant site of infection to the synovial membrane and then enter the joint cavity (*1*). They are deposited from the circulation into the subchondral bone with extension into the joint cavity (*2*). Microorganisms also can spread from an adjacent soft-tissue infection into the joint cavity (*3*). Microorganisms can be directly introduced into the joint by penetration through the skin (*4*).

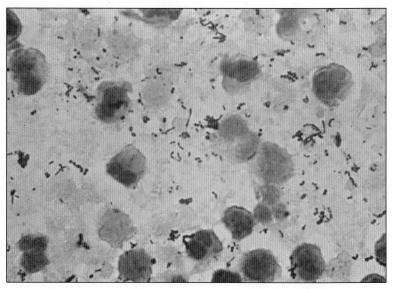

Figure 15-2 Gram stain of synovial fluid showing polymorphonu-clear leukocytes and gram-positive cocci, which on culture grew out *Staphylococcus aureus*. Patients presenting with recent onset of a warm, swollen, tender joint or bursa should have the joint or bursa aspirated immediately. The joint fluid should be examined for crystals, and Gram stain and cultures should be performed. Some of the fluid should be placed into an EDTA-containing tube for leukocyte count and differential. In bacterial arthritis, time is crucial because a delay in diagnosis and in initiating therapy may result in joint damage. (*Courtesy of* D. Stevens, MD.)

Septic Arthritis

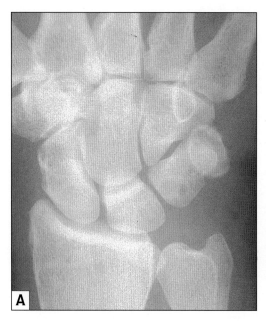
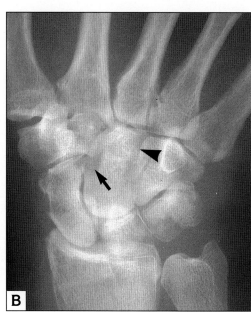
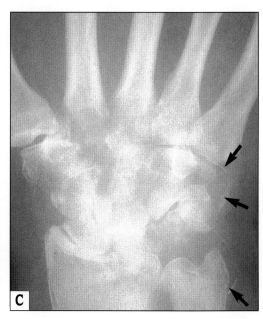

Figure 15-3 Septic arthritis of the wrist. Serial radiographs show progression of septic arthritis caused by *Staphylococcus aureus* infection of the wrist. This infection was hematogenously spread; however, a portal of entry could not be identified. The first sign of a septic joint is pain, quickly followed by swelling and redness of the overlying skin. The patient may experience fever and chills. The joint is exquisitely tender and painful. Arthro-centesis reveals cloudy fluid with cell counts of 50,000 to 100,000/mm^3 or greater that are predominantly polymorphonu-clear leukocytes. **A**, A radiograph on admission shows only soft-tissue swelling. **B**, Four weeks later, there is osteopenia of the carpal bones and proximal metacarpals. Joint space narrowing of the carpal articulations is present (*arrowhead*) and erosions can be seen (*arrow*). **C**, At 2.5 weeks later, diffuse destruction of the carpals and proximal metacarpals with extensive erosions is evi-dent (*arrows*). There is loss of joint space at the radial carpal, midcarpal, and common carpometacarpal articulations. (*Courtesy of* T. Gillespy, MD.)

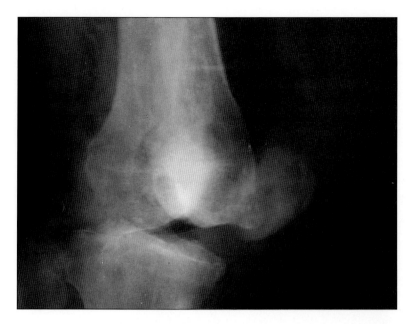

FIGURE 15-4 Septic arthritis of the knee. Lateral view of the knee showing intra-articular gas. Cultures from the joint, blood, and urine grew a gas-forming *Escherichia coli.* Erosions have not yet developed. There is underlying osteoarthritis manifested by joint-space narrowing, subchondral sclerosis, and osteophytes at the joint margins. Septic arthritis caused by gram-negative bacilli represents only 5% of joint infections and occurs most commonly in patients with chronic debilitating illness or those on immunosuppressive agents. Joint infection tends to affect previously damaged joints, as occurred in this patient. (*From* Gilliland BC, Caldwell JH: A splash in the joint. *West J Med* 1975, 123:58–59; with permission.)

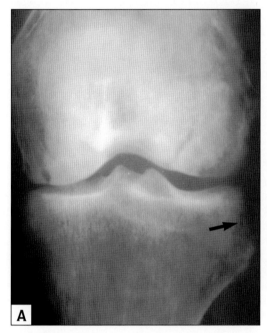

A

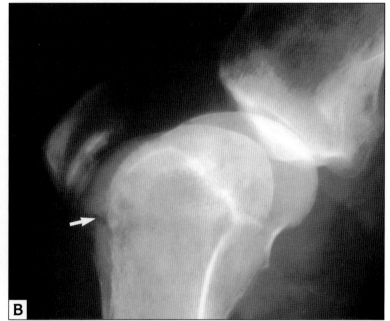

B

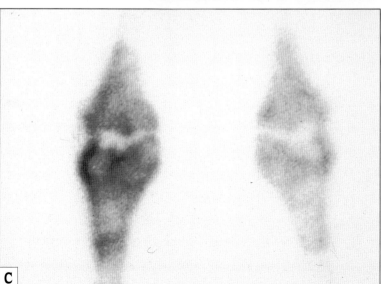

C

FIGURE 15-5 Septic arthritis of the knee due to *Serratia marcesens.* The patient was a 27-year-old woman who was an intravenous drug abuser. **A** and **B**, Radiographs show joint-space narrowing and bone erosions (*arrows*). **C**, A ^{99m}Tc bone scan shows increased activity in the right knee. Septic arthritis caused by *Serratia* is very uncommon and is seen most often in intravenous drug users and patients with debilitating and immune-compromising diseases including diabetes mellitus, rheumatoid arthritis, and systemic lupus erythematosus or following trauma. (*Courtesy of* M. Richardson, MD.)

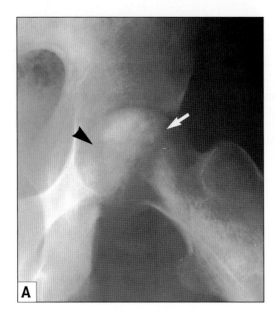 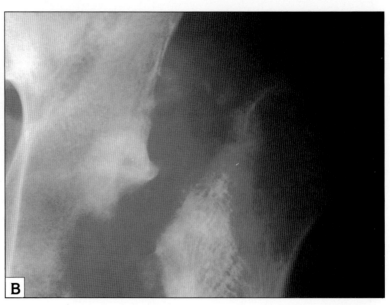

FIGURE 15-6 Septic arthritis and osteonecrosis of the right hip in a 25-year-old African-American man with sickle cell disease. The infection in this case was caused by *Staphylococcus aureus*. Patients with sickle cell disease are prone both to osteonecrosis and osteomyelitis. Septic arthritis is less common. **A**, Evidence for septic arthritis on this radiograph includes a bone erosion (*arrow*), joint-space narrowing, osteopenia and an effusion. A range of microorganisms have been described in septic arthritis, including *Salmonella*, *Staphylococcus*, *Streptococcus*, *Escherichia coli*, and *Enterobacter*. Of note, over half of the cases of osteomyelitis in patients with sickle cell disease are due to salmonellae, and in the remainder, gram-negative organisms predominate. Features of osteonecrosis in this radiograph are patchy sclerosis and lucency of the femoral head (*arrowhead*). **B**, The same joint after 2 months shows marked destruction of the femoral head. Decreased blood flow secondary to sickling of red cells may result in a poor response to antibiotic therapy in some patients. (*Courtesy of* T. Gillespy, MD.)

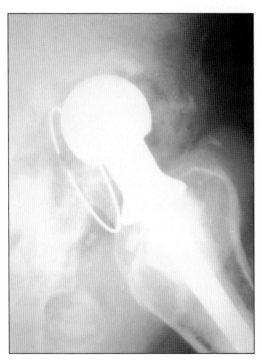

FIGURE 15-7 Prosthetic hip joint infected with *Staphylococcus epidermidis*. A radiograph shows loosening of the acetabular component, which has migrated inferiorly. Infection may cause loosening of either component or both. Loosening can also be the result of inadequate attachment of the prostheses to bone. In a total hip joint, clinical signs of infection may be minimal, and loosening of the prosthesis may be the first indication. Arthrography is a useful diagnostic procedure, and the joint fluid aspirated should be cultured for aerobes and anaerobes. The frequency of infection after total hip replacement is about 1%. Most infections appear within the first 2 years after surgery and are thought to represent latent infection. A small number of patients become infected later, which results from hematogenous spread. Although *S. aureus* is the most common cause of septic arthritis, infection with *S. epidermidis* appears to be more common in prosthetic joints, perhaps due to the effects of the prosthesis that allows a less virulent organism to survive. Rheumatoid arthritis patients with total hip replacement are especially at risk for infection. All patients with prosthetic joints should receive prophylactic antibiotics when undergoing potentially bacteremia-inducing procedures, such as dental extractions, teeth cleaning, urologic procedures, and colonoscopy. (*Courtesy of* M. Richardson, MD.)

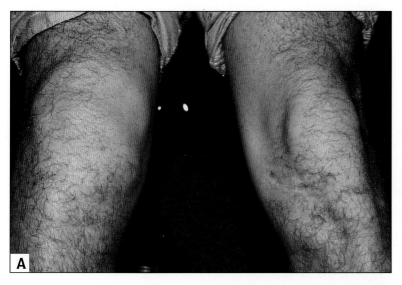

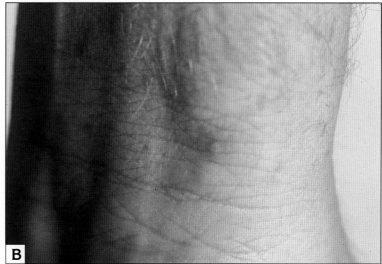

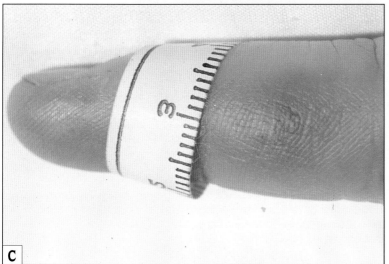

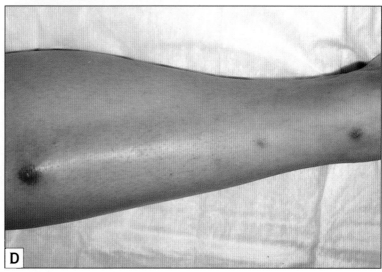

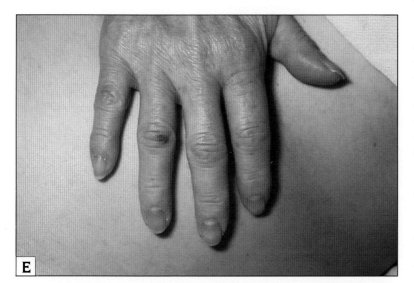

multiforme, or erythema nodosum. Tenosynovitis most often involves the wrist, ankles, and digits and helps to distinguish DGI from other forms of bacterial arthritis in which tenosynovitis is unusual. Suppurative arthritis develops in about 50% of patients with DGI and involves one or only a few joints. Arthritis is less common in disseminated meningococcal disease. Knees, ankles, and wrists are most often affected. Synovial fluid leukocyte counts range from 25,000–100,000/mm^3 with predominantly polymorphonuclear leukocytes. Unlike in other bacterial arthritis, Gram stains of synovial fluid show microorganisms in less than 25% of effusions. Blood and joint fluid cultures are positive in only about one third of patients. Cultures of the genitourinary track offer the best yield, and when positive along with clinical features of DGI, a presumptive diagnosis can be made. Cultures should also be obtained from the rectum and pharynx. Patients with DGI should be hospitalized and treated with parenteral antibiotics and adequate joint drainage. The antibiotic of choice is ceftriaxone, which should be continued until resolution of the disease. Individuals with hereditary deficiency of a complement component, particularly a late-acting C5, 6, 7, or 8 component, are susceptible to *Neisseria* infections. Patients with acquired complement deficiency, especially those with systemic lupus erythematosus, are also at risk for *Neisseria* infections. **A**, Swollen knee joint of a patient with DGI. (*Courtesy of* D. Stevens, MD.) **B**, Pustule on volar surface of wrist (DGI). **C**, Hemorrhagic papule on finger (DGI). **D**, Erythematous lesions with central ulceration (DGI). **E**, Hemorrhagic lesion in a patient with meningococcal infection.

FIGURE 15-8 Arthritis and skin lesions in disseminated gonococcal and meningococcal infection. Patients with disseminated gonococcal infection (DGI) present with fever, skin lesions, tenosynovitis, and migratory polyarthritis, and a similar clinical picture is seen in patients with disseminated meningococcal infection. Skin lesions occur in about two thirds of patients with DGI and can appear as pustules, hemorrhagic macules or papules, vesicles, bullae, erythema

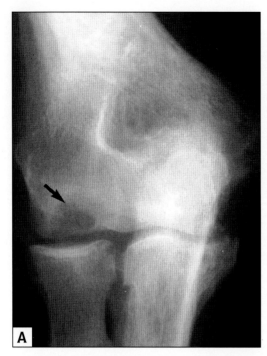
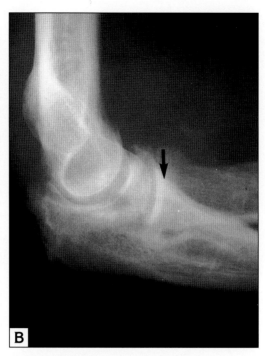

FIGURE 15-9 Tuberculosis of the right elbow. **A** and **B**, Radiographs of a Vietnamese man with a 3-month history of progressive pain and swelling of the right elbow show bone erosion (*arrows*) and some joint-space narrowing. A chest film showed no evidence of active pulmonary tuberculosis. Tuberculosis of peripheral joints is usually monoarticular, affecting most commonly the knees and hips. Infection usually reaches the joint by initially involving the subchondral bone and later eroding into the joint. On occasion, microorganisms deposit in the synovium. The onset of tuberculosis arthritis is insidious with low-grade inflammation; because of the rather unimpressive outward appearance of the joint, patients may go for weeks or months before the diagnosis is made. Synovial fluid shows a leukocyte count ranging from 10,000–25,000/mm³ with polymorphonuclear leukocytes predominating. Synovial biopsy has been reported to show histologic evidence of tuberculosis in 90% of cases. Cultures from synovium are positive in 90% of cases and from synovial fluid in 80% of patients. (*Courtesy of* M. Richardson, MD.)

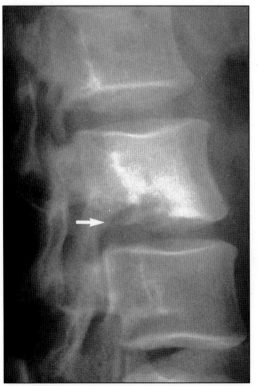

FIGURE 15-10 Tuberculosis of the spine. A radiograph shows osteolytic destruction in the body of L3 (*arrow*) extending into the disk and posteriorly into the isthmus of the inferior articular process. The adjacent disk space is narrowed. This patient experienced low back pain and low-grade fevers for the previous 2 months. Pain was aggravated by bending, straining, and lifting heavy objects. The patient was PPD positive, and a chest film did not show evidence of tuberculosis. The needle biopsy from the L3 area was nondiagnostic by microscopic examination but subsequently grew *Mycobacterium tuberculosis* on culture. Approximately 50% of skeletal tuberculosis involves the spine, with the thoracolumbar spine being the most common site. Active or even inactive pulmonary tuberculosis is not present in most cases; almost all patients are PPD positive. Mycobacteria reach the vertebral body by the hematogenous route. Infection initially involves the subchondral bone of the vertebral body, but may spread to other vertebrae beneath the anterior and/or posterior longitudinal ligaments or into the adjacent disk leading to disk space narrowing. Collapse of vertebrae and destruction of the disk may result in the development of kyphosis or a gibbous deformity and can cause cord compression and paraplegia. Infection can spread to the paraspinal tissue, forming a psoas abscess, which may extend into the groin and thigh. Paraspinal abscesses can also invade internal organs, such as the esophagus, bronchus, lung, and even aorta. Other sites of axial involvement include the sacroiliac joints and ribs.

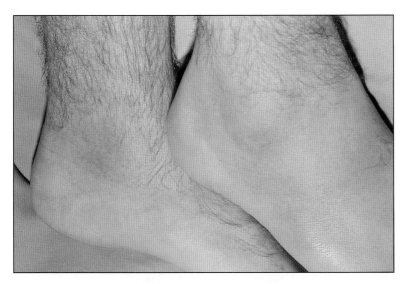

FIGURE 15-11 Arthritis of the ankles in a young man with hepatitis B. Patients may experience serum sickness symptoms of arthralgias, arthritis, and rash during the prodromal phase of hepatitis. Arthritis usually appears after the onset of prodromal symptoms of fever, sore throat, anorexia, nausea, and fatigue and is frequently accompanied by a maculopapular or urticarial rash. Each, however, can occur alone. The onset of arthritis is usually abrupt. Arthritis is often polyarticular and symmetric, and it involves hands, knees, ankles, shoulders, and elbows. On occasion, arthritis may be migratory. It subsides once jaundice develops, but in some patients arthritis may persist for several weeks or months. In anicteric patients, arthritis may resemble early rheumatoid arthritis. Hepatitis A infection can also present with arthralgias and rash. Chronic hepatitis B infection is found in approximately 20% of patients with necrotizing vasculitis (polyarteritis). Membranous glomerulonephritis and essential mixed cryoglobulinemia have also been associated with hepatitis B infection in some patients, but this association is greater with hepatitis C infection.

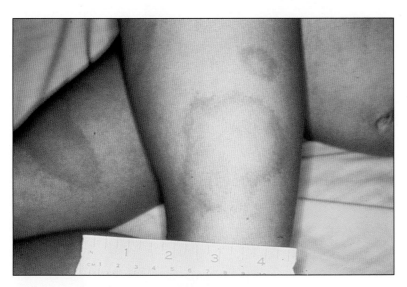

FIGURE 15-12 Lyme disease. A characteristic skin lesion develops at the site of a bite of the tick, *Ixodes dammini* or *I. pacificus* infected with the spirochete, *Borrelia burgdorferi*. Erythema chronicum migrans (ECM) begins as a macule or papule and after a few days expands into a large annular lesion with an erythematous border and partially clear center. Secondary annular lesions may follow. ECM is usually accompanied by a flulike illness with fever, chills, myalgias, arthralgias, and malaise. Greater than 50% of patients experience arthritis usually affecting one or two joints at any given time. Large joints, especially the knee, are most often involved, but small joints can also be affected. Onset of arthritis is usually abrupt, and attacks last weeks to months before subsiding. Episodes of arthritis recur for several years. Chronic destructive arthritis of large joints may develop in a few patients, especially those who are HLA-DR2 or DR4. (*From* Steere AC, Malawista SE, Hardin JA, *et al.*: Erythema chronicum migrans and Lyme arthritis: The enlarging clinical spectrum. *Ann Intern Med* 1977, 86:685–698; with permission.)

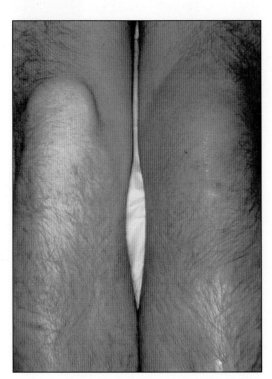

FIGURE 15-13 Acute prepatellar bursitis with cellulitis. Signs of acute inflammation can be seen in and around the knee. In > 50% of patients with septic bursitis an overlying skin infection is present, which may be an infected laceration, abrasion, or cellulitis. Distinguishing bursitis around the knee from septic arthritis or gout may be difficult. Useful distinguishing features include the anatomic localization of the signs of inflammation, including the amount and location of effusions, erythema, and tenderness. An inflamed bursa requires aspiration and examination for microorganisms and crystals. (*Courtesy of* the American College of Rheumatology.)

DIFFERENTIAL DIAGNOSIS

Crystal Deposition Diseases

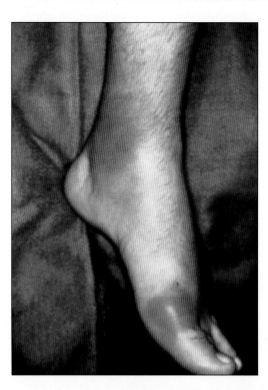

FIGURE 15-14 Acute gouty arthritis. Podagra (acute inflammation of the first metatarsalphalangeal joint) and inflammation of the ankle and posterior tibial tendon region. The intense inflammation may mimic cellulitis due to infection, as well as acute septic arthritis. Septic and acute gouty arthritis can coexist. Joint aspiration for culture, smear, and crystal examination can be used for rapid diagnosis. (*Courtesy of* the American College of Rheumatology.)

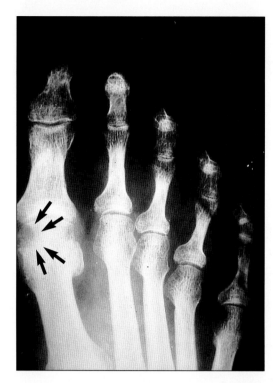

FIGURE 15-15 Metatarsophalangeal joint erosions due to tophi. The metatarsal head of the first toe, adjacent to the metatarsophalangeal joint, is eroded medially and laterally because of tophi. In comparison with erosions due to infections, the margins of the erosions are usually well demarcated, rather than indistinct, often with normal bone mineralization extending up to the eroded bone (*arrows*). (*Courtesy of* the American College of Rheumatology.)

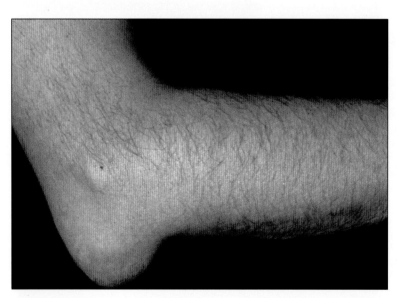
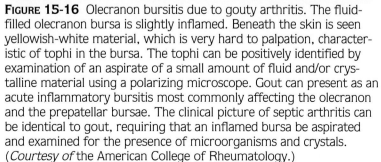

FIGURE 15-16 Olecranon bursitis due to gouty arthritis. The fluid-filled olecranon bursa is slightly inflamed. Beneath the skin is seen yellowish-white material, which is very hard to palpation, characteristic of tophi in the bursa. The tophi can be positively identified by examination of an aspirate of a small amount of fluid and/or crystalline material using a polarizing microscope. Gout can present as an acute inflammatory bursitis most commonly affecting the olecranon and the prepatellar bursae. The clinical picture of septic arthritis can be identical to gout, requiring that an inflamed bursa be aspirated and examined for the presence of microorganisms and crystals. (*Courtesy of* the American College of Rheumatology.)

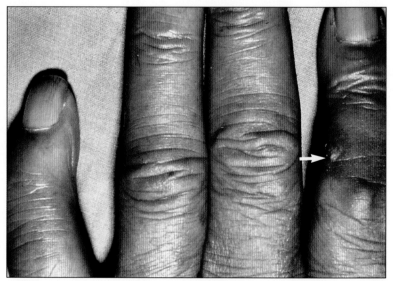

FIGURE 15-17 Tophus adjacent to the proximal interphalangeal joint of the second finger (*arrow*). A hard, yellowish deposit of sodium urate crystals appears in the skin. These are often asymptomatic but may become inflamed and/or drain chalky material. They tend to occur in cool locations, such as distal extremities or the ear. When not draining or inflamed, tophi are usually readily distinguished from abscesses or other nodular processes because of their firmness, characteristic appearance, and, usually, minimal tenderness. The chalky drainage is usually distinguishable from purulent drainage, but may be confusing. Microscopically, tophi are readily diagnosed by the presence of sheets of monosodium urate crystals. (*Courtesy of* the American College of Rheumatology.)

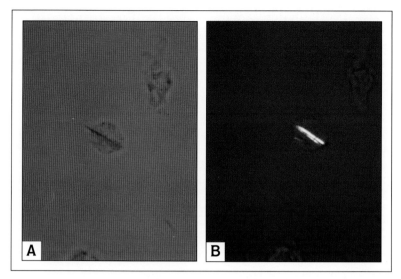

FIGURE 15-18 Intracellular monosodium urate crystal. Urate crystals are commonly phagocytized by polymorphonuclear leukocytes during acute gouty arthritis. **A,** Appearance of a wet preparation with routine transmission microscopy. The long, needle shape of the intracellular crystal is characteristic. Only a single crystal is clearly seen. **B,** Appearance of the same field using polarizing microscopy. Note that the needle-shaped crystal is very bright and can be identified as a doublet crystal. Furthermore, another smaller intracellular crystal is present. As demonstrated by the crystals in this example, some urate crystals are readily seen, and others may be harder to detect without polarizing microscopy. Synovial effusions during attacks of gouty arthritis are usually highly inflammatory, with polymorphonuclear leukocyte counts sometimes ranging up to the grossly purulent range seen in septic arthritis. Polarizing microscopy, preferably with use of a compensator (*see* Fig. 15-19) is necessary for absolute identification of urate crystals. (*Courtesy of* the American College of Rheumatology.)

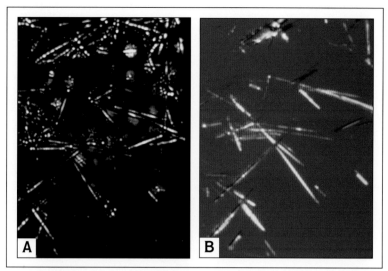

FIGURE 15-19 Monosodium urate crystals, as seen with a polarizing scope with and without compensator (first-order red plate). The long, thin, needle-shaped crystals of monosodium urate may be barely visible in joint fluid on routine electron microscopy. **A,** Because the crystals are strongly birefringent, they are usually readily seen with polarizing microscopy. The black background is caused by blockage of light transmission by the crossed polarizing filters. Because of rotation of the axis of light traveling through the crystals (birefringence), the crystals appear bright. **B,** Appearance of the crystals after a first-order red plate (compensator) is placed between the crossed polarizing filters. The urate crystals are yellow when aligned parallel with the slow axis of the compensator, and blue when perpendicular. This color pattern identifies the crystals as being negatively birefringent. Strong negative birefringence is a hallmark of urate crystals as they usually appear in synovial fluid and tophi. (*Courtesy of* the American College of Rheumatology.)

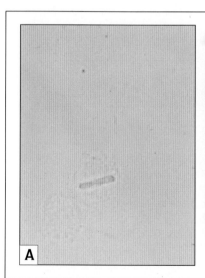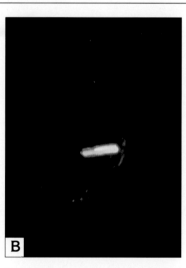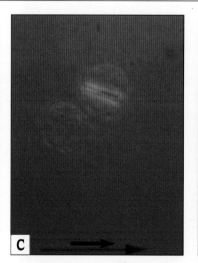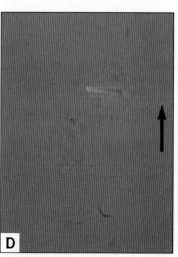

FIGURE 15-20 Calcium pyrophosphate dihydrate (CPPD) crystal in synovial fluid. Two leukocytes are shown, one of which contains a single crystal. **A,** Unstained synovial fluid is shown with standard bright-field microscopy. The crystal and cells are barely visible. **B,** Under polarizing microscopy, the background is dark, and the birefringent crystal is now readily visualized. The crystal is somewhat irregular, rhomboidal, or rod-shaped. CPPD crystals are relatively weakly birefringent, so they may be difficult to see even with polarizing microscopy. **C** and **D,** Polarizing microscopy with the compensator (first-order red plate). The slow axis of the compensator (*arrows*) is shown. In *panel 20C*, the slow axis of the compensator is parallel to the crystal, and the crystal appears blue. In *panel 20D*, the slow axis of the compensator is perpendicular to the crystal, and the crystal appears yellow. This color pattern demonstrates that the crystal is positively birefringent and is the reverse of what is observed with the negatively birefringent urate crystals associated with gout. (*Courtesy of* the American College of Rheumatology.)

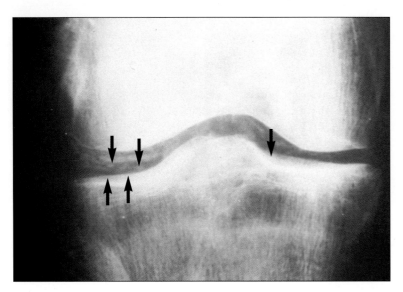

FIGURE 15-21 Chondrocalcinosis of the knee. Fine, irregular calcification of the knee cartilage is present (*arrows*). This pattern of calcification is usually caused by deposition in cartilage of calcium pyrophosphate dihydrate (CPPD) crystals. Patients with chondrocalcinosis may have a range of symptoms from asymptomatic to chronic or acute inflammation (pseudogout). Most common locations of chondrocalcinosis include the meniscus and joint cartilage of the knee, the wrist triangular cartilage (between the distal radius and ulna), the pubic symphysis, shoulders, and ankles. Chondrocalcinosis is relatively common in the elderly and rare in those under age 55 unless associated with a metabolic abnormality such as hyperparathyroidism or hemachromatosis. Acute flares of pseudogout must be distinguished from urate gout and from infectious arthritis. Pseudogout and septic arthritis may occur together. (*Courtesy of* the American College of Rheumatology.)

Noninfectious Inflammatory Arthritides

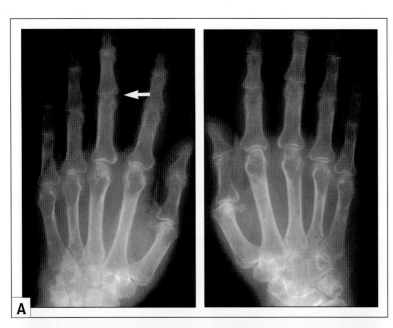

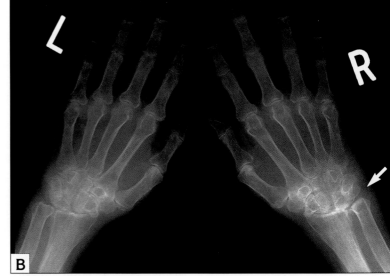

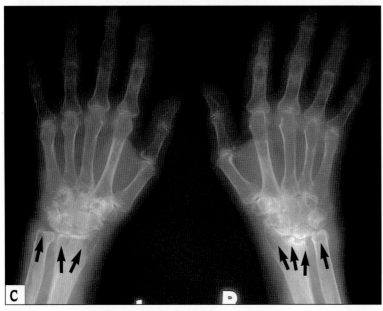

FIGURE 15-22 Rheumatoid arthritis. Progressive joint destruction documented by hand radiographs. **A,** Diffuse periarticular osteopenia, with early joint-space narrowing in the wrist and some erosions at the margins of the joints (*eg,* left third proximal interphalangeal joint, *arrow*), subluxation of right thumb metacarpophalangeal joint is seen. **B,** Three years later, progressive joint-space narrowing in wrist, metacarpophalangeal joints, and proximal interphalangeal joints is seen. Erosion and partial collapse of the wrist joints and erosion of the right ulnar styloid process are also seen (*arrow*). **C,** One year later, progressive destruction of wrist joint (more severe in right wrist) is seen, with loss of joint space, progressive collapse of carpal bones, and complete loss of the right ulnar styloid process. Severe erosions and cystic changes are present in distal ulna and radius bilaterally (*arrows*). Patients who are seropositive with long-standing severe erosive arthritis and particularly those on glucocorticoids are at risk of developing septic arthritis of one or several joints. Most infections are due to *Staphylococcus aureus.* The development of septic arthritis in a rheumatoid arthritis patient can be misdiagnosed initially as an exacerbation of rheumatoid arthritis.

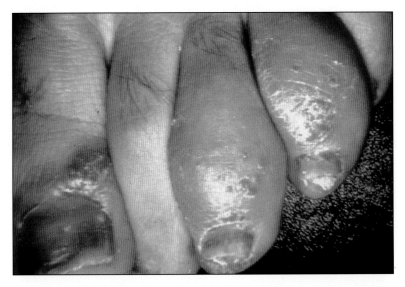

FIGURE 15-23 Psoriatic arthritis with digital dactylitis. Diffuse swelling of the second and third toes ("sausage toe") with erythema is seen. Papulosquamous cutaneous lesions are consistent with psoriasis. Note also dystrophic nail changes, characteristic of the onycholysis and onychodystophies that occur with psoriasis. The acute inflammation of the digit may be confused with septic arthritis or osteomyelitis, but the radiographic changes and clinical course allow differentiation from infection. Psoriatic arthritis may occur in patients with HIV infection. (*Courtesy of* the American College of Rheumatology.)

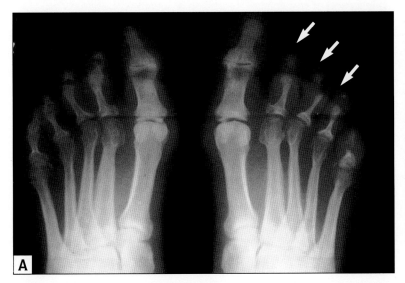

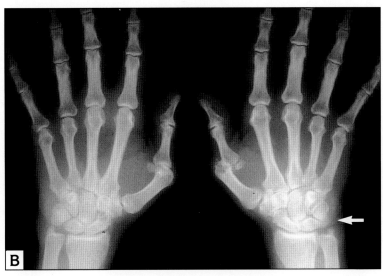

FIGURE 15-24 Psoriatic arthritis. **A**, Osteolysis of the toes. Several distal phalanges are totally resorbed (*arrows*), and middle phalanges are severely eroded. This very destructive pattern has been termed *arthritis mutilans*. **B**, Erosions at thumb metacarpophalangeal joints with subluxation. Erosions of right ulnar styloid

process are also present, giving a "whittled" appearance (*arrow*). This pattern of joint and bone destruction could possibly be confused with osteomyelitis. The absence of fever, presence of rash, and multiple joint involvement characteristic of psoriatic disease help to differentiate this disorder from infection.

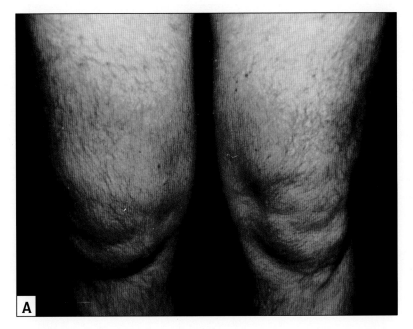

FIGURE 15-25 Reiter's syndrome and reactive arthritis. Reiter's syndrome is characterized by arthritis, urethritis, conjunctivitis, and mucocutaneous lesions, which are expressed in varying combinations and times. Reiter's syndrome is a reactive arthritis, which is defined as an acute immune-mediated inflammatory arthritis closely related to a preceding nonarticular infection caused by various organisms. The extra-articular features of Reiter's syndrome may not be present in reactive arthritis. Both are associated with HLA-B27, which is present in 60% to 80% of patients. Infectious agents that may trigger Reiter's syndrome/reactive arthritis include *Shigella, Yersinia, Salmonella, Campylobacter, Chlamydia, Ureaplasma,* and HIV. In the latter infectious agent, reactive arthritis and Reiter's syndrome appear to be more common in patients with AIDS-related complex and AIDS than in those who are only HIV-positive. Reactive arthritis follows *Streptococcus* group A infections and is considered to be an incomplete form of acute rheumatic fever. **A**, Acutely swollen knee in a patient with reactive arthritis. Typically, arthritis is an inflammatory, oligoarticular, asymmetric disorder, often beginning in the lower extremities before involving upper extremities. Sacroiliac joint and mild spinal involvement may occur. (*Courtesy of* the American College of Rheumatology.) (*continued*)

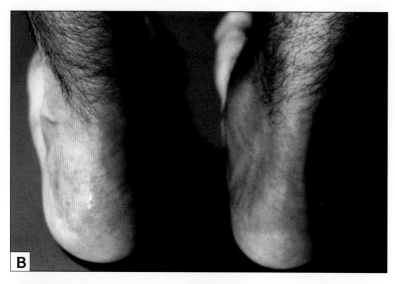

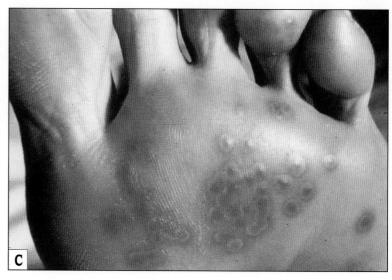

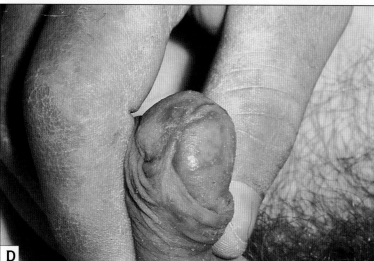

FIGURE 15-25 *(continued)* **B,** Swelling over the posterior calcaneus at the insertion of the Achilles' tendon in a patient with Reiter's syndrome. Inflammation at sites of ligamentous and tendinous insertions into bone is referred to as *enthesopathy* or *enthesitis* and is characteristic of the spondyloarthropathies, which include Reiter's syndrome, ankylosing spondylitis, and psoriatic arthritis. (*Courtesy* of the American College of Rheumatology.) **C,** Keratoderma blenorrhagica involving the sole. These are painless papulosquamous lesions that occur on the palms and/or soles and occasionally on the trunk and/or extremities. (*Courtesy of* the American College of Rheumatology.) **D,** Circinate balanitis in Reiter's syndrome. The lesion begins as a vesicle and evolves into a shallow, usually painless, ulcer or plaque. Superficial painless ulceration can also at times be observed on the tongue and palate.

MISCELLANEOUS INFLAMMATORY CONDITIONS

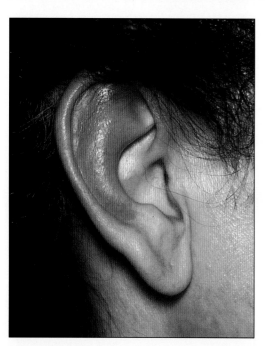

FIGURE 15-26 Relapsing polychondritis. The pinna or cartilaginous portion of the patient's ear is purplish-red and swollen. The soft ear lobe, which does not have underlying cartilage, is spared. The meatus of the external auditory canal in some patients may be swollen closed. As the inflammatory process progresses, the cartilage thins and loses its rigidity, and the pinna droops. Relapsing polychondritis is distinguished from cellulitis of the ear by the absence of inflammation of the ear lobe.

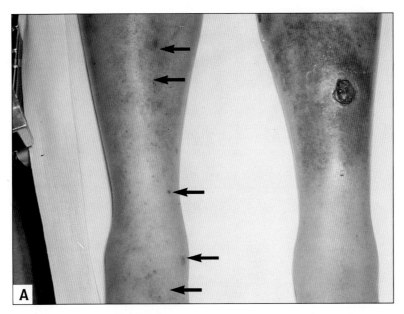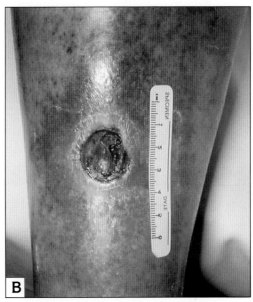

FIGURE 15-27   Mixed cryoglobulinemia due to hepatitis C. Vasculitic ulcers and cutaneous vasculitis. **A,** Confluent petechiae surround the large cutaneous ulcer on the left leg. Note also the scattered petechial rash on the right leg (*arrows*). Both legs are somewhat edematous, and the erythematous, swollen area surrounding the ulcer resembles cellulitis. **B,** The close-up demonstrates the erythematous margins of the ulcer, with a punched-out appearance of the ulcer. This patient had mixed cryoglobulinemia associated with hepatitis C as documented by both serology and the presence of circulating hepatitis C virus RNA. Clinical features included arthralgias, vasculitic rash, rheumatoid factor, and a mixed monoclonal IgM/polyclonal IgG cryoglobulin, but she lacked evidence of the glomerulonephritis frequently associated with mixed cryoglobulinemia.

SELECTED BIBLIOGRAPHY

Kelly WN, Harris ED, Ruddy S, Sledge CB (eds.): *Textbook of Rheumatology*, 4th ed. Philadelphia: W.B. Saunders; 1993.

McCarty DJ, Koopman W (eds.): *Arthritis and Allied Conditions: A Textbook of Rheumatology*, 12th ed. Malvern, PA, Lea & Febiger; 1993.

Resnick D, Niwayama G: *Diagnosis of Bone and Joint Disorders*, 2nd ed. Philadelphia: W.B. Saunders; 1988.

Espinoza L (ed.): Infectious Arthritis. *Rheum Dis Clin North Am* 1993, 19(2).

Winchester R (ed.): AIDS and Rheumatic Disease. *Rheum Dis Clin North Am* 1991, 17(1).

INDEX

Madura foot, 6.27–6.28
Maduramycosis, 6.27–6.28
Maggots, myiasis due to, 8.7, 10.2–10.3
Majocchi's granuloma, 6.12
Malignant syphilis, 12.6
Mandibular osteomyelitis, 14.28
Mayflies, 8.2
Measles, 7.9–7.10
Medullary osteomyelitis, 14.18, 14.19–14.20
Megalopyge opercularis, 10.4
Meningococcal infection, disseminated, 15.5
Microbiology *see also specific infections; specific microorganisms*
    clostridial, 13.2
    dog bite wound, 4.5
    human bite wound, 4.15
    streptococcal, 3.2–3.3
Microfilariae, *Onchocerca*, 10.5
Micrography, electron *see* Electron micrography
Microscopy, in syphilis, 12.3–12.4
Microsporum canis, 6.12
Milker's nodule, 5.6
Mites, 8.5, 10.4
    site of attachment of, primary lesion at, 9.8
    trombiculid, 9.12
Mixed necrotizing soft tissue infection, 13.7
Molluscum contagiosum, 7.2
Monkey bite wounds, 4.9–4.10
Mononuclear cells, peripheral blood, in leprosy, 11.17
Mononucleosis, 7.9
Monosodium urate crystals, deposition of, 15.8–15.9
Mosquitoes, 8.13–8.14
Mother yaw, 12.10
M-protein, 3.2
Mucocutaneous candidiasis, chronic, 6.6
Mucocutaneous leishmaniasis, 10.9
Mucocutaneous paracoccidioidomycosis, 6.26
Mucoid colony, *Streptococcus pyogenes*, 3.3
Mucous membranes, direct inoculation through, parasitic diseases acquired
        by, 10.15–10.16
Mucous patches, in secondary syphilis, 12.5
Murine typhus, 9.11, 9.13
Muscles, in myositis *see* Myositis
Mycetoma, 6.27–6.28
Mycobacterial infection, nontuberculous, skeletal, 14.33
Mycobacterium leprae, 1.4, 11.15–11.17
Mycobacterium marinum, in cellulitis, 1.4
Mycobacterium tuberculosis, 1.4
Mycobacterium ulcerans, 1.4
Mycoses *see also* Fungal infections; *specific type*
    deep, subcutaneous and, 6.23–6.28
Myiasis, 8.7, 10.2–10.3
Myonecrosis, 1.5, 13.3–13.5
Myositis, 1.5 *see also* Pyomyositis
    necrotizing, 1.5, 3.8

N ails

    fungal infections of, 6.13–6.15, 6.17
    in psoriatic arthritis with digital dactylitis, 15.11
    in trichinosis, 10.12
Nasal discharge, in congenital syphilis, 12.8

Nasal involvement, in yaws, 12.10
Necrolysis, epidermal, toxic, 2.8
Necroses
    epidermal, in boutonneuse fever, 9.7
    skin
        Rocky Mountain spotted fever and, 9.5
        spiders and, 8.6
Necrotizing fasciitis, 1.3, 1.5, 3.8
    spontaneous, *Clostridium septicum* and, 13.5
Necrotizing funisitis, in congenital syphilis, 12.8
Necrotizing myositis, streptococcal, 1.5, 3.8
Necrotizing soft tissue infections, nonclostridial, 13.6–13.8
Necrotizing vasculitis, hepatitis B infection and, 15.7
Nematodes, 10.12 *see also* Parasitic disease; *specific disease or nematode*
Neonatal herpes, 7.6
Nerves
    in leprosy, 11.12
        borderline tuberculoid, 11.5
        tuberculoid, 11.4
    in tabes dorsalis, 12.8
Neurocysticercosis, 10.14
Nikolsky's sign, in staphylococcal scalded skin syndrome, 2.8
Nodular lepromatous leprosy, 11.8
Nodular lymphangitis, 6.23–6.24
Nodular syphilis
    gummatous, 12.8
    secondary, 12.5
Nodules
    histoid, in lepromatous leprosy, 11.10–11.11
    milker's, 5.6
    onchocerciasis, 8.12
North Asian tick typhus, 9.7, 9.13

O cclusional human bites, 4.11–4.12

Oestrus ovis, 8.7
Olecranon, bursitis of, 15.8
Onchocerca volvulus, 8.11, 8.12
    microfilariae of, 10.5
Onchocerciasis, 8.11–8.13, 10.5–10.6
Onychomycoses, 6.13–6.15
    types of, 6.13
Oral chancre, in syphilis, 12.3
Oral infections
    candidiasis, 6.5
    herpes simplex virus, 7.5
Orf, 5.5, 7.11
Oriental rat flea, 8.11
Oriental spotted fever, 9.7, 9.13
Ornithosis, 5.8
Orthoptera, 8.2
Osteitis, goundou, in yaws, 12.10
Osteolysis, in psoriatic arthritis, 15.11
Osteomyelitis, 14.2–14.33
    anatomic types of, 14.18
    animal bite causing, 4.4
    chronic, 14.13–14.15
    clenched fist injury with, 4.13
    clinical types of, 14.2
    contiguous-focus
        with generalized vascular disease, 14.12–14.13